Private Acts, Social Consequences

AIDS and the Politics of Public Health

Ronald Bayer

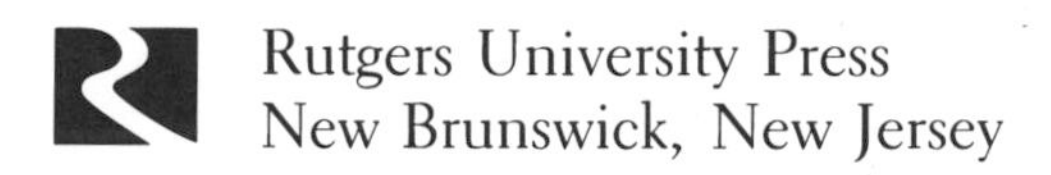

First published in cloth in the United States by The Free Press, 1989

First published in cloth in the United Kingdom by Collier Macmillian Publishers, 1989

First published in paperback in the United States by Rutgers University Press, 1991
This edition is reprinted by arrangement with The Free Press, a division of Macmillan, Inc.
Copyright © 1989, 1991 by Ronald Bayer

All rights reserved. No part of this book may be reproduced or transmitted in any form or by any means, electronic or mechanical, including photocopying, recording, or by any information storage and retrieval system, without permission in writing from the Publisher.

Manufactured in the United States of America

Library of Congress Cataloging-in-Publication Data

Bayer, Ronald.
Private acts, social consequences : AIDS and the politics of public health / Ronald Bayer.
p. cm.
Reprint, with a new afterword. Originally published: New York : Free Press, 1989.
Includes bibliographical references and index.
ISBN 0-8135-1624-2 (pbk.)
1. AIDS (Disease)—Government policy—United States. 2. AIDS (Disease)—Social aspects—United States. I. Title.
RA644.A25B39 1991
362.1'9697'9200973—dc20 90-42039
CIP

Material from Ronald Bayer, "AIDS, Power and Reason," reprinted from *Milbank Quarterly* (October 1986) by permission of the publisher. Material from Ronald Bayer and Jonathan Moreno, "Health Promotion: Ethical and Social Dilemmas of Government Policy," reprinted from *Health Affairs* (Summer 1986) by permission of the publisher. Quotations from Larry Kramer, *Reports from the Holocaust: The Making of an AIDS Activist* (New York: St. Martin's Press, 1989) by permission of Larry Kramer.

For Adelle Bayer, my mother,
and the memory of Max Bayer, my father

Contents

Acknowledgments

In 1983 Mathilde Krim, founding chairperson of the American Foundation for AIDS Research, but then director of the Interferon Laboratory at the Sloan Kettering Institution, approached The Hastings Center about what she saw as a critical problem. A new and deadly disease, AIDS, had begun to threaten gay men and others who were socially marginal. Nothing was known about its etiology. Epidemiological studies that would probe the most intimate details of the lives of homosexual and bisexual men and intravenous drug users were necessary. Yet, because of doubts about the extent to which confidentiality could be protected, fear of stigma, and the consequences of exposure, many were reluctant to participate in such research. It was out of this challenge—the need to protect privacy in the face of an unfolding epidemic—that my work on AIDS began at The Hastings Center.

Subsequently my colleague Carol Levine and I broadened our concerns to the many ethical challenges posed by the AIDS epidemic. To help us we brought together an extraordinary group of public health officials, physicians, philosophers, lawyers, historians, gay leaders, and civil liberties advocates to examine AIDS and the ethics of public health. They have been my teachers during the first years of the epidemic. This book, an outgrowth of my work at The Hastings Center, is a token of gratitude to them. A few foundations that understood how important it was to support the study of the ethical and social dimensions of a medical crisis made our studies possible. The Field, Norman, Gutfreund, Pearl River, Dana, and Pettus-Crowe foundations were critical at the outset. The American Foundation for AIDS Research assumed the preeminent role in making our work possible from 1986 to 1988.

In doing the research for this book I was assisted by many who were willing to share their time and personal archives with me. I especially want to thank Jeff Levi of the National Gay and Lesbian Task Force; Mervyn Silverman, former director of public health in San Francisco; Thomas Stoddard of the Lambda Legal Defense and Education Fund; Thomas Vernon, executive director of the Colorado Health Department; Michael Osterholm, state epidemiologist for Minnesota; and James Chin, now of the Global Program on AIDS at the World Health Organization.

At The Hastings Center I was assisted again and again by Marna Howarth, the librarian; Sara Swenson, the research assistant; and Lauri Posner, who could always bring order out of chaos. Virginia Wells and Bette Crigger typed from difficult handwritten manuscript pages with forbearance.

Allan Brandt, Larry Gostin, and Sheldon Landesman read an earlier version of this book and offered the balance of criticism and encouragement one can get only from good friends and tough colleagues.

My wife, Jane Alexander, brought to the reading of my manuscript the same critical eye for language that has always been invaluable to me.

Finally, I want to thank Joyce Seltzer, my editor, who always pressed me to go further.

Chapter 1

Private Acts, Social Consequences

Seven years ago the Centers for Disease Control reported the existence in California of a pattern of extraordinary illnesses among young gay men whose immune systems had been so compromised that they had lost the capacity to combat a host of lethal diseases. These were the sentinel cases of what has since become a pandemic of potentially catastrophic dimensions. In the years since AIDS was first discovered, America has been compelled to confront a challenge that is at once biological, social, and political. The epidemic will continue to make its demands felt for many years to come, since what some had believed might be a short-lived episode like toxic shock syndrome or Legionnaire's disease has proven to be quite different, and no end is in sight. Predictions of the ultimate toll in the United States over the next decades range into the hundreds of thousands. However this modern epidemic is brought under control, it is clear that no part of American social and political life will remain untouched.

It was in June 1981 that the Centers for Disease Control began to report the appearance in previously healthy gay men of diseases that in the past had occurred only in individuals whose immune systems had been severely compromised.[1] It was in that month that *Morbidity and Mortality Weekly Report*, the CDC's official publication, reported that between October 1980 and May 1981 five young men in Los Angeles had been diagnosed with pneumocystis carinii pneumonia. In an editorial note, the outcropping was termed "unusual." The *Report* suggested, by way of explanation, "an association between some aspect of homosexual lifestyle or disease acquired through sexual contact and pneumocystis pneumonia in this population. Based on clinical examination of each of these cases, the possibility of a cellular immune dysfunction related to a common exposure might also be involved."[2]

One month later, the CDC reported that in the prior thirty months Kaposi's sarcoma, a malignancy unusual in the United States, had been diagnosed in twenty-six gay men in New York City and California.[3] Eight of the patients had died within two years of diagnosis. In each of these cases two factors were striking: the youth of the victims—in the past, Kaposi's had been reported only in elderly Americans—and its "fulminant course."

On the first anniversary of the CDC's first report *MMWR* published an update that documented reports of 355 cases of Kaposi's sarcoma and/or serious opportunistic infections, especially pneumocystis pneumonia. Of these, 79 percent were either homosexual or bisexual. Among the heterosexuals, the dominant feature was a history of illicit intravenous drug use.[4] One week later *MMWR* reported on a single cluster of cases in Los Angeles and Orange counties, California, in which there was the suggestion of "possible [personal] association among the cases." A number of competing hypotheses were presented to explain the new syndrome, one of which involved an infectious agent.[5]

By mid-1984, the causative agent for AIDS was identified. Called HTLV-III by Americans and LAV by the French, the virus ultimately was to be named the Human Immunodeficiency Virus (HIV). A retrovirus, HIV had the capacity to integrate itself permanently into the genetic material of the cells it attacked, rendering the host individual infected for life. Years could elapse before the first clinical signs of disease. Yet in the asymptomatic state the infected individual could be transmitting HIV. Indeed, we now know that even before the first cases of AIDS had been discovered, a "silent epidemic" had commenced, many thousands having been infected and rendered infectious.

In June 1986, five years after the first AIDS reports, the United States Public Health Service estimated that between 1 and 1½ million Americans were infected with HIV.[6] How many would ultimately develop AIDS or be afflicted with AIDS-related complex (ARC)—a range of disorders which, though typically less severe than those associated with AIDS, could on occasion be fatal—could not be known. The PHS estimated that between 20 and 30 percent would develop AIDS by 1991.[7] Looking further into the future, the National Academy of Sciences and the Institute of Medicine predicted in 1986 that over the next five to ten years 25 to 50 percent of those infected would develop AIDS.[8] By 1991, most agreed, upwards of 270,000 cases of AIDS would have been recorded since the first cases were noted a decade earlier, and 170,000 deaths would have been attributed to the disease.

Made at a time when just over 20,000 cases had been counted, the projections foretold a staggering set of events within the next years. Absent an unanticipated breakthrough, the development of a vaccine capable of protecting the uninfected, or a therapy capable of preventing viral replication in those already infected, the statistics of 1986 thus carried a grim message. Like an approaching tidal wave first perceived at a great distance, the vast anticipated exaction in suffering and death had about it a tragic inevitability.

What the more remote future might look like was more difficult to foretell, depending very much on the pace of scientific progress and, as important, on the success of efforts to slow the rate of new infection. But many sober observers were willing to draw a picture of great severity. Thomas Quinn of the National Institute of Allergies and Infectious Diseases declared in early 1985, "This illness now ranks as one of the most serious epidemics confronting modern times."[9] In her fall 1985 address to the Institute of Medicine, June Osborn, dean of the School of Public Health at the University of Michigan, told her audience, "We in the United States have a world-class epidemic on our hands, which we have exported so effectively that the rest of the world is only a little bit behind us."[10] Speaking of the potential global impact of AIDS, the Institute of Medicine and the National Academy of Sciences estimated that worldwide infection could be as high as ten million.[11] In January 1987, Secretary of Health and Human Services Otis Bowen warned, "If we cannot make progress, we face the dreadful prospect of a worldwide death toll in the tens of millions a decade from now."[12] AIDS might indeed dwarf the earlier epidemics of smallpox, typhoid, and the Black Death. More apocalyptic was Stephen J. Gould, the popular but trenchant science writer and scientist who wrote in the Sunday Magazine of the *New York Times* that the AIDS epidemic could, before its end, fell one quarter of the globe's population.[13] Even when, within a year, the direst of these projections would be viewed as the product of undue alarm—at least for the advanced industrial world—none would deny that in the next years the United States would witness a grave medical and social challenge.

Like the epidemics of prior eras, AIDS has the potential for generating social disruption, for challenging the fabric of social life, for inspiring rash and oppressive measures, the more so since it has been indelibly marked in the United States by the social position of those who have borne the brunt of the disease in its formative period. Gay men and intravenous drug users have from the beginning comprised close to 90 percent of the cases. Increasingly a disease of the underclass, AIDS will in the future be affected by the cultures of the ghettos and will in turn have a profound impact on those cultures. As the disease spreads more rapidly among heroin users and their sexual partners, the color of those who fall victim will darken even further—as of 1987, 40 percent of all AIDS cases were black and Hispanic—thus adding another dimension to the perceived threat to society by the bearers of HIV infection, whether symptomatic or not.

In the face of this extended viral siege, American social institutions will be confronted with anxieties that may threaten the capacity to develop measured public policies based on reason and a scientific understanding of how HIV transmission occurs. The threat of AIDS may elicit Draconian measures and an unreasoned reliance upon coercion that could, while justified in the name of the public health, actually subvert the prospects of effective public health policy. Fear of how the rational exercise of public authority could ineluctably lead to repressive and counterproductive interventions may, on the other hand, immobilize those charged with the responsibility of acting to protect the public health. Will our capacity for social reason allow us to traverse a course threatened by irrational appeals to power and by irrational dread of public health measures? Will reason, balance, and a search for modest but effective interventions fall victim to a rancorous din? At stake is not only the question of how and whether it will be possible to weaken the viral antagonist, but the kind of society that America will become in the process. Statesmanlike leadership by public health officials based on a recognition of the importance of restraint in the exercise of their power will be critical. So, too, will the development of social policies that reflect a recognition of the collective responsibility for meeting the needs of those who fall victim to AIDS and pursuing vigorously the daunting scientific challenge posed by the AIDS virus. Only if this challenge is met can success be expected in eliciting the cooperation of those who are socially vulnerable and most at risk for HIV infection in the task of long-term behavioral change. Only if this challenge is met will it be possible to limit the toll of the epidemic in the years ahead.

Protecting the Realm of Privacy—Protecting the Public Health

The central epidemiological and clinical feature of AIDS, and the feature that makes the public health response to its spread so troubling for a liberal society, is that the transmission of HIV occurs in the context of the most intimate social relationships or in those contexts that have for nearly three-quarters of a century proved refractory to effective social control. The transmission of AIDS occurs in the course of sexual relationships, both heterosexual and homosexual, of childbearing, and of intravenous drug use. Fueled by the struggles of blacks, women, gay men, and lesbians, and the dedication and energy of civil rights and civil liberties organizations, over the past two decades the evolution of our constitutional law tradition, as well as our social ethos, has increasingly underscored the importance of privacy and of limiting the state's authority in these realms. Against this constitutional tradition and social ethos, AIDS has forced a confrontation with the problem of how to respond to private acts that have critical social consequences.

Starting with the landmark 1965 case of *Griswold v. Connecticut,* in which the Supreme Court struck down Connecticut's effort to prohibit the use of birth control devices by married couples, America's highest tribunal, as well as many of the most important appellate courts in the nation, began to chart a course that resulted in the flowering of a jurisprudence of privacy.[14] To those who sought to restrict the Court's concern to the married, Justice Brennan had declared, "If the right to privacy means anything, it is the right of the individual, married or single, to be free from unwarranted governmental intrusions into matters so fundamentally affecting a person as the decision of whether to bear or beget a child."[15] When the Court went on to protect the possession of pornography in the home, it declared, in the words of Justice Marshall, "Whatever may be the justification of other statutes regarding obscenity, we do not think they reach into the privacy of one's home. If the First Amendment means anything, it means that a state [may not tell an individual] what books he may read or what films he may watch. Our whole constitutional heritage rebels at the thought of giving government the power to control men's minds."[16] For those who sought to press the Court still further, it was not the sanctuary of the home itself that was critical but the intimacy of the acts combined with the effort to shield them from the view of those who might be offended that created the right to invoke the protective mantle of privacy. "Granting that society can proceed directly against the 'sexual embrace at high noon in Times Square' an appeal to such extremes should not provide the pretext for withdrawing all constitutional protections from sexual conduct whenever the participants fail to hermetically seal their actions," wrote Laurence Tribe, the liberal theorist of constitutional law.[17] Whatever the "threshhold of harm" required of the state when it seeks to intrude upon intimate acts in public, the threshhold rises "when the conduct occurs in a place or under circumstances that the *individuals involved* justifiably regard as private."[18]

Writing in 1980, fifteen years after the Griswold case, Kenneth Karst noted the sweep of the Court's efforts to protect privacy. More than fifty cases dealing with matters such as marriage, divorce, family relations, and decisions about whether to bear children had been decided. What linked the cases despite their diversity was a single theme, "the freedom of intimate association."[19] For Tribe, whose scope of interest went much further than that of Karst, what was so striking was the way in which the Court had searched the Constitution's language and spirit to provide justification for the expanding right of privacy. These rights had "materialized like holograms from 'emanations' and 'penumbras' . . . [and even] 'shadows' . . . of the First, Third, Fourth, and Fifth Amendments." But wherever the constitutional grounds had been rooted, "they [had] inspired among the most moving appeals in the judicial lexicon."[20]

This sweeping constitutional legacy, the product of a complex interaction of a liberal court, under the initial leadership of Earl

Warren, with the broader social challenges of the 1960s and 1970s, left unanswered the fundamental question of just how far the protective mantle of privacy might be extended. But just as the definition of privacy had emerged out of the political matrix of a reformist era, it was clear that a more conservative social climate and a more conservative judiciary would produce a less expansive conception of a protected realm for the individual.

The Supreme Court had not even in its most activist phase extended to homosexuals the protection against state intrusion. It is therefore not surprising that in June 1986 a conservative Court under the leadership of Warren Burger upheld Georgia's sodomy statute making homosexual acts a crime. Handed down by a bitterly divided tribunal in the fifth year of the AIDS epidemic, the decision in *Bowers v. Hardwick* denied that homosexuals had a "fundamental right . . . to engage in consensual sodomy."[21] Appeals to history, tradition, and the wisdom of the legislatures of the twenty-four states that outlawed homosexual conduct, even in private, were used to vanquish the claims of those who sought to extend the protections developed over two decades to gay men and lesbians.[22] In his concurring opinion, Chief Justice Burger wrote, "To hold that the act of homosexual sodomy is somehow protected as a fundamental right would be to cast aside millennia of moral teaching."[23] It was in the dissent, written by Justice Blackmun and joined by three additional justices, that the jurisprudence of privacy found its voice. "If [the right to privacy] means anything, it means that before Georgia can prosecute its citizens for making choices about the most intimate aspects of their lives, it must do more than assert that the choice they have made is an 'abominable crime not fit to be named among Christians.' "[24] What the Court's majority had failed to recognize was that "the right of an individual to conduct intimate relationships in the intimacy of his or her own home [is at] the heart of the constitution's protection of privacy."[25]

Paralleling the evolution of the Court's development of a robust doctrine of privacy in the 1960s and 1970s was a growing appreciation among many students of the criminal law that the very effort to enforce such sanctions with regard not only to consensual sexual activity but to the use of drugs as well, required that the state's agents engage in activities that were inherently corrupting. Filling jails with those arrested for the possession of drugs, alcoholics arrested for public drunkenness, and prostitutes had done little to resolve the problems besetting urban society but had strained severely the courts and prisons. The result was a "crisis of overcriminalization."[26]

Among liberal theoreticians an implicit ideology of restraint emerged to reflect the newer perspective on the limits of the criminal law, and on the capacity of all agencies of social control to compel adherence to standards of personal behavior where no complainant existed. When framed in the diction of sociology, this ideology focused on the unintended negative social consequences of "labeling" deviant behavior.[27] When framed by the concerns of law enforcement, it centered upon the "victimless crime."[28] Never fully and explicitly embraced, this perspective was, nevertheless, often reflected in the shifting strategies of social control and law enforcement. The sheer pragmatics of seeking to prevent the collapse of the criminal justice system under its own self-imposed burdens demanded such restraint.

While the law and jurisprudence of privacy evolved around sexuality, intimacy, and procreation, that centering on epidemic control remained largely frozen in time, the product of an earlier pattern of disease, a limited therapeutic capacity on the part of medicine, and a permissive standard of review by the courts when confronted by challenges to the exercise of the state's "police powers"—the constitutional basis for government interventions when threats to the public health were posed. In the face of tuberculosis, smallpox, scarlet fever, leprosy, cholera, bubonic plague, and venereal disease, public health officials had been able to offer little but the blunt instrument of isolation and quarantine when they attempted to limit the ravages of disease. When brought before the courts, officials were typically vindicated, regardless of the exactions on liberty demanded by their intercessions. Deference to legislative decisions and administrative findings was the hallmark of the era. Looking back on the court cases decided early in the century from the vantage point of contemporary standards of constitutional law, legal scholars have noted a marked "preference for social control over individual autonomy," in the earlier period.[29]

In 1901, for example, the Supreme Court of South Carolina, in a case that has become a celebrated instance of capitulation before unreasonable state authority, permitted the quarantine of an elderly woman suffering from anesthetic leprosy, though it acknowledged that there was "hardly any danger of contagion." The woman had lived in the community for years, had gone to church, taught school, and conducted her social life without ever having transmitted her illness to others. Yet the court decided that it was "manifest that the Board [of Health] were well within their duty in requiring the victim [of the disease] to be isolated given the 'distressing nature of her malady.' "[30] It mattered little that this woman would be deprived of her freedom—no less so than if she had been arrested, charged, and found guilty of a crime."The individual," held the Supreme Court of South Carolina, "has no more right to the freedom of spreading disease by carrying contagions on his person than he has to produce disease by maintaining his property in a noisome condition."[31]

In efforts to control venereal disease, state public health officials routinely detained prostitutes, subjected them to physical examinations, and often quarantined them on no greater showing of proof than that they were prostitutes and presumptively infected.[32] That the women were of "infamous character" played no small part in such decisions. But these women were not alone. Though there were some exceptions, most notably the refusal of a federal appeals court to uphold the quarantine of an entire neighborhood inhabited by Chinese in San Francisco as a way of containing an outbreak of plague,[33] the refusal of the courts to intercede in matters of public health followed naturally from the standard of judicial review applied.[34] A showing of some *reasonable* relationship between the public health measures adopted and the unimpeachable goal of reducing the spread of infectious disease was all that was required.[35]

Into the 1950s and 1960s, in the few cases involving tuberculosis control, the courts continued to demonstrate deference to the determinations of state health officials seeking to maintain authority over "recalcitrants" who refused to take the medication that rendered them noninfectious.[36] As late as 1966 a California court could grant the government plenary power in the face of disease by stating that "health regulations enacted by the state under its police power and providing even drastic measures for the elimination of disease . . . in a general way are not affected by constitutional provisions either of the state or national government."[37] But important changes in constitutional law would ultimately render such case law of limited precedential import. A radical transformation in judicial thinking, marked by a dramatic enhancement of due-process protection, would inevitably affect the willingness of the courts to tolerate restrictions on rights considered fundamental, even in the face of a modern epidemic.

Instead of deferring to legislative and administrative decisions, courts would exercise their power of review, demanding that government bear a heavy burden in justifying its impositions. Where "fundamental" rights were entailed, the standard of judicial examination that was to emerge would indeed be exacting. Under such circumstances the courts would apply the standard of "strict scrutiny" and would demand of the state that in seeking to achieve a "compelling state interest" it draw its restrictions "narrowly," relying upon the "least restrictive" alternative necessary.[38]

But despite the emergence of this standard, what would remain—had to remain — a matter of controversy was the scope of the rights to be defined as fundamental. As in the case of "privacy" the task of defining would be essentially political, the product of the interaction between prevailing judicial philosophies and the broader social climate. As the AIDS epidemic produced sharp encounters over the exercise of the state's public health authority, the courts would inevitably provide forums for struggles over the definition of the protected realm of fundamental rights. Precedent and the language of prior cases would structure the style and diction of the judicial decisions, but the outcomes would inevitably reflect the prevailing balance of political and ideological forces.

Reflecting the new willingness to challenge the imposition of restrictions in the name of health, a federal appeals court rejected—just two years before the CDC reported the first cases of AIDS—the effort on the part of the New York City Board of Education to isolate mentally retarded school children—among whom hepatitis B was endemic—from other pupils in public schools. Gone was the deference to determinations made by responsible public officials. "The School Board was unable to demonstrate that the health hazard . . . was anything more than a remote possibility."[39] Given the cost to the children involved—stigma and isolation—the court found the government's efforts unacceptable.

On the eve of the AIDS epidemic, Laurence Tribe had sought to capture the liberal constitutional conception of the powers of government when faced with a grave threat to the public health. "In an epidemic," he wrote, "it may be unquestioned that the state should require vaccination and quarantine." But that broad principle, he warned, could not be so construed as to justify the imposition of constraints or the deprivation of the fundamental rights of the weak in ways that bore no clear and demonstrable relationship to the legitimate concern for the protection of the public health. In each case when the state acted, Tribe asserted, it would be necessary to ask, "Who is being hurt? Who benefits? By what process is the rule imposed? For what reasons? With what likely effect as precedent?"[40] How far from the day—in 1900—when a treatise on constitutional law could declare that before the demands of public health, "all constitutionally guaranteed rights must give way"![41]

Personal Behavior and Social Burdens

This then was the legal-social context within which AIDS intruded upon America, forcing a consideration of how profoundly private acts with dire implications for the commonweal might be controlled.

The only effective public health strategy for limiting or slowing the further spread of HIV infection is one that will produce dramatic, even unprecedented, changes in the behavior of millions of men, women, and adolescents in this country, not only by those already infected, but also by those who are as yet uninfected. Such changes will require modifications in behaviors that are linked to deep biological and psychological drives and desires. Acts of restraint and even deprivation for extended periods, if not for the lifetimes of those infected and those most at risk for becoming infected, will be required if the AIDS epidemic is to be brought under control. Our collective fate is utterly dependent upon private choices, choices that will be made in the most intimate of settings beyond the observation of even the most thoroughgoing surveillance. We are ultimately dependent on the emergence of a culture of restraint and responsibility that will shape such choices. At a minimum such a culture would underscore the importance of preventing harm to others through HIV transmission and of preventing the birth of infants with AIDS. In a more robust form it would go further, stressing a communal concern over the extent to which individuals place themselves at risk for infection with the AIDS virus.

Like all grave social challenges, the AIDS epidemic thus imposes the necessity of transcending the self-interested perspective so characteristic of everyday life. It demands the emergence of a sense of communal responsibility, of the recognition of a moral obligation to desist from acts that may place others at risk. That it is the most private dimensions of daily life that are implicated in the transmission of HIV infection will make this transformation all the more difficult to accomplish. Vigilance and self-protection will, of necessity, remain critical. But the protection of others, of intimates, is the moral standard against which behaviors will have to be judged. Sexual practices, drug-using routines, childbearing decisions will require searching scrutiny in light of the threat posed by the AIDS virus.

The transmission of HIV has as its first and most obvious consequence a private tragedy: the infection of another human being. It is the intimacy of the transaction that has led some to warn against state involvement. "The disease's mode of contagion," has written Richard Mohr, a philosopher, "assures that those at risk are those whose actions contribute to their risk of infection. . . . It is the general feature of self-exposure that makes direct governmental coercive efforts to abate the disease particularly inappropriate."[42] But to conceive of the transmission of AIDS between consenting adults as belonging to the private realm alone and therefore beyond the legitimate concern of the state would be a serious mistake. Private choices involving the transmission of HIV infection cannot, and should not, be, like decisions about religious commitments, for example, a matter of public indifference. They have profound social implications. Each new carrier of HIV infection is a potential locus of further social contamination. When few individuals in a community are infected, the prospect of undertaking individual and collective measures designed to prevent the spread of AIDS is enhanced. When, however, the level of infection begins to reach a critical mass, when a level of saturation is approached, the prospect for adopting an effective program of prophylaxis is diminished.

In mid-1986 some epidemiologists estimated that more than 50 percent of the gay men in New York and San Francisco were infected with HIV.[43] In Los Angeles one study suggested that the level of infection was 31 percent among gay men.[44] Among intravenous drug users in New York City, the estimate of infection was over 60 percent.[45] At the end of 1987 one in sixty-one women who bore a child in New York City was infected with the AIDS virus.[46] There were, however, many regions of the country, especially in nonurban areas, where rates of infection were much lower. As a clinical intervention would seek to block viral replication in infected individuals, the challenge posed to the public health is to prevent the replication of New York and San Francisco.

Though there are differences because AIDS is an infectious disease, the problems posed by the new epidemic are similar in many ways to the problems posed by a host of behavior-related diseases—lung cancer, emphysema, cirrhosis—with which public health officials have had to deal since the surgeon general issued his first report on smoking in 1964. Ironically, at the very moment that an ethos of privacy was being enunciated, founded on philosophical individualism, the collective significance of every individual's acts began to assume greater currency in public debates.

The publication in 1975 of "A New Perspective on the Health of Canadians" represented a renewal of the public and official discussion of the role of government in modifying personal behaviors linked to disease and death.[47] In that report, Marc Lalonde, the minister of national health and welfare, bluntly stated, "Self-imposed risks and the environment are the principal or important underlying factors in each of the five major causes of death between ages one and seventy, and one can only conclude that unless the environment is changed and the self-imposed risks are reduced, the death rates will not be significantly reduced."[48] But even the pursuit of health had to be bounded by other considerations, especially when matters of liberty and privacy were at stake. Lalonde not only recognized the risks involved, but was alert to the nature of the opposition his challenge could well provoke: "The ultimate philosophical issue . . . is whether and to what extent government can get into the business of modifying human behavior, even if it does so to improve health."[49]

These themes found expression in the United States two years later with the publication of the widely read and debated essay, "The Responsibility of the Individual," by John Knowles, president of the Rockefeller Foundation. Though he noted the extent to which environmental and socioeconomic factors contributed to behavior with disastrous consequences for health, it was his striking comments on personal responsibility for morbidity that were so provocative. For Knowles, the social consequences of individual behavior in terms of the cost of medical intervention could no longer be tolerated: "The costs of individual irresponsibility in health have now become prohibitive. The choice is individual responsibility or social failure. Responsibility and duty must gain some degree of parity with right and freedom."[50]

The untoward social, but especially economic, consequences of individual behavior were to become the leitmotiv of the American debate over health, life-styles, and government policy. It clearly was central to Joseph Califano, secretary of the Department of Health, Education, and Welfare in the administration of President Jimmy Carter. In his introduction to *Healthy People*, the American analogue to the Lalonde report, Califano wrote, "Indulgence in private excess has results that are far from private. Public expenditures for health care are only one of the results."[51] While acknowledging that there might well be controversy and debate about the appropriate role of government in urging citizens to give up their pleasurable but harmful habits, Califano argued that "there could be no denying the public consequences of these private acts."[52]

For some, the tone of the literature on individual behavior and health was unacceptably moralistic. Critics on the left were especially acute in focusing on the "victim blaming" dimension of the arguments that seemed like so many poorly masked attempts to divest the government of any responsibility for caring for those who were ill and for the failure to focus on the social roots of the behaviors that were so clearly linked to illness and death.[53] Ultimately, however, there was a shared recognition that government had an important role to play in affecting disease-producing life-style decisions, that a failure to act would represent a dereliction of the responsibility "to promote the general welfare." But despite that common outlook, there remained sharp disagreements over the modes of intervention that might be relied upon by the state as it sought to shape individual health-related behaviors. Matters of liberty and the legitimate boundaries of public authority were at the heart of the debates. The specter of Big Brother, of the overbearing state intruding itself into the realm of privacy, and of Prohibition, America's disastrous Noble Experiment, haunted the encounters.

If the discussion of how health officials might act to modify cigarette and alcohol consumption as well as vehicular behavior could provoke such consternation, how much more intense would be the concern when the transmission of HIV infection was involved. In each of the former cases government could, if it chose to, radically affect the social context of private behaviors through product design, through pricing and taxation mechanisms, through the regulation and control of acts that take place in public. Invasions of privacy would be largely unnecessary. With the transmission of HIV, the public dimension of the acts that are critical for public health is exceedingly limited. The bedroom, not the highway or the commercial outlet for alcohol or tobacco, is involved. More important, sexual behavior and childbearing decisions are not the equivalents of smoking, drinking, and driving. They touch on intimate decisions that only the most totalitarian society could, without great trepidation, consider the realm of appropriate direct state regulation.

Politics, Public Health, and Civil Liberties

In the face of the AIDS epidemic the central problem before public health officials is how to change AIDS-related behaviors. The very privacy of the acts involved in the transmission of HIV infection imposes practical limitations; the importance of eliciting the cooperation of those most at risk for AIDS and of fostering the development of a culture of restraint and responsibility imposes political limitations; and the importance of privacy and civil liberties to American society imposes ideological limitations on the public health strategies that could be called on in the struggle against the epidemic. Rigorous surveillance and attempts at the regulation of the private acts linked to AIDS—were they possible—would not only entail morally repugnant invasions of privacy, evoking images from Orwell, but would be counterproductive as well. Both philosophical and pragmatic considerations thus dictate a common course within which the defense of public health and respect for civil liberties are joined. Yet it would represent a gross simplification to assert that in the effort to confront AIDS the claims of public health and civil liberties must invariably coincide.

The ethos of public health and that of civil liberties are radically distinct. At the most fundamental level, the ethos of public health takes the well-being of the community as its highest good and in the face of uncertainty—especially where the risks are high—would, to the extent deemed necessary, limit freedom or place restrictions on the realm of privacy in order to prevent morbidity from taking its toll. The burden of proof against proceeding from this perspective rests upon those who assert that the harms to liberty would, from a social point of view, outweigh the health benefits to be obtained from a proposed course of action.

From the point of view of civil liberties, the situation is quite the reverse. No civil libertarian denies the importance of protecting others from injury. The "harm principle" enunciated by John Stuart Mill is in fact the universally acknowledged limiting standard circumscribing individual freedom. For twentieth-century liberals and civil libertarians that principle has typically accorded considerable latitude to measures taken in the name of public health—indeed more so than some contemporary civil libertarians find comfortable. But since from a libertarian point of view the freedom of the individual is the highest good of a liberal society, measures designed to restrict personal freedom must be justified by a strong showing that no other path exists to protect the public health. The "least restrictive alternative" is now the standard against which civil libertarians measure any course that affects basic freedoms. When there are doubts, a heavy burden of proof must be borne by those who would act to impose restrictions.

These two abstractions, liberty and communal welfare, are always in a state of tension in the realm of public health policy. How the balance is struck in a particular instance in a function of philosophical and political commitments, and empirical matters: How virulent is a particular agent against which action is contemplated? With what degree of ease can it be transmitted? Are there therapeutic interventions that can blunt the consequence of infection? Does the epidemiology of transmission permit effective intervention? In the case of AIDS, the capacity of America to tolerate over an extended period the social stress engendered by a stark pattern of morbidity and mortality and the anticipation of ever greater losses in the future will determine how such empirical matters, philosophical concerns, and political perspectives are brought to bear on the making of public health policy.

In the fall of 1985—not long ago, but at a time when the number of AIDS cases was still relatively small—at the height of a wave of social anxiety and conflict about AIDS, an article entitled, "AIDS Isn't a Civil Rights Issue. It's a Genuine Plague" appeared in both East and West coast newspapers.[54] In his widely read challenge to the liberal community, Richard Restak wrote: "Plagues are not new. What is new are efforts by medically unsophisticated politicians and attorneys to dictate policy in regard to an illness that has the potential for wreaking a devastation such as has not been encountered on this planet in hundreds of years." Disturbed by efforts to defend the right of school children with AIDS to attend class as well as the employment rights of food handlers and medical workers afflicted by the disease, Restak asserted that what was of preeminent importance was the attainment of an understanding of "all the ways" in which the AIDS virus was transmitted. Prior to such a firm scientific understanding, "political posturing, slogancering, hollow reassurances and the inappropriate application of legal remedies to a medical problem can only make matters worse and potentially imperil the health of us all."

Restak's ideal of a public health strategy to combat AIDS that would be free of political and philosophical considerations is a chimera. Invoked here by an opponent of the broad interpretation of the requirements of civil rights and individual liberties, this vision paradoxically has also inspired those who have asserted that the advocates of more restrictive measures have permitted politics to intrude upon their outlook. The standard of a public health policy untouched by extrascientific considerations involves a profound misconception, a failure to apprehend the inherently political nature of all public health practice.

To speak of public health policy as if it could be apolitical represents an effort to mask the play of social forces appropriately called forth in the making of decisions affecting the communal welfare. Not to be confused with the reckless and irrational disregard of hard-won understandings of how specific diseases are transmitted or with the willful distortion of empirical findings, this perspective compels us to acknowledge that facts alone do not dictate the course of public health action. It is not simply that the inevitable uncertainties that confront decision makers require resolution, and that each such resolution requires a balancing of benefits and costs affecting the interests of men and women and the relationship between competing social values; more important, the body with which the public health is concerned is no mere passive organism upon which neat clinical maneuvers can be performed. Rather it is the body politic itself. Negotiation, trust, cooperation, and sometimes coercion, are always central to the practice of public health. These are especially important in the case of AIDS. It is only the retrospective reconstruction of the history of public health—involving a political amnesia — that permits contemporary critics to charge that we have become the victims of a modern disorder involving the distortion of all social practices by fractious considerations.

With AIDS, where the intimate behaviors of men and women have been implicated in the spread of a lethal illness, and where only the radical modification of these behaviors can alter the trajectory of morbidity and mortality, it was inevitable that political controversies touching the central values of a liberal society would be provoked. Because of the organizational and intellectual capacity of gay communities across America to compel attention to matters of privacy and the limits of the state's legitimate public health powers, the debates during the first years of the AIDS epidemic took on their unique public character. How different the situation would have been if AIDS first and overwhelmingly had struck black and Hispanic heroin users and their sexual partners. The profound issues raised by government efforts to control an epidemic spread by private and typically consensual acts would not have changed, but certainly they would not have been given the same salience.

Now that the role of heroin users and their sexual partners in the spread of AIDS has begun to arouse so much concern, the contours of the public health debate will inevitably change, affected as much by factors of class, race, and ethnicity as by some of the unique problems raised by the heterosexual transmission of HIV infection.

No issue will more dramatically underscore the tension between the rights of privacy and the demands of the public health than that posed by the transmission of the AIDS virus by largely impoverished black and Hispanic women to their offspring. The importance of preventing the birth of infants who will go on to develop AIDS will force a confrontation over how HIV-infected women ought to exercise their hard-won reproductive rights, and may, given the social status of the women involved, threaten the very existence of those rights. Furthermore, the color and social status of those who become infected with the AIDS virus as a result of intravenous drug use may evoke repressive policies that are not only inimical to civil liberties but destructive of the prospect of establishing a bond between public health officials and men and women already profoundly distrustful of public authority. If public health officials are seduced by the allure of power or are driven to coercion by the pressure of politicians, they will be unable to pursue those policies most likely to contribute to the emergence of a culture of restraint and responsibility among those whose life circumstances make the prospect for such a culture so problematical. They will have failed to meet the challenge of AIDS.

In the next years AIDS will impose sharp demands on American political and social institutions. To meet them effectively, not only health officials but the broader public must examine the history and legacy of the first years of the epidemic. An understanding of the forces called into play by AIDS, the costs of false starts, the errors of omission and commission in facing the threat of HIV transmission, and the fragility of the achievements in limiting the spread of the viral antagonist will be critical if the challenges of a maturing epidemic are to be met forcefully and with due regard for the preservation of the important social values at stake.

Chapter 2

Sex and the Bathhouses

The Politics of Privacy

Because from the beginning of the AIDS epidemic, homosexuality had been so starkly identified with the new fatal disease, it was inevitable that deep antipathies would be tapped as American social institutions began to respond to the crisis. It was also inevitable that dread that antihomosexual forces might be mobilized in the name of public health would frame the reaction of gay political organizations that since the 1960s had been engaged in a struggle for civil rights and social toleration. In the course of that struggle, and working against the legacy of fear, the defense of privacy became a central feature of gay political ideology. In the era of homosexual repression, secrecy was the only safeguard. In the era of gay self-affirmation the demand for a right to privacy became the touchstone of a social movement that drew ideological support from the much broader movements of the 1960s and the evolving jurisprudence of sexuality in the United States. Since the state had criminalized homosexuality it was only natural that gay political groups would adopt as part of their strategic posture the civil libertarian's suspicion of government.

What a bitter irony, then, that the very survival of gay men during the AIDS epidemic would require a strategy that would subject their most intimate behaviors to close scrutiny and necessitate calls by public health officials and gay leaders alike for the radical transformation of sexual conduct. Historically rooted antagonisms to the agencies of government would have to be confronted and overcome if effective interventions were to be developed.

For public health officials, whose legacy of anti-venereal disease campaigns included periodic sweeps of red-light districts and closure of houses of prostitution and whose control of epidemics had historically relied upon coercive state power, the ultimate challenge was to develop a language and practice of public health that would encourage the participation, rather than the resistance, of gay men. They would have to press for changed sexual behavior without appearing to don the robes of moralism. Collaborative relationships with gay organizations would have to be built without antagonizing conservative social forces that would consider such efforts a public sanction of immorality. Finally, it would, at times, be necessary to exercise public health authority in opposition to the most articulate forces in the gay community.

These challenges would present themselves dramatically, first in San Francisco and then in New York, in the furious and deeply divisive debate over gay bathhouses. Commercial enterprises that permitted and facilitated multiple and often anonymous sexual encounters, the baths had emerged in the 1970's as a singular expression of bold gay sexuality. That they existed so openly was evidence of a changed sociopolitical climate of sexuality, at least in the most cosmopolitan American cities. Their fate would be brought into question by the AIDS epidemic, when the demands of public health confronted the claims of an inviolate domain of privacy. Would the intimacy of the sexual encounters that occurred within the baths transform their public character? Would the public character of the baths divest the sexual encounters that occurred within them of their private and protected status? As these issues were encountered, they would reveal profound differences over the very definition of privacy and the appropriate claims of the community when faced with an epidemic.

AIDS, Sex, and the Gay Community

In the first year of the AIDS epidemic, as the number of new cases continued to mount, case control studies undertaken by epidemiologists began to identify what was believed to be a subset of homosexual men who were more likely to be at risk for developing Kaposi's sarcoma and the other opportunistic infections associated with immunosuppression.[1] These men were more likely to have had many anonymous sexual partners, to have had a history of a variety of sexually transmitted diseases, and to have engaged in sexual practices that increased the risk of exposure to small amounts of blood and feces. Early on, the director of the Centers for Disease Control noted that "the most important variable was that AIDS patients had more male sexual partners than the controls, an average of sixty per year for patients compared to twenty-five per year for the controls."[2]

As each new report documented the outcropping of the pattern of lethal opportunistic infections and Kaposi's sarcoma among gay and bisexual men, concern mounted in gay communities across the country, but especially on the East and West coasts. The suggestion that there might be a link between sexual lifestyle and the likelihood of falling victim to the disorders reported by the CDC in its accounts of the unfolding epidemic forced some gay commentators to ask disturbing questions about the pattern of sexual behavior that seemed responsible for the still inexplicable and fatal diseases. But concern and rising anxiety were, even in the first months of the epidemic, balanced by efforts to contain the panic that could be socially and psychologically disruptive to gay men and that, it was feared, might spark a wave of antigay outbursts from those who would be threatened by the "gay cancer," first called "gay-related immune deficiency."

Writing in the *New York Native*, a local gay newspaper, just months after the CDC's first reports of pneumocystis carinii pneumonia and Kaposi's sarcoma, Lawrence Mass, a gay physician, explored the question of whether an infectious agent or some environmental factor could best account for the immunological suppression of the men who had fallen ill.[3] He also noted the possible contributory roles of anal trauma and of multiple sexual partners. Thus did gay men begin to traverse the treacherous sociomedical terrain that was to open the question of what it was about gay culture and gay sexual practice that could be responsible for the new diseases. Characteristically, this article, designed to meet the needs of a nonprofessional audience, both acknowledged the possibility of a grave medical threat and stressed the need to contain anxiety. Citing an early AIDS researcher, the article ended on a strangely antialarmist note. The new disease might represent the beginning of a "significant epidemic" but "this is no reason to panic, to respond to this news with alarm."

But despite such efforts to preserve a concerned, cautious, and watchful stance, some writers in the gay press believed that alarm was appropriate and that, at the very least, a direct confrontation with the behavior of gay men was required. Larry Kramer, the successful screenplay writer, who would later author *The Normal Heart*, a bitter play about the social response to AIDS, sounded the tocsin in the fall of 1981.[4] Noting the rising number of cases—though in retrospect they were still so few—he wrote, "It is difficult to write this without sounding alarmist or too emotional or just plain scared. . . . The men who have been stricken don't appear to have done anything that many New York gay men haven't done at one time or another." In the face of scientific uncertainty, he cried out, "We're appalled that this is happening to them and terrified that it could happen to us." Responding some months later to those who were critical of his emotional tone and to his suggestion that what gay men did to themselves or with each other was responsible for the spread of AIDS, Kramer wrote, "But *something* we are doing *is* ticking off a time bomb that is causing a breakdown in immunity in certain bodies, and while it is true that we don't know what it is, specifically, isn't it better to be cautious until various suspected causes have been discounted rather than reckless?" In Los Angeles the publisher of the *Advocate*, David Goodstein, echoed Kramer's sentiments—but in a far more restrained manner—when he wrote in early 1982, "Whether we like it or not, the fact is that aspects of the urban gay lifestyle we have created in the last decade are hazardous to our health. . . . Our lifestyle can become an elaborate suicidal ritual. Our safety and survival depend on each of us and our individual behavior."[5] Nathan Fain, who provided much of the *Advocate*'s reporting on AIDS in 1982, underscored the tension that informed the emerging debate about AIDS and sexuality, a tension between the importance of sexual caution and the specter of moralism. "One word is like a hand grenade in the whole affair: 'promiscuity.'"[6]

The tentative manner in which the gay press addressed these matters early in the epidemic reflected both profound disagreements within the gay community and deep anxieties about how the open discussion of gay sexual culture and practices might create an ideological climate within which the hard-won advances of greater sexual tolerance in America could be swept away in the name of public health. Writing of these two dimensions of the debate, Lawrence Mass said, "Outside the gay community the current epidemic is already inspiring the kind of medical-moral speculation that swept England a century ago. Within the gay community, a parallel crisis of ideology is threatening to explode. With much confusion on all sides, advocates of sexual 'fulfillment' are being opposed to critics of 'promiscuity.' "[7]

Out of this crisis began to emerge a consensus on the part of physicians caring for gay men and those nonphysicians who monitored the scientific literature for the readership of gay newspapers and magazines. By mid-1982 the voice of sexual moderation began to assume the characteristics of an orthodoxy demanded by health, the health of each gay man as well as the health of the gay community. Physicians, many of them gay, began to urge their patients to exercise caution, to choose fewer partners, those in good health. "It is not sex itself as the moralists would have it, but the number of different sexual encounters that may increase risk."[8]

The growing recognition that engaging in sex with many anonymous sexual partners increased the risk of AIDS cut across the controversy over whether such behavior was itself hazardous or whether it was hazardous because it enhanced the prospect of coming into contact with an as-yet-to-be-discovered infectious agent. Among the most articulate antagonists of the pattern of behavior involving multiple anonymous sexual partners was Joseph Sonnabend, a physician who treated many early AIDS patients. He rejected the suggestion that a specific infectious agent could account for AIDS. It was "promiscuity" itself, with the attendant multiple and repeated bouts of sexually transmitted diseases, that produced such catastrophic clinical consequences. Sonnabend propounded his thesis in medical journals and the gay press. Fully aware of how provocative his use of the term "promiscuous" would be, he used it precisely for that reason. "There can be no equivocation. Promiscuity is a considerable health hazard."[9] Alert to how his message might be appropriated by moralists who opposed homosexuality, he assumed the mantle of a value-free medical scientist. "This is not a moralistic judgment, but a clear statement of the devastating effects of repeated infections." While he avoided attributing blame to those who in the past had engaged in promiscuous behavior, he was harsh in what he had to say about physicians, including himself, who had failed to speak clearly and bluntly about the toll taken by sexually transmitted diseases. "A desire to appear nonjudgmental, a desire to remain untinged by moralism, fear of provoking ire, have all fostered a conspiracy of silence. . . . Gay men have been poorly served by their medical attendants during the past ten years. . . . For years no clear message about the danger of promiscuity has emanated from those in whom gay men have entrusted their well-being."

Sonnabend's thesis, measured in its tone, was put even more forcefully by two gay men, Michael Callen and Richard Berkowitz, in an essay published in the *New York Native*.[10] Assuming full responsibility for the diseases that now afflicted them, they warned the gay community about the necessity for radical behavior change. The unwillingness to acknowledge the consequences of sexual excess had silenced the gay community, "but deep down we know who we are and why we are sick." Situating the explosion of sexual activity in the 1960s and 1970s in the context of a rebellion against a "sex-negative culture," they warned that what had been proclaimed as "healthy" self-affirmation "now threatens the very fabric of urban gay male life." With foreboding, they portrayed the prospect of state intervention if the gay community did not assume a direct role in effecting a radical modification of the pattern of promiscuity that was responsible for AIDS. But more, they warned about survival itself. "The motto of promiscuous men has been so many men, so little time. In the 1970s they worried about so many men; in the 80s we will have to worry about so little time. For some, perhaps, homosexuality will always mean promiscuity. They may very well die for that belief."

Paired with this angry cry in the same issue of the *Native* was Peter Seitzman's "Good Luck, Bad Luck: The Role of Chance in Contracting AIDS."[11] A physician, and member of the gay and lesbian medical group, New York Physicians for Human Rights, Seitzman centered his argument on the existence of a transmissible agent and then suggested that just as was the case with hepatitis B, with which gay men were so familiar, there were probably asymptomatic carriers of the yet-to-be-discovered agent. The conclusions he drew were dire. "You can control promiscuity. But your one partner may be infected. Is this fair? No. Is it possible? Yes."

Despite the radical disjunction between the two etiological perspectives, Seitzman believed that there was the basis for a common practical approach to meeting the crisis posed by AIDS. It centered on the recognition of the risk associated with promiscuity. "They believe promiscuity is the *cause*. I believe promiscuity allows the *spread*. We all seek to curtail promiscuity itself." But given the common goal, Seitzman believed it nevertheless critical to distance himself from the accusatory tone that was so central to the article written by Callen and Berkowitz. Guilt, he asserted, could only confound an already tragic situation. "No one has done anything wrong or immoral. . . . It's no one's fault . . . it's simply a nightmare come true. . . . We are victims and not the guilty, and if we can't convince ourselves of that, then how can we expect the rest of society to see us that way?"[12]

Moralism was not only a threat because of the rationalization it could provide for those all too ready to launch an antihomosexual crusade but because of the resistance it would provoke within the gay community to the "lessons" now painfully being learned from the unfolding pattern of morbidity and mortality. But the brutal truth of the consensus on the risks of sexual encounters with many anonymous partners did in fact provoke expressions of opposition, some that reflected the desperation of those who viewed their culture as under attack, others of a more personalistic kind.

The calls for restraint were sometimes seen as nothing more than thinly disguised demands for a return to sexual conventionality. Once again, it was argued, physicians were seeking to establish their dominance over homosexuality, now with the collaboration of those who carried their message in the gay press. In a particularly extreme example of the antagonism provoked by medicine's warning, Michael Lynch wrote in the *Body Politic*, a Canadian gay journal, "Gays are once again allowing the medical profession to define, restrict, pathologize us." To follow the advice of physicians would involve a renunciation of "the power to determine our own identity," and would represent "a communal betrayal of gargantuan proportions" of gay liberation founded upon a "sexual brotherhood of promiscuity." Doubts about the scientific foundations, on the basis of which the cautionary advice was being proffered, inspired others. "I feel that what we are being advised to do involves all of the things I became gay to get away from. . . . So we have a disease for which supposedly the cure is to go back to all the styles that were preached at us in the first place. It will take a lot more evidence before I'm about to do that."[13]

It mattered little, at times, whether the calls for sexual moderation and caution were presented as a requirement of prudence or as a moral imperative. Writing in response to the cautionary advice that appeared in the *New York Native,* one correspondent asserted that the risks involved in hailing a taxi were a greater threat than sexual relations with a stranger.[14] Faced with constraints that would follow from the warnings about promiscuity—"they are actually asking us to avoid all casual sex"—he preferred to take his chances. "I refuse to blight my life in order—supposedly—to preserve it." Even when the risks of AIDS were not disputed, hostility surfaced when the provision of information took on an instructional tone. So antagonistic were some to the overt efforts to modify sexual behavior, by those who saw it as their professional or communal responsibility to warn about AIDS, that they responded as if a threat to privacy and "self-determination" were at stake. "One must regulate one's life based on enlightened thinking, not on hysterical fear. I really do not think it appropriate for any doctor, any victim, or *anyone*, to tell me what I ought to do; just give me the facts, and I'll decide, thank you."[15]

Such resistance drew the response of Larry Kramer in "1,112 and Counting," a dramatic call to arms published in the *Native* in 1983.[16] Like his appeal to the gay community published a year and a half earlier this article thundered its message of alarm. "Our continued existence as gay men upon the face of this earth is at stake. Unless we fight for our lives, we shall die. In all the history of homosexuality, we have never been so close to death and extinction before. Many of us are dying and are dead already." A demand for more money for research into AIDS, a denunciation of government officials who failed to respond because it was the lives of gay men that were at stake, this jeremiad also pointed a finger of accusation at gay men who refused to change their sexual lives. "I am sick of guys who moan that giving up careless sex until this blows over is worse than death. How can they value life so little and cocks and asses so much? Come with me, guys, while I visit a few of our friends in intensive care. . . . Notice the looks in their eyes, guys. They'd give up sex forever if you could promise them life."

It was in the context of such wrathful outbursts, growing anxiety, dread among gay men, and an appreciation of how advice about changing sexual behavior might take on the quality of moralism that efforts to gain the confidence of those at risk for AIDS took shape. Most remarkable was the frequent adoption of the diction of responsible but private choice, a diction that explicitly rejected any impression that a *demand* was being made for change in private behavior. Early in 1983 the Kaposi's Foundation, one of the early West Coast organizational responses to AIDS, asserted, "[We] must walk a tight rope by providing information to high risk gays, while not appearing to be 'moralistic' about the factors believed to be associated with AIDS, including promiscuity. . . . We want to educate the public not spread alarm. We are not a morals board and we want to create a presence that can be trusted. . . . We are not here to judge you. But here's what's known. Draw your own conclusions."[17]

The recommendations being urged upon gay men in this period already went far beyond those that stressed the importance of reducing the number of different sexual partners. In its advisory on "AIDS and Healthful Gay Male Sexual Activity," the American Association of Physicians for Human Rights, a small but prominent national gay and lesbian physicians' organization, urged that AIDS be thought of as a sexually transmitted disease and that eliminating those sexual practices linked to such diseases might also reduce the risk of developing AIDS.[18] Thus AAPHR urged the avoidance of one-time encounters with anonymous partners and group sex; oral-anal contact ("rimming"); the insertion of the fist into the rectum ("fisting"); active or passive rectal intercourse; fecal contamination ("scat"); and mucous membrane (mouth or rectum) contact with semen or urine. The use of condoms during intercourse was presented as possibly providing some protection. AAPHR recognized that such changes would prove difficult to many men, since they would involve giving up familiar and deeply desired sources of pleasure. It acknowledged, furthermore, that such recommendations were based on very incomplete scientific data. But the seriousness of AIDS demanded that as physicians they be "perhaps overly cautious in [their recommendations rather] than to find out later [that] we have not been cautious enough." Concerned that it be viewed as "too judgmental" the association of gay physicians noted, "We too have experienced these diseases and are trying to practice what we preach."

Accompanying the repeated calls for caution were attempts to encourage the exploration of forms of sexual intimacy and pleasure that did not involve the risk of AIDS. This message was conveyed to the gay community not only through its own media and self-help organizations like the Gay Men's Health Crisis in New York City, but by some public agencies as well. In May 1983 the San Francisco

Department of Public Health published a brochure directed at the gay community that incorporated both warnings about the importance of avoiding life-threatening sexual behaviors and a message of hope. "Part of the responsibility for ending this epidemic (or at least reducing our own risk of developing AIDS) lies with each of us as individuals. Quite simply, we must face the reality of AIDS in our community and our individual lifestyles. . . . None of [the] suggestions for risk reduction preclude a rich and exciting social and sexual life for any gay man in San Francisco. The reality of the AIDS epidemic in our community may, however, cause many of us to examine exactly how we are treating ourselves and each other."[19] Not only self-defense but an obligation to protect others was called for by the communal medical threat.

Privacy, Sex, and the Bathhouses

As the public health dimensions of the AIDS epidemic increasingly took center stage, the limitations of those perspectives that were focused solely on the decisions of gay men as private individuals were to become ever more apparent. This was the context within which the question of the gay bathhouse was to become the subject of an acrimonious controversy that would divide the gay community and force a confrontation over privacy, sexual behavior, and limits of state intervention in the name of public health. As early as March 1982 David Goodstein of the *Advocate* was to broach the issue, in the most cautious of ways. "It could be that the sex palaces which encourage orgies and lack adequate showers are public health hazards. And I shudder at the political implications of this notion."[20] Randy Shilts, the gay San Francisco *Chronicle* reporter who was to emerge as a strong antagonist of the bathhouses, the sexual culture they fostered, and the timidity of gay political leaders in confronting the public health implications of the continued operation of such establishments, was sharper and more blunt when he wrote in the *New York Native*, "By the mid 1970s promiscuity was less a lifestyle than an article of faith. . . . Before long an entire subculture and business network emerged catering to drugged out alcoholic gay men with penchants for kinky promiscuous sexual acts." And so in cities across America bathhouses opened their doors, "unprecedented in that they were businesses created solely for the purpose of quick multiple sexual acts, often accomplished without speaking so much as one word."[21] Because of the visceral antagonism to anything that resembled the moralism that had made of homosexuality itself a despised form of love, none of this was ever questioned.

But in the face of the AIDS epidemic and with wide-scale recognition that promiscuity posed a grave health hazard to the gay community, the bathhouse could no longer avoid scrutiny. For some the solution was to mandate the posting of warnings in the bathhouses. Reflecting how difficult it was to consider even such a modest move and expressing the dominance of a posture that came close to equating warnings about dangerous sex with moralism was the observation of Dan William, a gay physician in New York: "Deep in my heart I'm a civil libertarian . . . [but] it may even be appropriate to mandate warnings as we do with cigarettes. (I would support the right to smoke. But we [gay physicians] have a duty to warn)."[22] Thinking about a bleaker future he even hinted at the possibility of greater restrictions, stipulating, however, that the gay community would have to be involved in formulating necessary guidelines.

Despite the occasional public suggestion that the gay community might have to collaborate with public health officials in regulating the bathhouses or in limiting the activity permitted to occur within them, the dominant ideological voice projected by the gay press was antistatist, hostile to the claims that the defense of the public health by government officials might rightfully entail restrictions on commercial establishments serving the sexual desire of their gay clientele, even hostile at times to the suggestion that the gay community act to force changes in those institutions that provided a setting for anonymous sexual encounters that could well lead to the further spread of AIDS. Indeed, despite the language of community that filled the columns of the gay press, a radical, almost asocial individualism inspired much of the early rhetoric about the bathhouse. In 1983, Lawrence Mass, often a voice of sober reflection in the unfolding AIDS crisis, thus wrote in the *New York Native*: "What we decide to do about these health hazards will depend on how we decide to deal with them as individuals. . . . The issue is not where we have sex, but with whom and with how many. If the baths were to be closed or transformed, it should be because the market has changed, not because of vigilante impulsivity."[23]

The specter of an intrusive paternalistic state haunted Mass's vision. Closing the baths could inevitably lead to "laws that would eliminate opportunities to have casual sex." Such restrictions might in turn be just one small step from legislation that would control smoking, alcohol consumption, and homosexuality itself. As his rhetorical pitch rose, Mass concluded, "To demand that the bathhouses be shut down would probably do little to limit the spread of the disease, but could significantly hasten the no-longer creeping pace of fascism against minorities in this country." Writing one year later in the *Advocate*, Nathan Fain also demonstrated a profound commitment to self-determination. Those who continued to attend the bathhouses could, he argued, be considered to have chosen a suicidal course. "The real question is, is their suicide any business of society?" For Fain there really was no doubt about the answer.[24]

The arguments about the public health benefits that might follow from regulating or closing the baths and about the rights of those who chose to engage in high-risk sexual activity in commercial establishments were to appear again and again in the public debate over the next year. But the abstract discussion of principles and epidemiological judgments took on concrete form in San Francisco, where, beginning in mid-1983, the gay community, the city government, and the public health authorities were to become embroiled in a fifteen-month confrontation over how to respond to the bathhouses in the face of the AIDS epidemic.

San Francisco and the Battle of the Baths

Two years after the onset of the AIDS epidemic, in mid-1983, little had changed in the operation of the San Francisco bathhouses. Despairing of the possibility that the proprietors would ever undertake modifications that would affect their commercial interests and impatient with those who had failed to grasp the significance of the epidemic, some gay activists believed it time to move beyond voluntarism and to engage the power of the state to foster changes in the sex establishments.[25] And so they began to urge the director of the city's Department of Health, Mervyn Silverman, to use his authority to elicit the agreement of bathhouse owners to post warnings about unsafe sexual practices. Others believed that warnings were not enough. In the summer of 1983 Mayor Dianne Feinstein made it clear to Silverman that she wanted him to shut the bathhouses.[26] A demand for dramatic action was to come from at least one politically prominent gay figure, Larry Littlejohn, a veteran of the early years of the gay liberation movement and a leader in the struggle of the early 1970s to eliminate homosexuality from American psychiatry's classification of mental diseases.[27]

In his response to Littlejohn, Silverman demonstrated a remarkable caution that was to make him the target of the mayor's ire and win for him the admiration of most politically vocal elements in the gay community. Alone among public health figures across the country, Silverman was to be forced in this period to confront openly the cross-pressures of those who viewed the bathhouses as dangerous to the public health and those who saw them as important because of their potential role in educating the sexually active about the risks to which they were exposing themselves and their symbolic significance in the struggle for the defense of the freedom of the gay community. In a letter to Littlejohn written in mid-May, Silverman seemed utterly opposed to any moves that would entail coercive intervention.[28] Closure was unjustified on public health grounds, would be politically unacceptable, and would represent an unwarranted restriction of civil liberties. Though he was aware that AIDS was a sexually transmitted disease and was cognizant of the activities that took place within the baths, he refused to term them a threat to the public health. "Because the facilities of most bathhouses do not present a public health hazard I feel it would be inappropriate and in fact illegal for me to close down all bathhouses and other such places that are used for anonymous and multiple sex contacts." Furthermore, such a move would entail a political insult, an insult to the "intelligence of many of our citizens." Finally, closure would represent an "invasion of . . . privacy." Rather than undertaking such repressive measures, Silverman stressed the importance of educating the gay community about the risks of AIDS and suggested therefore the "voluntary" posting of warnings in the bathhouses.

Four months later, Silverman responded to another of Littlejohn's demands for action, again noting the civil rights issues involved in closure.[29] He went on to argue (there was in fact little basis for his very sanguine picture) that the effort to seek the cooperation of bathhouse owners for the posting of warnings had met with compliance, that bathhouse attendance had decreased, and that there was "little orgy activity" in evidence at those establishments that had drawn Littlejohn's antagonism. Finally, Silverman argued that closure might in fact be counterproductive. "I do not share your impression that the subculture who use bathhouses would not immediately switch to other locations where we would have less access to post warnings and provide some education."

The threat of bathhouse closure was further underscored by Pat Norman, the coordinator of gay and lesbian services at the health department and an activist in the city's lesbian community. Closure, she said, would be a "largely meaningless gesture" from a public health perspective. Norman viewed the pressure on the gay community to shut the baths as a political price being demanded by a hostile society—a ransom to prove the moral worthiness of those at risk for AIDS, a demonstration that the funds requested for research and medical care would be well spent. "Has the debate shifted from the containment of the disease to the containment of a people?"[30]

As the controversy continued to fester in San Francisco, no visible public health official appeared willing to adopt publicly the position being pressed by Larry Littlejohn and privately by some physicians concerned by the spreading epidemic. Speaking to a joint meeting of the American Association of State and Territorial Health Officials and the U.S. Conference of Local Health Officers, Edward Brandt, Jr., the assistant secretary of health and the federal official most responsible for national policy on AIDS, deferred to local authorities. "There are few issues more volatile than human sexuality and privacy. They are not issues for the [Department of Health and Human Services]. It is important that the gay community and public health officials clear that [discussion up] and fast."[31] When Randy Shilts reported in the San Francisco *Chronicle* in February 1984 that James Curran, head of the AIDS Activity Office, at the Centers for Disease Control, believed the bathhouses should be closed, Curran went to some lengths to state that he had been misquoted and misrepresented. What he believed and hoped was that the bathhouses would close for lack of business. He had never suggested state intervention. In language reflecting the public timidity of the period, he went on to say, "I [don't] see a role for government in legislating sexual behavior or legislating change." For Shilts, a critic of Silverman's unwillingness to act, Curran's clarification was nothing more than an effort to amend his remarks in response to the "political heat" they had generated.[32]

With no public support for closing the baths by the nation's health officials and with apparently only isolated individuals within the gay community calling for closure, Silverman continued to stress throughout the first three months of 1984 that any action directed against the bathhouses would have to come from gay organizations. Extremely sensitive to how a misstep on his part might disrupt the effective working relationship he believed he had developed with gay groups and which he felt was critical to his overall strategy for containing the AIDS epidemic, he refused to take steps "that might make me look good to a lot of straight people in the community."[33] The lessons of history were clear to San Francisco's chief health official: government was not an effective agent for getting people to change their sexual behavior.

By mid-March of 1984 Larry Littlejohn, frustrated by his inability to press the Department of Public Health to take aggressive measures against San Francisco's bathhouses and despairing of his ability to mobilize the leadership of the city's gay community behind such a move, decided upon a dramatic course—one that would fundamentally alter the nature of the bathhouse debate. Littlejohn planned to launch a petition campaign that would place an initiative on the November ballot requiring the city's Board of Supervisors to prohibit sexual activity in the baths.[34] Justifying this move with its obvious risks of stirring local and national antihomosexual sentiments, Littlejohn cited the empirical evidence of failure of the city's modest educational efforts to modify the behavior of those who attended the bathhouses. Health promotion campaigns had failed to solve the problem of drug abuse and drunk driving, had not succeeded in gaining compliance from drivers to wear seat belts, had not prevented unwanted pregnancies. "We must not fool ourselves. There are no educational programs that will effectively change high risk for AIDS sex habits of bathhouse patrons to safe sex."[35] To stop the spread of AIDS would require not only clear statements but appropriate action as well.

Aware that he would be charged with calling upon the state to violate the realm of privacy in a way that was anathema to the political outlook of the organized gay community, Littlejohn drew a sharp distinction between public settings and the home. "If people want to continue dangerous sex activities in the privacy of their homes—so be it, that is their right. They are foolish to do so. However, bathhouses are public places. They are licensed by the city; they are the proper subject of public policy considerations." There were for Littlejohn "no real civil liberties issue[s] here." For those who might accuse him of a betrayal of the cause of gay liberation, he asserted the preeminence of saving gay lives. "I care more for my gay brothers. I care enough to speak out even if that should make me unpopular with some persons."[36]

When Littlejohn's plans were made public at the end of March the pace of debate intensified. Mervyn Silverman met with several gay physicians who spoke to him about the medical consequences of failing to close the bathhouses.[37] The director of health underscored his concern that any action to be taken on the bathhouses have the support of the gay community. Without such support he could not move despite the threat of Littlejohn's efforts. And so a small group of prominent gay individuals met to plan the mobilization of that support. Motivated by the dread of an electoral battle over the baths, the fear that the gay community's major achievements would be lost in the process, as well as by the toll being taken by AIDS, all but two of those attending the session agreed to sign a letter to Silverman calling upon him to close the baths.[38] In addition to lending their own support to a move on Silverman's behalf, each of the participants agreed to seek the support of others—in all approximately one hundred prominent figures in the gay community were targeted for this effort.

But the enthusiasm of those who believed they could organize broad-scale gay community backing for closure—a condition set by Silverman—was not shared by others. Not only did they fail to generate additional signatures, but their effort generated significant political and professional opposition.[39] The National Gay Task Force issued a statement that, though warning of the risks associated with "anonymous sex with multiple partners," expressed unalterable opposition to state intervention.[40] "NGTF feels most strongly that personal behavior should not be regulated by the state, which historically has been an instrument of our oppression. Furthermore, state closure of such establishments would be largely symbolic, a largely symbolic gesture that would provide a false sense of security that the AIDS epidemic had somehow been contained." From the faculty of the Institute for the Advanced Study of Human Sexuality, a group that included Wardell D. Pomeroy, a well-known former colleague of Alfred Kinsey, a letter was sent to Silverman warning of the consequences of closure. Sexual activity driven from the bathhouses would shift to other locations and would hinder any "scientific and professional approaches" to the problem. Without rational justification, bathhouse closure could only be viewed as "short-sighted, simplistic, and obvious in its political rather than humanitarian motivation."[41]

In San Francisco itself resistance was reflected at a meeting of gay leaders on the evening of March 29. At that session, it became clear to Silverman that given his requirement of gay community support he would be unable to act.[42] And so on March 30 Silverman appeared before a planned press conference and announced that he would need more time to formulate the health department's policy.[43]

Even for some who had signed the original letter calling for closure, there was a sense of relief that so dramatic a move had not been forced in three days as the result of the announcement of Littlejohn's effort. Frank Robinson, a writer who had signed the call, stated, "I'm personally pleased that there is more time for more input, for more discussion on the subject."[44] He hoped that bathhouse owners would, in the time available, "board up the glory holes . . . close the orgy rooms, turn on the lights," provide a condom to every customer, and a copy of the safe sex education pamphlet "Let's Talk." But he also urged the gay community to acknowledge that "the biggest threat to the gay community is not that some people want to close the bathhouses. The biggest threat is a hideous, disfiguring, terminal disease called AIDS." Alluding to the March 29 meeting, at which it became clear to Silverman that he could not expect broad-scale support from the gay community for closure, Robinson lamented, "At Thursday's meeting . . . there were 172 ghosts who were not heard from, but if they could have spoken I think they would have reminded us of the terribly bitter fact that many of us seem to have forgotten. AIDS is something we give to each other."

Very different was the tone of an editorial that appeared in a gay newspaper, the *Bay Area Reporter* (*BAR*). Listing the names of the sixteen individuals, including the "traitor extraordinaire," Larry Littlejohn, who supported closure, the *BAR* equated each of these indiviuals to Marshal Pétain.[45] "The people would have given away our right to assemble, our right to do with our own bodies what we choose, the few gains we have made in the past 25 years. These sixteen would have killed the movement—gladly handing it all over to forces that have beaten us down since time immemorial."

In the period immediately following the March 30 press conference, Silverman was praised by civil liberties and gay rights groups for his restraint, his unwillingness to capitulate to political pressure from pro-closure forces, his determination to assert the primacy of what they considered the requirements of public health over expediency, and his respect for the critically important values of civil liberties. Most forceful in its articulation of the importance of shielding the right of adults to conduct their sexual lives free of state interference, even in the face of decisions that could lead to illness and death, was a letter to Silverman from Neil Schram, president of the American Association of Physicians for Human Rights.[46] Drawing upon the antistatist and individualistic themes of gay political thought, Schram linked the debate over the bathhouses to those that had raged over other behaviorally related diseases—those caused by smoking, alcohol consumption, and overeating, and to the risks associated with motorcycle riding without helmets. Ignoring the powerful public health appeals that had, in fact, often provided the grounds for broadly supported government regulations, Schram asserted that the state should adopt a laissez-faire perspective. Personal freedom was at stake. Physicians had an obligation to educate and warn about high-risk behavior. But it was not for the medical community or the state in its public health role "to try to force behavioral change. . . . The closing of businesses to protect people from themselves cannot be accepted. . . . Ultimately each individual is responsible for himself." To permit the closure of the bathhouses would be to permit an assault on an institution "where it is safe to meet other gay people without fear of arrest and harassment," and would represent the "beginning of the end." The logic of closure led to disastrous consequences. Underscoring a theme that would surface again and again, he warned of the ineluctable course that would lead from the public bathhouse to the private bedroom. "Why could people not argue next that since 'gay sex causes AIDS' prevent gay people from meeting each other, so close the bars and finally outlaw sex in the bedroom again?" The memories of oppression were all too fresh. Repeating the leitmotiv of virtually every pronouncement in the organized gay medical community, Schram concluded, "There should be no misunderstanding. AAPHR strongly discourages sexual contact with multiple anonymous partners. But we cannot and will not support any effort to enforce that viewpoint."

Silverman was made aware not only of the vociferous opposition to closure by important elements in the gay community, but of his isolation within his own profession as well. Indeed, in anticipation of a March 30 closure announcement some public health officials sought to reassure the gay communities in their own cities. An initial draft statement prepared for the commissioner of health of New York City stated, "The city does not plan to close any establishments that serve lesbian and gay customers. . . . There is no reason to do so in New York."[47] The director of New York City's Office of Gay and Lesbian Health stressed, "There is no science to support the closing of the bathhouses." For Roger Enlow education of the community at large as well as within the bathhouse was the "only effective means of behavior change."[48] Similarly, a draft statement prepared by the Philadelphia Health Department stated, "The Department . . . considers such action to be unwarranted at this time. . . . [we] probably do not have the authority to take such action. We view this as probably an infringement of civil liberties."[49]

But despite pressures to refrain from action, the forces set in motion by Larry Littlejohn's initiative, the insistent pressure of Mayor Dianne Feinstein, the persistent though often private warnings of many gay physicians associated with the treatment of AIDS patients, and Silverman's own changing perception of what was required to confront the AIDS crisis in San Francisco made it certain that the aborted announcement of March 30 would not end with a complete about-face. Action against the baths was inevitable.

In the face of such pressures, Silverman was warned by the city attorney's office that closure solely on health grounds would not withstand legal challenge.[50] This, of course, was Silverman's nightmare: to take the fateful step of closing the bathhouses as a way of reinforcing the message about the risks of unsafe sexual activity and to have such a move overruled by the courts.[51] The result would be a deep fissure between the health department and the gay community, as well as a confused public message about the dangers of high-risk sex.

This was the context within which Silverman convened a meeting of local, state, and federal health experts to discuss the future of the bathhouses.[52] Among those involved were James Curran, director of AIDS activity for the CDC, James Chin, chief of infectious disease for the state of California, Dean Echenberg, Silverman's deputy for communicable diseases, local medical leaders, and a number of prominent gay physicians. On April 3 the group met for hours, and at last a consensus was reached. Instead of closing the baths, the group settled on a regulatory approach. "There should be no sex between individuals in public facilities which would lead to the spread of AIDS."[53] The decision to prohibit all sex between individuals at the bathhouses was fateful because of its rejection of the distinction between safe, possibly safe, and unsafe sex so central to the educational efforts being undertaken by both the city and gay health organizations. In explaining that decision, Silverman said, "There was no way, really, that we could inspect to see if someone was wearing a condom, if they had put it on correctly—talk about infringement—that would have been incredible."[54]

Six days later Silverman addressed the press. Flanked by gay physicians, he reported the unanimous conclusion of his advisory panel that "all sexual activity between individuals be eliminated in public facilities in San Francisco where the transmission of AIDS is likely to occur." While he underscored the role his action would have on the course of the AIDS epidemic, he stressed that his move was only part of a much broader program of education.[55] Among the most visible gay physicians supporting Silverman's move were Don Abrams and Marcus Conant. Both were haunted by visions of their dying patients, and by the toll being taken by AIDS. Abrams viewed the bathhouse as uniquely contributing to an environment within which the disease could spread. Dismissing the objections of physicians who opposed this course, he noted that many were psychiatrists who had never seen "what AIDS does to its victims. . . . We're talking about life and death."[56] Conant was moved by the knowledge that some of his own patients continued to attend the baths. "They have no moral problem with it. Clearly, any public health measure ever taken limits people's civil liberties. . . . A year ago I opposed bathhouse closure because I felt gay men would stop going out of fear."[57] They had not.

The picture of Silverman supported by gay physicians provoked the ire of authors and editorial writers in the gay press on both coasts. A betrayal of a central tenet of the gay political culture was involved. Writing in the *Advocate*, published in Los Angeles, Nathan Fain asserted, "What is shocking about the San Francisco news is the alacrity with which a significant number of gay men and lesbians acted to urge their city to make criminals of some of their own people. However sincere the motivation behind the action, it broadcast an alarm to the rest of the world. The message: in San Francisco gay trust broke apart, one tribe willing to sell the other back."[58] David Goodstein, publisher of the *Advocate*, admitted his own perplexity in the face of the bathhouse issue but concluded that the risks of regulation were too serious. "On the one hand, if one life is saved by closing the places, it makes sense to protect the fools from themselves. On the other hand, the most important freedom in the world is the freedom to be a damned fool. We fought hard to open those places. God only knows to what length our persecutors will go if we give them permission to shut them down."[59] On the East Coast, the editor of the *New York Native* denounced the collaboration of those gays who supported Silverman's moves. "Why," he asked, "would we who almost physically restrain our friends from going to the baths now speak so vociferously against restricting sex inside them?" He warned of "well-intentioned evils" that might be done "in the name of public health." The inevitable outcome of even "minor infringements," he asserted, would be disastrous for the gay community. "First you shut down the baths; then you shut down the bars. First you impede the sexually active; then you impede the gay couple." To those who argued that in the face of a health emergency it was permissible to act aggressively and then to worry about civil liberties, he responded, "Where civil liberties are concerned, very often there is no 'later.'"[60] Capturing the tenor of the criticism directed at those who rejected the equation of the commercial bathhouse and the private bedroom, of those who believed that public health officials had no alternative but to enforce restrictions on institutions that fostered a lethal promiscuity, Randy Shilts suggested that a "homosexual McCarthyism" had descended upon San Francisco's gay community.[61]

To those who had struggled to protect the bathhouse from state control, Silverman's decision represented a grave defeat with critical implications for the privacy rights of gay men, not only in San Francisco but across the nation. What made the decision all the more troubling was that its potential impact on halting the spread of AIDS was not at all certain. The health department's decision seemed, despite the effort to provide medical and epidemiological justifications, important primarily because of its symbolic value. But the costs to privacy would be anything but symbolic.

The issues were sharply cast by Thomas Stoddard, legislative director of the New York Civil Liberties Union, who was to become the executive director of the gay Lambda Legal Defense and Education Fund. In an urgent letter to Dorothy Ehrlich, executive director of the Northern California Civil Liberties Union, he urged her to move swiftly in the face of Silverman's decision.[62] For Stoddard any effort to regulate conduct in the bathhouse had to be viewed as antithetical to the principles of civil liberties. "There are two principles at stake here: the right of sexual privacy and the right of gay people to the equal protection of the laws." Acknowledging that the bathhouse might indeed promote conduct implicated in the spread of AIDS, he nevertheless underscored his opposition to state interference. "To admit that we confront a problem of grave significance, disease related sexual conduct at public bathhouses is not the same issue as whether government should be the means by which we solve the problem. That is, it seems to me, a fundamental precept of civil liberties. . . . Civil libertarians are naturally distrustful of government. . . . Therefore, they turn to the state only when there is no real alternative." Action on the part of the gay community, picket lines outside the bathhouses, would be an acceptable method of pressing the bathhouses to change. The specter of sodomy statutes haunted Stoddard's communication. "With the history [of sodomy laws] and with consensual sodomy still a crime in nearly half the states, it hardly seems appropriate to invite the state to regulate private sexual conduct when now it does not." For Stoddard the issues went beyond San Francisco. "Let me also state that I have an ulterior motive in writing this letter. San Francisco is being watched by those in New York, Illinois, by those in Texas, and by those in every other part of the country. If San Francisco—the mecca of gay culture—chooses to close down or regulate public bathhouses, it will give incentive to other cities . . . and in those places, I can virtually assure you, the actions taken will be far harder to keep within reasonable limits. . . . San Francisco will have given succor and encouragement to bigots and homophobes throughout the country to regulate, restrict and punish gay people."[62]

In the face of Silverman's announcement, the Gay Rights Chapter of the Northern California Civil Liberties Union moved with great speed and at its May meeting passed a resolution calling upon the Northern California Civil Liberties Union to adopt a policy statement consistent with its longstanding condemnation of government restrictions on the private sexual behavior of consenting adults.[63] Central to the conceptual foundations of the proposed policy was the definition of the private. Rejecting the distinction between commercial and noncommercial space, the policy sought to bring within the orbit of protection all acts performed under conditions that would be unlikely to be observed by "persons likely to find them offensive." Presented at the May 10 board meeting of the Northern California Civil Liberties Union, the gay chapter's draft was, after some debate, adopted.[64]

At least one board member, however, was distressed by the tone of the resolution and wrote of her concerns. "Though the ACLU's mandate is the protection of civil liberties, it surely needs to balance the requirements of the public as against private rights and to recognize the difficulty in striking a balance, rather than taking for granted that such a balance falls against government in this case."[65] For this critic, the uncertainties of the case, given the gravity of AIDS, demanded careful attention to the requirements of public health.

By May the lines of ideological conflict were sharply drawn. Civil liberties groups and gay rights and gay medical organizations saw in the anticipated regulations an unwarranted intrusion upon constitutionally protected privacy rights. Those supporting regulations saw in them a legitimate and rational exercise of the public health authority of the state. There were sufficient grounds for action. The limits imposed by uncertainty were not a warrant for inactivity. In the confrontation and controversy that were to fester over the next six months, these diametrically opposed perspectives would be played out in a complex series of bureaucratic encounters. Framing the entire imbroglio was the open and lingering clash between Mayor Dianne Feinstein, who in both private and public settings accused the health department of dragging its feet on the bathhouse issue, and Mervyn Silverman, who saw himself as trying to chart a judicious and effective course, one that would have an impact on the course of the AIDS epidemic in San Francisco, one that would not alienate the gay community.[66]

In the face of repeated challenges to the public health justification for his proposed course of action, yet a new and more serious threat to Silverman's goal of regulating the bathhouses was to emerge in the summer of 1984, this time from an utterly unexpected source, the Centers for Disease Control. In a letter from William Darrow, a senior research sociologist with the AIDS Activity Office at the CDC, to Dean Echenberg, the epidemiological relationship between AIDS and bathhouse attendance—the very foundation of the public health case for regulation or closure—was brought into question. Although an earlier national case control study had showed evidence of such a relationship, Darrow found no such association in his just-completed examination of data derived from the San Francisco Clinic cohort study. "Although numbers of partners and AIDS are significantly related, and men who go to bathhouses tend to have greater numbers of partners, bathhouse attendance [itself] is *not* significantly associated with AIDS."[67]

Though bathhouses still emerged as a locus for the pattern of sexual activity linked to AIDS, Darrow's letter clearly served to minimize their significance. Without reference to the heated political battle then in progress in San Francisco or to the conflict in which the public health department found itself embroiled, Darrow had in fact entered the fray. Silverman and Dean Echenberg, his deputy for communicable diseases, were furious and indeed would expend some effort to force a modification of the letter's conclusions by protesting to Darrow's superiors at the CDC.[68] Ultimately, they were successful in wresting a new analysis, with conclusions that were more compatible with the effort to justify the regulation of the bathhouses.[69] But that was not to be for three months. In the summer of 1984 they had to confront the inevitable political consequences of the new CDC findings as gay leaders seized upon the Darrow letter in an effort to force a retreat.

Silverman resisted such pressure and continued to bridle under the bureaucratic restraints that had thwarted his plans to regulate the baths. To break the stalemate, he once again called together the advisory group that had urged the regulation of bathhouse activity. But this time consensus eluded the group. Five supported closure of the commercial establishments at the earliest possible moment; five sought to give the gay community additional time to develop an effective strategy for dealing with bathhouse behavior.[70] Faced with this failure, Silverman chose to do what he had resisted doing for more than a year. He decided to close the baths.

Having made that decision, Silverman sought the advice of the city's attorney on the most appropriate course of action, one that would be sustained in the anticipated court challenges that would greet his effort. Most important in the response he received was the recommendation that the occurrence of high-risk behavior in the city's bathhouses and sex clubs be established as a matter of proof. "Therefore, you should utilize city health inspectors, volunteer medical professionals and conceivably private investigators to irregularly surveil [sic] the suspect establishments on five to ten separate occasions for purposes of determining if high risk behavior is taking place."[71] Such an effort would require that Silverman replicate an effort earlier undertaken by the mayor that had created an outcry against the use of "sex spies." Once having established the existence of high-risk behaviors in the bathhouses, Silverman could then use his authority to close them as public nuisances.

Following the city attorney's advice, Silverman authorized the surveillance of the bathhouses and sex clubs. What made the reports of the city's investigators remarkable was not only the vivid detail with which they described—often in the clumsy language of those unprepared to describe sexual encounters among men, frequently involving more than two individuals—the results of their surveillance, but the fact that they would become part of the public record as affidavits in the city's case against the bathhouses. Some of what was described, acts of mutual masturbation, for example, did not involve "high-risk sex." Some did.

One investigator described darkened hallways in which groups of men would gather "and masturbate themselves or someone else." Then he provided a graphic picture of multiple sexual encounters, and an orgy involving fellatio. "At approximately 10 P.M. two white males knelt on their knees in a darkened hallway next to the orgy room and committed fellatio on a tall white male wearing a black cowboy hat and vest. They would alternate. One would suck the penis while the other would lick the testicles and inner thigh areas. This activity attracted approximately five or six other males to the area to watch and participate. The two men who were doing the fellatio to the cowboy would periodically switch and begin sucking other erect penises that were nearby. The male wearing the cowboy hat ejaculated in the mouth of the small dark man. . . . It appeared the sperm was swallowed."[72]

This report and those prepared by the other investigators achieved the desired impact. Whatever the actual tabulation of safe, unsafe, and possibly safe sex acts observed might have revealed, the descriptions portrayed the existence of activity that would serve to shock the sensibilities of the conventional and disturb those concerned with the transmission of a deadly disease.

With evidence in hand to buttress the decision he had already made, Silverman moved directly against fourteen sex establishments, declaring them public nuisances. Involved were six baths, four gay sex clubs, two gay movie theaters, and two gay bookstores. On October 9 Silverman issued the following announcement: "The places that I have ordered closed today have continued in the face of this epidemic to provide an environment that encourages and facilitates multiple unsafe sexual contacts, which are an important contributory factor in the spread of this deadly disease. When activities are proven to be dangerous to the public and continue to take place in commercial settings, the Health Department has the duty to intercede and halt the operation of such establishments."[73]

Thus did Silverman reject the claims of those who sought to protect the bathhouse by the invocation of the principles governing the state's relationship to private sexual behavior between consenting adults. The very commercial nature of the establishments involved removed, for him, the protective mantle and provided the warrant for intervention. Responding to whose who he knew would charge that his actions represented a profound assault on the interests of gay men, and a reversal of the social and legal advances attained by San Francisco's homosexual community, Silverman ended his statement by declaring, "Make no mistake about it. These fourteen establishments are not fostering gay liberation. They are fostering disease and death." Gone were the concerns about privacy that had been so prominently featured in Silverman's responses to Larry Littlejohn when the health department first had been pressed to move against the baths. Having obtained what he believed was the political support of important elements in the gay community for closure, he could discard the rhetoric of individual liberty.

The city's move provoked an expected series of protests. The Board of Directors of the California Branch of the National Organization of Women expressed "grave concern about the civil rights implications of closures."[74] Brett Cassens, president of the American Association of Physicians for Human Rights, wrote to Silverman about how "deeply disturbed" his association was. "Despite the feeble attempts of several health officers to rationalize the public health need for ending bathhouse sex, it is recognized that this decision is rooted in prejudice and emotion." Sounding an oft-repeated theme he asked, "Were no lessons learned from Prohibition?"[75]

Despite the protracted debate over the bathhouses, the city's move produced a very modest public demonstration attended by only three hundred protestors.[76] Though they were few, their anger was manifest. Banners read "Keep the City Out of Our Sex Lives," "Personal Rights vs. Public Hysteria," "Closure Feeds Bigotry," "Self-Control Not State Control." Randy Stallings, chair of the rally, declared, "What you are seeing in this city in 1984 is an attack on gay male sexuality and that has nothing to do with the worst tragedy we have ever faced. While they attack our sexuality and our rights to assemble, people are dying of AIDS." Jim Geary, director of the Shanti Project, which provided psychological and social support to AIDS patients, went further. "The closure does not save gay lives—but gives license to antigay violence and suffocates our sexual and emotional nature. We are being portrayed as uncontrollable animals without a conscience."

Ultimately Silverman's decision transformed the political struggle that had been waged for more than a year into a legal confrontation to be fought out in the courts. The dispute did not thereby lose its political dimensions, but the lines of argument, the strategies of the contesting parties, and the very language of the encounter were demonstrably affected by the change in venue and the dictates of the adversarial system of justice. The stage now was set for a full and direct confrontation over the constitutional issues raised by the exercise of restrictive state actions in the midst of an unfolding public health crisis, a confrontation that would reveal how the traditional powers of the state to protect the public health would fare in the face of the jurisprudence of privacy and the protections afforded by due-process constraints upon governmental actions.

As it moved to defend its decision in a San Francisco court, the city argued that the least exacting standard of judicial review should be applied. Nothing more than a demonstration of a reasonable relationship between closure and the public health goal of interdicting the spread of AIDS should be required.[77] Unlike those who would assert that the regulations entailed so critical a restriction on personal freedom that the most searching and demanding standard of review should be imposed, the city sought a grant of authority to exercise great discretion in the pursuit of the public health. No more burdensome a standard of review was called for since the privileged realm of privacy was not, for the city, under challenge. Borrowing from the language of legal precedents that sought to hinder state intervention when important freedoms were at stake, the city asserted, "The right to operate a business in a manner contributing to the spread of a fatal disease cannot be deemed 'fundamental' or 'implicit in the concept of ordered liberty,' so as to be included in the right of personal privacy." What appeared to be a rather technical legal question of the appropriate standard of judicial review was, in fact, quite critical. A relaxed standard would make it quite easy for the city to bear the burden of proving its case. A more demanding standard, the application of judicially defined "strict scrutiny," would have meant virtual defeat.

Silverman's declaration, appended to the city's brief, provided the public health rationale for the city attorney's legal strategy of persuading the court to defer to the conclusions drawn by those responsible for the defense of the community's health. Gone was the earlier and forcefully expressed concern about the potential impact of closure on civil liberties. Whatever his private beliefs, a declaration in an adversarial proceeding was not the place for the public health director to voice his doubts. "As a public health officer, I consider it my duty to fashion and implement public policies designed to . . . bring to an end [the operations of] commercial enterprises that involve exploitation for profit of an *individual's willingness* to engage in potentially lethal forms of recreation." Stressing the public setting within which such behavior occurred—with dire consequences for the spread of "virulent disease" and losses to the community measured in the cost of providing care and in the premature death of those who might otherwise have been expected to contribute to the public well-being—he asserted, "Altering sexual activity is a matter of individual privacy; when that sexual activity takes place in a commercial setting, this government has the prerogative and duty to intercede."

In addition to Silverman's declaration and the reports of the investigators who had been sent into the bathhouses, the city's case was supported by the declarations of leaders in California's medical establishment. Some, like Don Abrams and Marcus Conant, had already figured prominently in the controversy. Abrams noted that in the histories of patients cared for at the San Francisco General Hospital, the bathhouse repeatedly appeared as the point of contact with sexual partners. Conant's declaration told of AIDS patients who planned to return to the bathhouses for future sexual contacts. "Since they got [AIDS] there, they did not feel guilty about giving it back." Conant did not share the fear of many gay leaders about the national impact of bathhouse closure in San Francisco. Instead, he saw such action as providing a salutory model for the nation. "If San Francisco was willing to face this problem and close down those businesses that exist solely to promote high risk anonymous sex . . . similar facilities throughout the nation will look to that action and close down too. I believe that this will have a dramatic impact nationally in terms of reducing the incidence of AIDS." A less global assessment of the positive impact of bathhouse closure was given by James Chin, chief of infectious disease for the state of California, who asserted that he "had no doubt that the closure of the bathhouses would be a positive step in reducing the incidence of AIDS in San Francisco." Other declarations stressed the social impact of the private acts that would be impeded by closure. Merle Sande, chief of medical services at San Francisco General Hospital, underscored the growing burden on his institution of caring for AIDS patients. William Atchley, president of the hospital's medical staff, stated that "when the sexual behavior of the individual starts to wreak havoc on the health of the community . . . it is up to doctors and health organizations to try to stop it [by eliminating] the source of contagion."

Perhaps most remarkable in the city's well-prepared case was the failure to obtain a clear declaration of support for closure from any nationally known epidemiologist involved in the study of AIDS and the patterns of sexual behavior among gay men. For Dean Echenberg, it was clear that investigators dependent upon the cooperation of the gay community feared that collaboration with the San Francisco authorities would result in a rupture of professionally critical relationships of trust.[78] And so Echenberg's own declaration had to incorporate epidemiological data that would prove persuasive. "I was not writing a paper for [the journal] *Science*. I was trying to convince the public and the courts. . . . That is how we organized the depositions." It was not the bathhouses per se that posed a health hazard, stated Echenberg. They were important "because they facilitate . . . high numbers of sexual contacts. . . . These facilities flourish and profit by culturing a medium ideally suited for one main purpose, which is encouraging and facilitating high numbers of sexual contacts."[78] How effective would closure be? How many lives would be saved? Echenberg chose not to answer these questions which would be so central to the arguments of his opponents.

The case presented by the bathhouse owners challenged the city's case on both empirical and constitutional grounds. "The issue is whether the plaintiff has carried its burden of proving that [closure] will be sufficiently effective to justify the obviously serious intrusion on property rights, privacy rights, and associational rights." Because closure involved the infringement of fundamental rights, the most searching standard—"strict scrutiny"—was required.[79]

Citing statements made by Silverman when he was resisting pressure to close the baths, the defendants stressed that even the city's chief public health officer had grave doubts about the impact of such a move on the spread of the AIDS epidemic. "The simple fact . . . is that closure of a few locations will simply move bath patrons elsewhere." Both the CDC's data (William Darrow's letter to Dean Echenberg that questioned the independent contributory role of bathhouse attendance in the spread of AIDS was noted) and the city's own research findings were used to demonstrate that closure would do little to control the spread of AIDS. Furthermore, the city's assertion that the baths were the venue of demonstrably unsafe sexual activity was rejected. While denouncing the reliance upon the city's investigators to obtain evidence about bathhouse behavior as "government snooping in the extreme," the defendants argued that a close examination of their reports failed to substantiate the city's claims. "The evidence reveals that over the course of at least eight visits . . . and untold hours of surveillance . . . the total number of unsafe sex incidents equaled two from one premise and three from another."

But such empirical challenges were preliminary to the central constitutional arguments upon which the defendants chose to rest their case. It was here that the radical distinction between those who sought to define a broad realm of privacy and those who defined the bathhouse as public space, appropriately subject to public regulation, was most sharply drawn. But unlike those who had argued that bathhouse intervention would ineluctably lead to control over the bedroom, that there was a grim inevitability to the movement from interventions to control private acts in public settings to interventions that would seek to control private acts in the most private of settings, the proprietors argued that there was no conceptual distinction between the bathhouse and the bedroom. The commercial nature of the establishments, so central to the city's case, was deemed legally irrelevant. "There is simply no legal basis to distinguish the right to engage in consensual sexual activity in defendants' premises from the right to engage in consensual sexual activity in hotels or private homes. [There is] no difference between someone who rents a cubicle in a bathhouse and someone who makes a mortgage payment on his house."

For purposes of protecting sexual activity from state intervention "private no longer means 'alone' or completely hidden from view," argued the proprietors. Drawing upon the case law on sexual privacy and pornography, they asserted that neither the numbers present nor the ability of members of the willing public to gain access to such activity was critical. Instead, it was the likely presence of individuals who could be offended and the awareness of the participants in sexual conduct that viewers were likely to be offended, that defined the conditions under which state intervention would be constitutionally permissible.

In a separate memorandum submitted to the court on behalf of bathhouse patrons, the ideological commitment to freedom from state interference was presented forcefully, all the more so because it acknowledged that moves designed to restrict the liberty of gay men might actually be effective in combating the epidemic. "Precious freedoms are at stake here. A dreaded disease is on the move. People are dying and it is incumbent upon government to stop the devastation that is taking place. The action which government decides to take, however, cannot be based on guesses or unproven assumptions. The liberties at stake are too precious to risk. [The patrons] are not only in jeopardy of losing their constitutional liberties if the [city] succeeds in closing [the baths], they are in addition precisely the men who are at risk of losing their lives if truly effective measures against AIDS are sacrificed out of too great deference to their associational and privacy rights. They are willing to take that chance."

To buttress their case, the bathhouse owners included declarations from epidemiologists, public health officials, physicians associated with the care of AIDS patients and the defense of gay rights, as well as a social historian. The centerpiece of the defense came from Alan R. Kristal, director of the Office of Epidemiological Surveillance for the New York City Health Department. Based upon estimates of the number of gay men still patronizing San Francisco's bathhouses, he sought to demonstrate that closure would have virtually no impact on the AIDS epidemic. The maximum overall reduction in AIDS cases from bathhouse closure would be less than 1/4 of 1 percent. Could such an impact provide the basis for rational, not to speak of constitutional, public health policy? For Kristal, the answer was clear. "No public health official would institute a public health intervention based upon such a tiny expected benefit, and I know of no comparable *public* health crisis where similar intervention was attempted based on such a tiny expected benefit." Both the associate deputy director of the Communicable Disease Control Programs for Los Angeles County, Shirley Fannin, and Martin Finn, medical director for Public Health Programs for the Los Angeles County Department of Health Services declared their opposition to closure, thus highlighting the isolation of their San Francisco colleagues. Fanin declared, "Just as closing houses of prostitution has never been an effective method for controlling other sexually transmitted diseases, it is predictable that closing bathhouses will not significantly help in the control of AIDS." Finn, using arguments that Silverman had himself made in the early days of the debate, stressed the importance of using the bathhouse for safe sex education, engaging those who might be dispersed and made unreachable by closure.

Finally, the case against closure was set in the context of the long history of attacks on gay institutions. Among the declarations provided by the defense was a lengthy social history of the baths by Allan Berube. Unlike those who sought to portray the baths solely as reservoirs of infection, Berube saw their emergence and survival as "an integral part of gay political history." In the face of stigmatization and persecution the "bathhouses represent a major success [of gay people] in a century-long political struggle to overcome isolation and develop a sense of community and pride in their sexuality, to gain their right to sexual privacy, to win the right to associate with each other in public and to create 'safety zones' where gay men could be sexual and affectionate with each other with a minimal threat of violence, blackmail, loss of employment, arrest, imprisonment, and humiliation." For the general public the closure of the baths might simply be viewed as a public health measure involving a minor restriction in the face of an epidemic. For the gay community, argued Berube, such an effort would evoke the memory of the long and bitter history of bathhouse raids. Appealing to the prudence of those charged with protecting the public health, he warned that closure would foster mistrust of government and a lack of compliance with government health programs.

On November 28, Judge Roy Wonder issued his long-awaited order. The city's move for closure was rejected.[80] Instead, the court ordered bathhouse owners to hire monitors to prohibit "high-risk" sexual activity, as defined by the private San Francisco AIDS Foundation. The ruling also prohibited proprietors from renting or operating "any and all private rooms." The doors to the individual video cubicles, booths, or rooms were to be removed. Thus to the question of whether the closed booth represented private and protected space, the judge responded by eliminating the possibility of retreating behind the closed door. Finally, acknowledging the argument that the bathhouses could serve as centers for safe sex education, Judge Wonder mandated that they undertake such programs.

Wonder's order, which came close to Silverman's initial April proposals for regulation, was denounced in the press, by those involved in the litigation, and by San Francisco's mayor. The San Francisco *Examiner* termed the decision "the epitome of judicial folly" and called upon the Board of Supervisors to enact an emergency decree closing the establishments.[81] The San Francisco *Chronicle*, in an editorial entitled "Putting Spies in Sex Clubs," declared, "The order defies common sense. It is something like selling tickets to a swimming pool and forbidding anyone to get wet."[82] Mayor Feinstein, long a bitter opponent of the bathhouses, and a critic of what she had viewed as Silverman's vacillation, remarked, "Most importantly, the ruling allows the continued exposure . . . to AIDS."[83] Thomas Steel, attorney for the bathhouses, asserted that the orders entailed a judicially mandated invasion of privacy.[84] Silverman, who acknowledged the order as being close to his own earlier regulatory proposals, was primarily concerned with how the new rules could be enforced.[85] Modifications in the judicial order made one month later conceded to the city on all matters that were deemed critical from Silverman's perspective.[86]

And so nine months after Mervyn Silverman had first proposed the regulation of bathhouse behavior, with the unanimous support of his expert panel, such regulations were in place as a result of a court-ordered modification of a move to close the establishments. Commenting on the extraordinarily complex and lengthy political process that had produced this final outcome and the tentativeness with which he had made his first moves, Silverman stressed that his concern for preserving an open and collaborative relationship with the gay community had been a critical factor. "If it had been a heterosexual disease, I'd have closed them immediately."[87] Though his restraint has been denounced as the reflection of timidity and fecklessness, Silverman had, in fact, been constrained by his understanding of the political and social context within which he had been pressed to respond to AIDS and the specter of political isolation from those he sought to influence. He had thus charted a prudent, if modest, course. From the perspective of public health, if he had erred, it was because he had relied initially on the language of the rights of privacy to justify his refusal to move against the baths. Having asserted that principle rather than pragmatic concerns limited the course available to him, he had lost an early opportunity to engage in a forthright public debate over the role of his department in shaping the culture of sexual behavior in the context of the AIDS epidemic.

New York City and the Baths

The furious debate over the bathhouses in San Francisco, the shifting posture of its director of health, and finally the response of the court to the city's attempt at closure were watched carefully by the gay community as well as by public health officials in New York City, the epicenter of the American AIDS epidemic. Nevertheless, matters developed more slowly there in large part because of the continued refusal of public health officials to consider closure a legitimate intervention. And when closure was attempted, it was imposed upon the city and the local gay community by state health officials responsive to a different set of political imperatives from those that prevailed in New York City itself.

When compelled by events to address the bathhouse issue, health officials in New York assumed a remarkable posture of restraint. That Roger Enlow, responsible for gay and lesbian health affairs for New York City's Department of Health, would denounce all talk of bathhouse closure as threatening a "gross infringement on individual choice and freedom" was less striking than the blunt rejection of such a course by the commissioner of health, David Sencer, who, unlike Mervyn Silverman, would never shift his position on the matter.[88] In one interview he stated, "I can see no reason why we would close the bathhouses. I don't think that changing the habitat is necessarily going to change the behavior. . . . To try to legislate changes in lifestyle has never been effective. Public education through the route of organized groups who are at risk is the most important thing."[89] Sencer went further, and indeed sought to interdict efforts from within his department to bring pressure on the bathhouses by some increasingly alarmed elements in the gay community. The commissioner of health for the state of New York was no more inclined to consider closure, though he was asked to consider the option by Governor Mario Cuomo, who was ultimately to play a critical role in the outcome of the New York bathhouse controversy.[90] This reluctance persisted until October 1985 despite advice in mid-1983 from the general counsel of the State Health Department that "the reported multiplicity of sexual contacts, especially among strangers, in baths patronized by homosexuals suggests that closing them will significantly reduce the risk of exposure of homosexual and bisexual males to AIDS."[91]

The unwillingness of the public health authorities to assume any leadership on the bathhouse issue and the apparent failure of the preeminent community-based AIDS service organization—the Gay Men's Health Crisis—to speak clearly about the responsibility of bathhouse owners produced an environment in which, despite the growing concern over AIDS, business as usual was the order of the day. At a meeting called by Roger Enlow to discuss the matter—at which the National Gay Task Force, the Gay Men's Health Crisis, and People with AIDS were all in attendance, it was reported that on some nights one could witness crowds of individuals awaiting entry to the St. Marks Baths.[92] Efforts by one physician—Joseph Sonnabend—to issue a warning about the possibility of meeting patrons with AIDS at the baths was countered by those who asserted that "fear and anxiety are not lasting [behavior] modifiers." For the National Gay Task Force (NGTF), the growing tension within the gay community and the increasingly vocal calls for action against the baths by some was cause for concern. "We oppose efforts to close any gay establishment. . . . Still this spring we may see baths and bars prohibited. We may witness, as one man suggested, a wholesale assault on such businesses through harassment under fire and police code violations brought to the authorities' attention by gay zealots. We may see, indeed, a form of gay civil war unless Enlow and others similarly concerned prevail."[93]

This public pronouncement masked, however, growing concern within the NGTF over a vacuum of leadership in the face of the challenge being launched by "gay zealots." In a memorandum to Virginia Apuzzo, executive director of the organization, John Boring, responsible for AIDS activities, wrote, "Is there anything else we can or should be doing to discourage people from going to the baths that we haven't already been doing?" Fearful that "coming down too hard" on the baths would "play into the hands" of antihomosexual forces and would exacerbate strife within the gay community, he nevertheless urged stronger support for risk reduction campaigns. "It is important that we appear forthright in our position. We cannot equivocate or appear as though we are running scared from a difficult public health issue (GMHC [Gay Men's Health Crisis] conveys the opposite image). At the same time we must resign ourselves to the fact that a vocal emotional minority within our community . . . will accuse us of using civil liberties as a cover for protecting the business interests of the bathhouses."[94]

In New York, as in San Francisco, civil libertarians attempted to seize the initiative, thus holding at bay those committed to closing down the bathhouses. Just as he had urged forceful efforts on the part of the Northern California Branch of the ACLU, Thomas Stoddard of the New York Civil Liberties Union sought to press his anti-interventionist perspective on the gay community and public health officials. "This is a gay problem and the gay community should turn to its own resources for the resolution of the problem." As he had done before, Stoddard warned of the ultimate risks of state intervention. "Homophobes and perhaps more well-meaning health officials will ultimately push the logic to its ultimate extreme—if bathhouses, why not movie houses, and if movie houses, why not gay bars, and if we close all these dangerous places, why not criminalize the underlying conduct?"[95] The logic of closure led ineluctably to the reenactment of sodomy statutes. The force of Stoddard's argument and the receptivity of the gay community to such claims created a climate within which few were willing to openly advocate closure, fewer certainly than was the case in San Francisco, where by the fall of 1984 the commissioner of health, supported by prominent gay physicians, had moved against the baths.

The first full airing of the issue within a public health framework took place before the State Health Department's AIDS Institute Advisory Council in December 1984.[96] There Michael Callen—a vigorous critic of sexual promiscuity in the gay community—took up the challenge of arguing the case for "temporary closure." "I believe that commercial sex establishments play a central role in stoking the raging fire of AIDS in our community. I believe that closing them down will have a significant beneficial effect on reducing the incidence of AIDS." Aware of the civil liberties implications of his proposals, he wrote, "It is a difficult task to measure principles against the price of real human life, but that is the task which faces us." Closure, Callen stressed, could have both direct and symbolic effects. To those who dismissed the latter as of little public health moment, he responded that closure would send a message to all gay men that the epidemic was so critical that drastic action was required. But the impact would be more than symbolic. Though he did not deny the possibility that high-risk behavior might move to other venues, Callen suggested that this argument missed the point. "The logic behind temporary closure of commercial sex establishments is not to make it impossible for gay men to engage in high-risk behavior—but to make it much more difficult."[97] Even were three out of four bathhouse patrons to reproduce their behavioral patterns in other settings, one would not. Wasn't saving that life "worth the hypothetical risk" to civil liberties posed by business closures? Unlike Stoddard and other civil libertarians who equated the bathhouse with the private home, Callen stressed the commercial and public nature of the institutions he was subjecting to scathing attack. But despite his passionate arguments for closure, Callen could not bring himself to embrace state intervention. The task had to be borne by the gay community. A failure to meet the challenge would not only provoke a condemnatory stance by the broader community—the charge of irresponsibility—but the necessity for state action itself.

Peter Vogel, the gay co-chair of the Advisory Council, presented the case against mandated closure, emphasizing instead the potential role of commercial pressure. "I would like to see the bathhouses closed because people stop going."[98] Alternatively, he would have preferred to see them changed so that they "don't function in the same way." And so despite the apparent clash between Callen and Vogel there was a shared reluctance to countenance closure by state fiat. So powerful was the legacy of distrust of the government among gay men that even in this crucial encounter recourse to unofficial pressure—either by the "community" or the market—was the preferred strategy for change.

Despite the public denunciations of state threats, there was a growing, if rueful, recognition by some gay leaders that in the absence of government pressure, the bathhouse owners would at best reluctantly cooperate with efforts to use their settings to educate patrons to the risks of AIDS and make modifications in commercial practices that would discourage high-risk behavior. In an internal memorandum of the National Gay Task Force following the Advisory Council meeting, John Boring was compelled to acknowledge that there was little education taking place in the baths and that patrons continued to engage in unsafe sexual practices. "Perhaps," he concluded, "the threat of government intervention [would be] useful in 'jawboning' the owners into action." But despite his bow in the direction of "jawboning," Boring too believed that the needed changes had to be the result of pressure by the gay community.[99]

The extraordinary anxiety with which the issue of bathhouse regulation, not to speak of closure, was approached was reflected in the limited scope of the recommendations issued in January 1985 by the Coalition for Sexual Responsibility, a small group of gay activists committed to facing the bathhouse issue head on. Emphasis was placed on using commercial sex establishments as places to educate and warn, and on structural changes that would limit the possibility of multiple anonymous sexual encounters. What the coalition had explicitly refused to endorse, however, was more far-reaching changes: the elimination of private rooms and stalls; the removal of doors from such private enclaves; and the eviction of those engaged in high-risk sexual activity, defined as anything other than masturbation.[100]

For those who believed that the continued operation of the bathhouses during the AIDS epidemic represented a serious threat to the survival of the gay community, these recommendations were utterly inadequate. Most significant in this regard was Stephen Caiazza, president of the New York Physicians for Human Rights. Called upon by the Coalition for Sexual Responsibility to negotiate the acceptance of its recommendations with bathhouse owners, he responded by stating, "I feel it impossible for me to have any role in negotiating with the bathhouses short of presenting a demand for their immediate closure and their continued closure during the AIDS crisis." In an impassioned letter to David Nimmons, chair of the coalition, Caiazza was to stake out a posture that would ultimately isolate him from the organized elements of New York's gay political constituency. "Since I cannot outright cure the disease, my obligation as a doctor is to prevent it. . . . As part of the endeavor it is my obligation to remind gay men as loudly and as stridently as I can that the practice of contagion-free sex necessarily involves avoiding all establishments that encourage high-risk sexual behavior. This means that gay men have a duty and responsibility not only to themselves but to their brothers and to the people of the city in general to boycott and condemn the baths. As a corollary, leaders of the gay community have an obligation to be in the vanguard of all efforts to curtail the use and the existence of the baths while AIDS remains a menace." Caiazza had no illusions about the impact that bathhouse closure would have on the gross configuration of the AIDS epidemic, and he fully acknowledged the likelihood that whatever was done to the baths, the incidence of the disease would continue to "climb geometrically." But his was not primarily the calculus of epidemiology, nor ironically, that of public health. Rather, it was the cry of outrage of the clinician confronted with his own impotence. "It is medically undeniable that if the baths close some lives, how many we do not know, will certainly be saved, and as a physician, my primary and ultimate duty is to save lives regardless of how many or how few lives I am dealing with."[101]

To those who viewed closure under state edict as anathema, and for whom the recent San Francisco court rulings permitting close inspection and regulation of sexual activity in the bathhouses represented a grave violation of civil liberties, the need to find an accommodation with the bathhouse owners was increasingly apparent.[102] Failure could only set the stage for a reenactment of the events that had transpired on the West Coast and would at the same time represent an abdication of the responsibility to foster behavioral modifications on the part of those who chose to attend the baths.

The urgency of this effort for the political leadership of the gay community was underscored by David Axelrod, commissioner of health for New York State. Speaking before the New York Physicians for Human Rights, he reiterated his opposition to state-mandated closure. Public health would not be served and civil rights would be violated if the government pursued a course of "edict and

. . . interference." Action on the part of the gay community was preferable. But he warned, "Unless there is voluntary compliance and unless you can assist us in dealing with the issue, the pressure for governmental intervention will undoubtedly increase."[103]

But the gay community was neither prepared for nor capable of action. Immobilized by their distrust of the state, gay political leaders could only hope that the bathhouses would yield to persuasion. The state's AIDS Institute Advisory Council, upon which gay leaders had considerable influence, could do no better. Charged with the task of enunciating a policy for the bathhouses, it could, after about six months, only endorse the recommendations made in January by the Coalition for Sexual Responsibility and urge the gay community to take on the task of addressing the bathhouse issue.[104] Peter Vogel explained the dilemma faced by the council: "Everybody has said . . . they don't want the government to directly intervene. They want the community to try to clean up its own act. . . . The community on the other hand does not have the leverage with the establishments to force them to clean up their act. That's the final irony."[105] And so the first state encounter with the bathhouses had ended with a "half step"—an official endorsement of the weak recommendations of a gay community group. But like the state health commissioner, Vogel warned that time was running out. Political pressure to move against the baths was mounting. "Yes, there has been some pressure [within the governor's office for closure]. I don't think that the governor or the commissioner are prepared to act at the present time, but I think it would not be fair to say that there was not something lurking in the background."[106]

By the end of September, the constellation of political forces had indeed changed, forcing an abrupt shift in the state's policy of laissez faire and reliance upon voluntary change fostered by the gay community through its negotiations with the proprietors of commercial sex establishments. On September 30, during a meeting of his senior staff, Governor Cuomo called upon Health Commissioner Axelrod to reexamine the state's policy on the bathhouses. Concerned about the rising toll being taken by the epidemic, the transmission of the disease to the wives of bisexual men "who did not know of their husband's proclivities," and about the birth of children with AIDS, the governor had grown impatient.[107]

Discussions about the bathhouses took on a sharply political character when, one day after the Governor's private request to his health commissioner, the Republican candidate for mayor of New York, Diane McGrath, called publicly for the immediate closure of bathhouses, bars, theaters, and pornography shops serving a gay clientele, as part of a broad-scale assault on what she perceived to be the inadequacy of the city's response to AIDS.[108] Her call for mandatory AIDS virus antibody screening of teachers, food handlers, health care workers, barbers, beauticians, and prostitutes, and the dismissal of those found positive would be quickly swept aside as without scientific merit. But her demand for bathhouse closure "to protect these people from themselves" was to force the issue onto the political stage, where the sole advocate of closure had been the mayoral candidate for the Right to Life Party, Rabbi Lew Y. Levin.[109] Had the health commissioners of both New York City and State adopted an openly critical stance toward the bathhouses, they could have asserted the claims of the public health while cautioning against precipitate moves to closure. But they had not, and thus they fueled the very opposition they sought to neutralize.

To those who had grown restive, the defense of civil liberties and privacy so central to the pronouncements of the health commissioners of both city and state were nothing more than rationalizations for an unacceptable posture of restraint. The carefully nurtured relationship between health officials and the gay community—viewed by the former as critical to the containment of the AIDS epidemic—was threatened by those who believed the consequences of such collaboration to be a perilous betrayal of the public health and a subordination of communal well-being to political expediency.

As the political climate was shifting, the Coalition for Sexual Responsibility issued a report that underscored its very limited success in fostering changes in bathhouse operation. Three separate inspections dating from May 1985 had been undertaken, the most recent of which found only two of the city's ten bathhouses in "full compliance" with its modest set of recommendations. "The gay community has made its effort to work from within without unnecessary state intervention. But the response of the bathhouses has been, for the most part irresponsible and disappointing."[110]

This report fueled the demands for closure and compelled those who had struggled to prevent such an outcome to maneuver desperately to thwart what by mid-October 1985 increasingly seemed inevitable. David Sencer, commissioner of health for the city of New York, remained unalterably opposed to closure and unlike Mervyn

Silverman—who had offered and had had his assistance rejected—was uninterested in whether at least some sectors of the gay community could be called upon for support.[111] Alan Kristal, director of the Office of Epidemiological Surveillance and Statistics, who with Sencer's approval had joined the case against closure of the San Francisco baths a year earlier, wrote in a memorandum to the commissioner that closing the baths would have little impact on the AIDS epidemic. Too few gay men still attended them. But more critical, a new element was added to the argument. In San Francisco a central question had been whether bathhouse attendance facilitated multiple sexual contacts, which everyone acknowledged increased the risk of AIDS. Now the relevance of promiscuity itself was subjected to scrutiny. "The prevalence of infection [with the AIDS virus] in the sexually active gay population is already so high that the environment from which one selects sexual partners has little relevance."[112] Thus, by implication Kristal had suggested that whatever bathhouse closure might have achieved at an earlier date, such an intervention was too late for New York.

In a letter that reflected a sense of resignation, the Lambda Legal Defense and Education Fund called upon Axelrod to respect the efforts of the gay community to use the bathhouses for risk reduction education and to foster the adoption of the recommendations of the Coalition for Sexual Responsibility. But in a major strategic shift designed to forestall the possibility of outright closure, Lambda acknowledged that state intervention would be called for "in the event that private establishments refuse[d] or fail[ed] to self-regulate." Under those circumstances the legal defense group would "support your effort to impose such education and regulations through state regulatory means short of closure."[113]

Opposition to closure also came from the *New York Times*, which had sought to chart an antialarmist course during the epidemic. Noting that closer inspection might be called for by the city, the editors warned that policies "inspired by public morals" might not be wise from the vantage of public health. "The bathhouses offend many people's sensibilities, but if society's purpose is to slow the spread of AIDS, it may be more prudent to keep them open under closer watch."[114]

Finally, in an attempt to reassure Mayor Koch of the soundness of his resistance to closure, David Sencer wrote the mayor on October 22 that shutting the baths not only would contribute little to controlling the spread of AIDS, but might actually be counterproductive. This conclusion, he asserted, was shared by the state's health commissioner, David Axelrod. Echoing the concerns voiced by Mervyn Silverman before he was able to elicit support for closure from elements of San Francisco's gay community, and refusing to strike out in any way that would promote a public health perspective offensive to the most vocal elements of the gay community, Sencer warned, "Control of this disease, as in most diseases, is predicated on voluntary cooperation with public policy. If we resort to individual coercion will this lead the public to shun cooperation on more important issues?"[115]

Two days later, despite Sencer's reassurance to Mayor Koch, David Axelrod, flanked by the state's governor, announced at a press conference held by the two state officials that he had concluded that bathhouses permitting or promoting "sexual activity that produced blood to blood or semen to blood contact" were a "serious menace to the public health and must be prohibited."[116] Reviewing his efforts dating from July 1983 to obtain voluntary cooperation from bathhouse owners and his own "initial optimism" about educational approaches, he now asserted that the "desired results" had not been achieved. To avoid the impression that "politics" rather than "science" had dictated the shift in public health policy Axelrod and the governor both asserted that new evidence on the bathhouse situation had come to light. "I was responding," said Axelrod, "to absolute frustration in attempting to minimize the transmission of [the AIDS virus] and the problem of an absolutely fatal disease. . . . I was not responding to pressure from the governor." In fact, the evidence was no different from that which had been available for some time. What had changed was the political willingness to tolerate a situation that many viewed as unacceptable in the face of the AIDS epidemic. To soften the implications that this move was directed at the gay community alone, Cuomo asserted that an as-yet-to-be-specified set of recommendations to be placed before the New York Health Council would apply to "any establishment that catered to dangerous heterosexual or homosexual sex."

On the next day, Axelrod presented his recommendations to the State Public Health Council, asking it to adopt them by exercise of its emergency powers so that they would become effective immediately rather than after a more extended bureaucratic process. And so after more than two years of refusing to consider closure, the commissioner believed that not a moment should pass before action was taken. "Every day we wait there are additional individuals who are being exposed either within the homosexual, bisexual, or heterosexual community. . . . I think it is incumbent upon us after having attempted for two years to achieve voluntary compliance . . . to move forward and not to wait and expose additional innocent persons. . . . I do believe we have an obligation to be concerned about one individual or several individuals or a group of individuals."[117] But the emergency was not simply one created by the need to protect gay men from themselves. Bisexual men who attended the baths would infect their unsuspecting female partners who would in turn become sources of further infection. These women would bear children destined to die of AIDS. At this critical juncture it was necessary to invoke the specter of the general threat of AIDS and the image of dying children.

The resolution adopted by the council with only one dissenting voice found that "sexual practices that result in the introduction of semen into the rectal or oral cavity of another are high risk sexual activity, and while use of a condom or withdrawal prior to ejaculation may mitigate such risk, it is impossible as a practical matter to ascertain whether either preventive action is being taken."[118] As a result, the council resolved that "places which are used as establishments [by those] engaging in high risk sexual activity must be regarded as public health nuisances, [and] dangerous to public health." Local health officials and local boards of health "may close such facilities or establishments."

Only Victor Sidel, long identified with left-wing causes in health policy, and president of the American Public Health Association, voiced his opposition, stressing the precipitate nature of the action and the failure to provide adequate opportunity for gay groups to present their views on the language and scope of the resolution. Requesting only a delay of a few days, he challenged those who accepted the commissioner's interpretation of the prevailing situation. As Axelrod had sought to justify his new stance by presenting a grave picture, Sidel sought to thwart the move by an antialarmist characterization of the situation. The data suggested that the epidemic curve was "now flat." But Sidel stood alone, as he would sixty days later when the council met to ratify its emergency act of October 25.

Though the decision affecting commercial sex establishments would have its primary impact on New York City, the final determination to adopt the new health rules was taken without seeking the prior approval of Mayor Edward Koch and certainly demonstrated little concern for how the policy would affect New York City's Department of Health, which in most health-related matters operated with a high degree of autonomy from the state. When city health officials and the mayor said it might take some time before they could implement the state's new rule, the governor warned that he would move against the bathhouses directly.[119] And so under pressure, the city was compelled to act.

On November 7 the Mine Shaft—a back-room bar with a notorious reputation for flouting every recommendation for reducing high-risk sexual activity—was closed by court order and indeed was defended by virtually no one.[120] Some sex-oriented establishments posted warnings announcing the health department's ruling: "It is illegal to have anal or oral intercourse in public." Others required patrons to sign pledges that they would engage in only safe sex. Some closed.[121]

What began as an effort to create a narrowly tailored rule covering commercial sex establishments had potentially far broader implications, however, since the term "establishment" had been defined by the Public Health Council as "any place in which entry, membership, [and] goods or services are purchased." Thus, when pressed, Axelrod acknowledged that "if we find that a hotel . . . is catering to that kind of activity, then I think we will have reason to take action and if necessary a warrant to go into rooms."[122] At last, in an unguarded moment, in an incautiously worded remark, a health commissioner had said what gay leaders and civil liberties opponents of bathhouse closure had warned about from the very outset of the debate over regulating sex in public settings. And if the state could regulate the hotel room, might it not extend its surveillance and supervision to the bedroom? Indeed, the Coalition of Lesbian and Gay Rights charged that the Health Council's rule had granted local health officials the power to "inquire into every homosexual man's apartment and/or living accommodation where 'entry is purchased.' "[123] Stressing that a radical disjunction existed between the private and the public, the coalition asserted that the council had gone beyond its authority, which was limited to the protection of *public* health. To the coalition the private included sexual encounters between men at the baths.

When the emergency regulations were brought to the Public Health Council on December 20 for final action, there was no reason to believe that the earlier ruling would be reversed. Victor Sidel challenged his colleagues, warning of the political implications of the council's actions. "If the only measure that we take is closing certain kinds of commercial establishments in which dangerous behavior takes place, I think that we have no choice [but] in subsequent meetings to talk about commercial establishments in which cigarette smoking takes place . . . where liquor is sold, after which people drive. . . . I think we are treading on extremely dangerous ground."[124] At this meeting, Sidel again stood alone.

By this time, however, the center of conflict had shifted from the Public Health Council to the courts, where as a result of New York City's closure of the St. Marks Baths, widely acknowledged as being among the most cooperative establishments in terms of the recommendations of the Committee for Sexual Responsibility, a legal challenge had been brought. Here, as in California, the demands of the adversarial process dictated the form and content of the arguments placed before the court, sharpening the constitutional divide that separated the parties.

In its case, the city relied on the affidavits of investigators from the Department of Consumer Affairs—the city's Health Department had been bypassed for political reasons—to substantiate its case that despite a reputation of cooperation the St. Marks Baths was in fact a setting for high-risk sex.[125] After noting that inspectors had witnessed nearly fifty instances of oral and anal sex, the city asserted, "One can reasonably conclude that far more high-risk activity took place behind many cubicle doors and publicly . . . when city inspectors were not present."

"Society is not defenseless," stated the city, "in its efforts to combat [this] fatal disease when only prevention is available to interrupt the spread of infection."[126] Drawing upon the language long used by public officials seeking to exercise their discretionary authority and citing the wide berth accorded to the state in the exercise of its police powers, the city argued that acts that were "rationally related to the furtherance of important public health objectives" should be sustained even if they "impinged to some degree" on the exercise of personal freedom. Faced with an epidemic like AIDS the authorities could "err on the side of prevention and caution." Rejecting the claim that a commercial establishment, within which sexual conduct could be observed in open spaces by paying patrons, could seek protection in the name of privacy, the city drew a sharp distinction between the home and the bathhouse. Equally significant, it stressed the importance of using public health powers in a manner consistent with the limitations imposed by a principled respect for privacy as well as the pragmatics of public policy. "The high value placed on the sanctity and privacy of the home may well mean that as a practical matter much sexual conduct which may spread AIDS is not affected by the new regulation and would be reduced primarily through public education efforts. This does not mean, however, that a responsible government should forgo regulating the conduct where constitutionally permissible and where it is practical to do so in order to save lives through such efforts."

Like the defense of the San Francisco bathhouses, the arguments put forth to protect the St. Marks Baths stressed broad constitutional principles of privacy and the rights protected by the First Amendment. "The closing of the bathhouses would trespass not only upon the 'penumbral' right of privacy protected by the Ninth Amendment but the express right of association protected by the First Amendment."[127] It was not, as the city asserted, the privacy of the home that the long line of cases involving sexuality and even pornography involved, but the behaviors themselves when performed in settings that were beyond the public view, beyond the view of those who might be shocked and offended.

The affidavits presented by the St. Marks Baths in support of its case were like those submitted by opponents of closure in San Francisco. Public health officials Shirley Fannin, associate director of the Communicable Disease Programs in Los Angeles County, who had testified against the San Francisco Health Department, and Bailes Walker, Jr., commissioner of public health for Massachusetts, argued that bathhouse closure would have no impact on the spread of AIDS. Sociologists and historians, including Allan Berube, whose long history of the baths had been part of the San Francisco case against closure, spoke of the protective function of the baths for gay men and especially for those who used them as a setting for "coming out." Finally, in a move that proponents of closure viewed as emblematic of the corruption of the city's gay leadership, the Gay

Men's Health Crisis asserted that the St. Marks Baths had indeed cooperated with its program of risk-reduction education. Absent but informing many of the arguments was the voice of the New York City Health Department, which for political reasons could not enter the case on the side it had so forcefully sought to defend in the months preceding the decision of Commissioner Axelrod.

On January 6, 1986, Judge Richard W. Wallach of the New York Supreme Court upheld the city's action against the St. Marks Baths. In the face of conflicting evidence regarding the potential impact of closure on the spread of AIDS, the court deferred to the state's judgment, rejecting the appeal that it substitute its own evaluation of the evidence at hand. "The judicial function is exhausted with the discovery that the relation between means and end is [not] vain and fanciful, an illusory pretense."[128] In a decision that was not unmindful of the privacy interests that were at stake, but which was nevertheless deferential to the determinations made by the government, the court found that the city had met the burden of proof required to sustain a public health measure taken in the face of an epidemic with a death rate like that associated with AIDS. Most important in the decision, and framing the court's perspective, was the rejection of the claim that bathhouse closure was equivalent to the invasion of the privacy of the home. "The privacy protection of sexual activity conducted in a private home does not extend to commercial establishments simply because they provide an opportunity for intimate behavior or sexual release." Had the two been viewed as indistinguishable the balance might well have shifted against the state.

As the bathhouse controversy continued to play itself out in New York and San Francisco, the Executive Task Force on AIDS of the United States Public Health Service looked on with a concern that reflected the growing sense of alarm about the course of the epidemic and indicated a developing recognition of the importance of taking forceful measures to interrupt the spread of infection by the AIDS virus.[129] On November 7, 1985, a circular letter to state and territorial health officials from Donald Hopkins, the assistant surgeon general, placed the Public Health Service publicly and formally on record as "endorsing state and local action to regulate or close these establishments when taken on the basis of information indicating that these facilities represent a risk to public health."[130]

The action by Donald Hopkins followed by less than a month the overwhelming approval by the House of Representatives of a largely symbolic legislative amendment, introduced by arch-conservative California Representative William Dannemyer, that authorized the surgeon general to use funds to "close or quarantine as a public health hazard any bathhouse or massage parlor which in his judgment can be determined to facilitate the transmission or spread of the AIDS epidemic."[131] For Dannemyer, who was eventually to propose legislation that would deny federal revenue sharing funds to cities that did not close their bathhouses, legislation was necessary as a "small step toward doing something to help people who in many cases seem unable or unwilling to help themselves."[132] It was also a step that, he believed, posed no threat to civil liberties. Openly antihomosexual, Dannemyer declared, "Sodomy committed in public should not be raised to the level of a protected civil right. Therefore, closing bathhouses is not an infringement on anyone's rights."

Support for closure was also to come eventually from the usually conservative House of Delegates of the American Medical Association, after a floor debate in which the well-worn arguments over whether such establishments could be used effectively as points of sex education or whether they represented an imminent threat to the public health were repeated. The resolution that passed "easily" by voice vote declared "communal sex establishments such as bathhouses, brothels, sex clubs, sex bars, and adult bookstores that provide facilities for sexual intercourse—function as reservoirs for the spread of sexually transmitted diseases."[133]

Support for closure or stringent regulation of the baths came not only from those who were clearly identified with conservative political postures, however. In a report prepared for the Centers for Disease Control that was highly critical of the failure of public health law to reflect the changing conception of what the Constitution required in terms of due process protections, it was argued that "it would be irresponsible if public health departments were knowingly to countenance *unsafe* activity in premises over which [they had] control, even if some percentage of that activity would occur in more private forums."[134] It was clearly possible to acknowledge the importance of civil liberties and privacy without subscribing to the positions adopted by gay political organizations and the American Civil Liberties Union.

But despite growing support for bathhouse closure or careful regulation and the apparent willingness of some courts to defer to action taken under broadly defined powers of the state to protect the public health, moves to close or regulate the baths did not meet uniformly with success. The refusal of the San Francisco superior court to countenance closure, and its effort to mandate regulation instead, was but one indication of the capacity of the courts to force public health officials to tailor their measures with some regard for the privacy interests at stake. In New York State the attempt to shut a Buffalo bathhouse failed when the court found that the public health authorities had not conducted a thorough investigation of the establishment they sought to close and that they had, therefore, not borne the necessary burden of proof.[135]

More striking was the refusal of a superior court in Los Angeles to permit the strict regulation of the bathhouses in a way that would have put an end to virtually all sexual activity among patrons. At the end of August 1986, Judge John Cole ruled against such restrictions because he believed that "the county could not prove that its regulations would reduce the spread of AIDS." Indeed, he was convinced by evidence brought before him that the baths, which provided safer sex educational material and condoms, were in fact less hazardous than other venues where sexual contact between gay men occurred.[136]

But it was not only court action that prevented the wholesale closing or strict regulation of bathhouses across the country. Restraint was fostered by the recognition on the part of public health officials, as well as municipal and state officials, that efforts to impose restrictions and closure inevitably entailed costly encounters with local gay communities at a time when collaborative efforts at preventing the spread of AIDS seemed so critical. Prudence and political judgment were integral to rather than deviations from the principles of public health. Mayor Dianne Feinstein of San Francisco was thus unable to obtain support for a resolution favoring closure from the AIDS Task Force of the U.S. Conference of Mayors of which she was chair.[137] More striking, some public health officials who were publicly identified with very aggressive postures on intervention in the AIDS epidemic and who had been critical of those who had failed to adopt traditional public health measures, chose not to target the baths. Kristine Gebbie, chair of the AIDS Task Force of the Association of State and Territorial Health Officials and administrator of the Oregon Health Department, did not press for closure from her Oregon HIV/AIDS Policy Committee.[138] Michael Osterholm, state epidemiologist for Minnesota, who fought a hard-won battle for the use of sexual contact notification to warn the partners of HIV-infected individuals about their exposure, despite the opposition of gay and civil liberties groups, stated that while he could not "condone" the bathhouses, he believed the effort that would be required to shut them would not be "cost beneficial." "It would be a visible act but would it accomplish enough?"[139]

For those who believed that public health officials had both the legal and moral authority to shut baths where unsafe sexual activity occurred, the failure to do so represented nothing less than a failure of nerve. The willingness to countenance the continued operation of commercial sex establishments and tolerate private booths designed to shield sexual activity from view in those bathhouses where such conduct was prohibited in public rooms seemed an almost inexplicable refusal to exercise the power vested in public health officials and exercised in virtually every other circumstance where disease threatened the community's well-being.

The tenacity with which some local health officials—most prominently David Sencer in New York City—refused to consider either closure or regulation of the baths; their incorporation of the diction of civil liberties and privacy in public pronouncements on the appropriate public health course; their reluctance to deploy their considerable powers to cajole bathhouse owners to adopt radical modifications in the operation of their businesses; their unwillingness to confront the leadership of gay communities over the failure to mobilize pressure against bathhouse proprietors—all contributed to the dismay with which they were perceived.

That local health officials did not move more forcefully to close or regulate the bathhouses in the first years of the AIDS epidemic was in part a consequence of the political constraints imposed by having to chart a course compatible with a broad strategy of cooperation with gay men, who viewed with profound suspicion all agencies of the state. Public health officials were also restrained by the impact of liberal political values—the centers of the AIDS epidemic were also cosmopolitan cities with political cultures of relative tolerance—and the recognition that bathhouse behavior was but a very small part of the larger problem of a pattern of sexual behavior that occurred in settings beyond the reach of the state. Prudence dictated an appreciation of all these factors.

Too often, however, the result was timidity and a failure to appreciate the ways in which a public culture of sexual restraint and responsibility could be fostered by the interventions of health officials. If regulating or closing the baths could not directly affect the course of the epidemic—the number of gay men who attended them was relatively small—the symbolic significance of such public health measures could nevertheless have served as a powerful statement about the dangers of promiscuity, about the importance of self-protection and the protection of others. In an epidemic where educating millions about the necessity of radical changes in private behavior was widely acknowledged as fundamental, the failure to appreciate the importance of symbolic measures was a profound misjudgment. It was a misjudgment conditioned by the political forces evoked by the AIDS epidemic.

Chapter 3

Blood, Privacy, and Stigma

The Politics of Safety

For the first year of the epidemic AIDS remained almost exclusively a disease of the marginal—gay and bisexual men, intravenous drug users, recent immigrants from Haiti. However threatening such an epidemiological pattern was to the broader community, it provided at the same time a reassuring message. Virtually all heterosexuals who did not engage in socially aberrant behavior had little to fear. But on July 16, 1982, a report in CDC's *Morbidity and Mortality Weekly Report* was to shatter the illusion of security.[1] Three cases of pneumocystis carinii pneumonia had been reported among patients with hemophilia A, the most severe form of the disorder. Two had died; one remained critically ill. All three were heterosexual. None had a history of intravenous drug use. In commenting on these cases, the CDC stated, "Although the course of the severe immune dysfunction is unknown, the occurrence among the three hemophiliac cases suggests the possible transmission of an agent through blood products."[2] If this was true, the implications for both hemophiliacs treated with Factor VIII, a clotting agent that in concentrated form is derived from the pooled plasma of large numbers of donors, and for transfusion recipients, could be disastrous.

If the bathhouse debate had focused on the clash between the demands of sexual privacy and the protection of the public health, the controversy over how to protect the blood supply from those who might infect it centered on questions of social stigma—the consequences of identifying whole classes as the potential sources of contamination. Just as the threat to blood—symbolic of life itself—galvanized communal anxiety, the threat of exclusion from the blood donor pool represented a profound threat to the social standing of those who would be classed as a danger to the public health. In addition to concerns over privacy so central to the bathhouse controversy, the debate over the blood supply thus placed into question the gay struggle for social integration. If the bathhouse controversy forced those drawn into the debate to confront the problem of how much evidence of how much benefit was necessary before the state might legitimately exercise public health powers that restricted liberty, the debate over the blood supply compelled antagonists to ask about the level of evidence required before discriminatory policies designed to protect the public health might be enforced. Finally, the conflict over how best to protect the blood supply forced a confrontation over the role of explicit rules and expectations, of public norms of behavior, in fostering a sense of social responsibility among those whose acts could have dire consequences for the well-being of others. On each level of conflict blood bankers, public health officials, and representatives of the gay community confronted each other under the watchful eyes of the constituencies to which they were responsible.

Toward a Restrictive Donor Policy

Concerned that the CDC's report on AIDS among hemophiliacs would produce anxiety and clinically unwise decisions, the National Hemophilia Foundation sought to reassure patients dependent on Factor VIII concentrate. "It is important to note that at this time the *risk* of contracting this immunosuppressive agent is *minimal* and the CDC is not recommending any change in blood product use."[3] But despite these words of reassurance there were those who believed that the three case reports were sufficient to warrant extraordinary concern about the safety of the blood supply. They also believed that it was appropriate to consider more exclusionary blood donor policies in order to prevent the inadvertent transmission of the as-yet-to-be-discovered agent responsible for the severe assault on the body's immune system.

A few gay physicians felt that the situation required the withdrawal of some homosexual men from the donor pool. While emphasizing that homosexuality itself was not a risk factor, Dan William warned in an interview published in the *New York Native* in August 1982 that "promiscuous gay men" with a prior history of multiple sexually transmitted diseases not give blood until more information was available.[4] Nevertheless, for the political leadership of the gay community the potential for a socially catastrophic turn in public policy was all too easy to discern. Speaking on behalf of the Fund for Human Dignity at a meeting in mid-July, Virginia Apuzzo warned against a return to the "bad old days . . . when a recurrently scapegoated minority could be sweepingly restigmatized for the taint of bad blood."[5] Indeed because it feared the development of policies that would place the onus of a contaminated blood supply on the gay community, New York's Gay Men's Health Crisis called upon gays to "cover the costs of blood transfusions for AIDS victims" by increasing their own donations.[6]

But for those who saw in the new threat of AIDS a matter of gravity requiring drastic measures, fears about invasions of privacy and the prospects of stigma paled as matters of significance. Though in its public posture the National Hemophilia Foundation remained silent about the desirability of pursuing the option of excluding all gay men from the donor pool, it quietly began to press for such a course within the blood banking community. On October 3, 1982, the Foundation's Board of Directors adopted a resolution put forth by its medical and scientific advisory committee that urged "all sources of Factor VIII products to exclude from plasma donation all individuals who were homosexual, intravenous drug users, or recent residents of Haiti."[7] A month later, in a letter to the president of the American Blood Commission, an association of blood banking and related professional organizations, the foundation wrote, "We recognize that this request is made on the basis of incomplete information, but in our view it is prudent as a precautionary measure until we get a better understanding of the nature of the disease. . . . As we are all aware, this is a sensitive issue and we do not want to cause any undue alarm. . . . We are communicating directly with you in the hope that we can move forward to work at the best way to deal with this problem."[8]

But the sense of alarm was indeed growing. At a December 4 meeting of the Blood Products Advisory Committee of the Food and Drug Administration, Bruce Evatt of the CDC reported five additional cases of AIDS among hemophiliacs. He also reported an ongoing investigation of five AIDS cases that might well have been linked to blood transfusions received within the prior eighteen months. In one case an infant had received a donation from a gay man who, though apparently healthy at the time of donation, had developed AIDS seven months later. "So I think that transfusion-associated AIDS is coming very rapidly, and I think will probably follow the same course that we have seen with hemophilia patients." Evatt was especially pessimistic about the prospects for hemophilia patients because of the possible contamination of whole lots of Factor VIII concentrate. "So if it is in the concentrate, and if it is transmissible in the concentrate, then you have a large proportion of the hemophilia population already exposed and you can expect that, no matter what you do at this point." Some at the meeting, like Louis Aledort of the National Hemophilia Foundation, responded by seeking the removal of potential carriers from the donor pool. Others, however, like Joseph Bove, of the Yale–New Haven Blood Bank, warned that "there are unbelievable problems with trying to screen out any subset of potential donors based on sexual habits." He made that acknowledgment despite the recognition that AIDS worried him "because the potential for a catastrophy seems to be present and because I don't really know what to do about it."[9]

Six days later *Morbidity and Mortality Report* made public the additional cases of AIDS among hemophiliacs as well as the case of the twenty-month-old child who had died of AIDS following multiple transfusions, one of which had come from an apparently healthy donor who subsequently developed AIDS.[10] In its editorial comment CDC stated, "This report and continuing reports of AIDS among persons with hemophilia A raise serious questions about possible transmission of AIDS through blood and blood products. The Assistant Secretary of Health is convening an advisory committee to address these questions."[11]

In the face of the accumulating evidence and the *MMWR* report of December 10, the officials of the blood banking community responded with the voice of reassurance and with what from the perspective of only a few more months would seem to be extraordinary caution. The American Red Cross, "share[d] its deep concern" about the possibility that AIDS might be caused by a blood-borne agent. Since there were no tests to identify those who might be the carriers of such an agent, "policies for acceptance of blood donors [were] being reviewed to develop a prudent approach to donor selection."[12] Kenneth Woods, president of the Council of Community Blood Centers, went further. Though he described the available data as "far from conclusive, fragmentary, and as yet entirely too notional," Woods suggested as a precaution that "organized groups known to be comprised largely of individuals at higher risk than the general population should not donate blood for transfusion or plasma for coagulating factors." Homosexually promiscuous men were specifically identified as among those who should desist from blood donations. Nevertheless, Woods warned that explicit predonation questions about "sexual habits would be an ineffective way for forcing such exclusion. . . . The small number of prospective blood donors to whom such questions would apply frequently do not respond in sufficient candor."[13] Finally, in the wake of the December 10 CDC report, the Board of Directors of the American Blood Commission rejected the earlier and privately communicated proposal of the National Hemophilia Foundation that explicit efforts be made to exclude members of high-risk groups from blood donations. "The Board believes that there is still not sufficient information available to formulate a policy." Faced with scientific uncertainty the blood bankers had elected not to act.[14] Institutional concerns, including fears about the disruptive consequences of fashioning explicit exclusionary policies, rather than concerns about stigma and privacy, were at work, though the latter would ultimately be called upon to justify a policy of restraint.

Despite the public rejection by the blood banking community of proposals to screen out those who were considered most at risk for transmitting an as-yet-unidentified AIDS agent, leaders of the gay community viewed the evolving discussion and an impending CDC conference to be held on January 4, 1983, with great concern. Writing in the *New York Native,* Larry Bush, a political commentator, noted, "Nearly every one responsible for addressing [the blood issue] has demonstrated extraordinary restraint and sensitivity to the potentially hostile public reaction that might be created by a few incautious words. . . . Because they are fraught with such anti-gay consequences, one almost hesitates to put any speculation on the issue before the public. . . . The real gravity underlying these questions—in addition to health, which concerns us all—is that we still live in a place and time in which it is [possible] to treat gays unfairly on the basis of outrageous and mistaken assumptions. As of this writing that form of maltreatment has not yet pervaded this area of public health planning, but one certainly can appreciate why it is that gays must respond with extraordinary caution."[15]

Just a week before the planned CDC conference, James Curran, head of AIDS activities at the Centers for Disease Control, expressed his fears about how divisive and volatile the session might become and cautioned that the gay community might best respond to the challenge posed by the available evidence about the risk of AIDS in blood products by seizing the "political initiative with a call for voluntary withdrawal of gays from the donor pool."[16] Whatever the role of self-defense in the protection of individuals from sexual exposure to the threat of AIDS, recipients of transfusions were defenseless in the face of contaminated blood. Gay leaders were uniquely situated to underscore the obligation to act responsibly in the face of the threat of AIDS. They could shape the perspectives of gay men who were uncertain about the implications of the scientific evidence, and of the moral burdens imposed by the available data. Curran warned that a failure to take such action might produce the very reaction so feared by those concerned about the danger of stigmatization. "The thing is, people are dying. The medical problem is more important than the civil rights issue."

It was against this background of politically charged anxiety and a publicly announced decision on the part of the Alpha Therapeutics Corporation, a major supplier of commercial plasma products, that it would begin to exclude gay men and other high-risk individuals from its collection pool, that the January 4 meeting was held.[17] Present at the session—the Workshop to Formulate Recommendations for Prevention of Acquired Immune Deficiency Syndrome—were representatives of the CDC, the National Institutes of Health, the Food and Drug Administration, the American Red Cross, the American Association of Blood Banks, the Council of Community Blood Centers, the National Hemophilia Foundation, and private manufacturers of blood products. Bruce Voeller represented the National Gay Task Force, of which he was the former executive director, and Roger Enlow attended on behalf of the American Association of

Physicians for Human Rights.[18] Despite the presentation of CDC evidence about the risk of AIDS, some representatives of the blood banking community maintained that the data were insufficient and all talk of exclusionary policies was premature. Most articulate in pressing the case for restraint were Aaron Kellner of the New York Blood Center and Joseph Bove of Yale, both of whom were haunted by the institutional implications of acknowledging the blood-AIDS linkage. Kellner argued, "Don't overstate the facts. There are at most three cases of AIDS from blood donations and the evidence in two of the cases is very soft. And there are only a handful of cases among hemophiliacs."[19] Despite Bove's anxiety—expressed a month earlier at the FDA's blood products safety meeting—he dismissed as precipitate the call for action. "We are contemplating all these wide-ranging measures because one baby got AIDS after transfusion from a person who later came down with AIDS, and there may be a few other cases."[20]

To these voices of skepticism, CDC officials responded with a sense of dismay and urgency.[21] In the face of alarming evidence and a grave threat to communal well-being, those concerned about public health had characteristically chosen to err on the side of safety. The insistence upon scientific certitude thus represented a striking deviation, a posture antithetical to the principles of public health practice, an empirically cloaked subterfuge whose purpose was to avoid the discomfiting need for action. The assistant director of Public Health Practice for the CDC and chair of the meeting asserted, "To bury our heads in the sand and say 'let's wait for more cases' is not an adequate public health measure."[22] Donald Francis expressed his exasperation by challenging, "When will there be enough cases to act upon?"[23] For David Sencer, former director of the CDC and commissioner of health in New York City, there was no question. "Does anyone doubt that we are dealing with an infectious agent that is transmitted by blood and sexual contacts?"[24]

Representatives of the gay community forcefully opposed every suggestion that blood banks follow the lead taken by Alpha Therapeutics in questioning prospective donors about their sexual orientation and practices. Such questioning would not only represent an invasion of privacy, but would fail to achieve its purported goal. Bruce Voeller, speaking on behalf of the National Gay Task Force, sought to draw a distinction between those gays at high risk for AIDS and homosexual men more generally. "So-called fast lane gays are causing the problem, and they are just a minority of male homosexuals. You'll stigmatize, at the very time of a major civil rights movement, a whole group only a tiny fraction of whom qualify as the problem we are here to address."[25] Roger Enlow sounded a theme that was to become central to the early gay political perspective on the blood problem. It was blood, not donors, that should be screened.[26] Testing to detect surrogate markers that would suggest the presence of increased risk was called for. Opposition to donor screening also came from David Sencer[27] and Donald Armstrong of the Sloan Kettering Institute in New York—both of whom had no doubt about the threat posed by infected blood, but who found the prospect of questions about sexual orientation an objectionable practice.

For those who had hoped that a clear consensus would emerge from this meeting—which was widely reported in both medical and lay press—the day-long session was a profound disappointment. Officials within the Public Health Service, who would be responsible for preparing recommendations for a national blood policy in the face of the challenge posed by AIDS, were left with an openly divided world of blood bankers and commercial plasma collecting organizations. In contrast, for gay leaders who perceived in the prospect of open questioning about sexual orientation a grave threat to privacy, the stalemate represented a success.

From the perspective of the gay community even greater success was achieved at a meeting of the Committee on Transfusion Transmitted Diseases of the American Association of Blood Banks held two days later. Though asserting that the evidence for the transmission of AIDS by blood transfusions was "weak," the committee nevertheless believed it critical to "respond to the possibility that a new and infectious illness" had surfaced.[28] Its recommendations urged physicians to consider with caution the decision to use blood products, suggested the use of autologous blood transfusions in the case of elective surgery, and noted the importance of screening donors for symptoms of AIDS or exposure to AIDS. In terms of the politically charged issue of the relationship of the blood banking world to the gay community, the committee asserted that those responsible for donor recruitment extend the practice adopted by many blood bankers years earlier because of the threat of hepatitis B among gay men. They were urged "not [to] target" groups that "may have a high incidence of AIDS." Furthermore, blood bankers were called upon to support "the leadership of groups which include some individuals at high risk of AIDS" in their efforts to educate their constituencies about the dangers of blood donation. Stressing education and voluntary self-deferral by those at risk, the committee explicitly rejected the direct questioning of donors about sexual orientation. "There is currently considerable pressure on the blood banking community to restrict blood donations by all gay males. Direct or indirect questions about a donor's sexual preference are inappropriate. Such an invasion of privacy can be justified only if it demonstrates clear-cut benefit. In fact, there is evidence that such questions, no matter how well intended, are ineffective in eliminating those donors who may carry AIDS."[29]

The committee's decision was hailed by the gay community. Roger Enlow, who had worked so doggedly to achieve the results, saw in them a victory of "scientific and medical" fact over "cultural and personal bias."[30] A precedent had been established with the full cooperation and participation of gay community representatives and the "portion of our health care system under direct fire. We've preserved not just gay rights but human rights and the primacy of individual choice." In language that revealed an overriding commitment to individualism, even in the face of a challenge to the collective well-being, he stressed the dangers of public actions that by the articulation of public norms would impinge upon private choices.

With only minor changes this committee report was adopted one week later, on January 13, 1983, by the three major blood banking organizations—the American Association of Blood Banks, the American Red Cross, and the Council of Community Blood Centers.[31] It was this position that compelled the American Hemophilia Foundation to make public the policy it had quietly pursued since the fall of 1982. On January 14, its Medical and Scientific Advisory Committee issued twelve recommendations, among which was one that stressed the importance of identification by direct questioning of individuals "who belong to groups at high risk of transmitting AIDS, specifically male homosexuals; intravenous drug-users; and those who have recently resided in Haiti."[32]

Stung by this announcement, the National Gay Task Force and more than fifty other gay political, social, and medical organizations issued a denunciation of the Hemophilia Foundation.[33] "The concern of the NHF has been the safety of the blood products upon which the survival of hemophiliacs is based. But to single out any segment of our society as a source of unsafe blood is divisive and dangerous. . . . Above all it is incumbent upon blood industry and government agencies that regulate blood donor policy to refrain from suggestions or implementation of a blood donor screening program which, by whatever means, or under whatever name, amounts to a political solution to a medical problem. Pitting victim against victim will serve only to divert attention from the vital medical and ethical concerns that lie at the heart of this health crisis."

The allied gay organizations took the opportunity to challenge the structure of the blood banking system, especially its commercial components, and in lieu of a strategy of exclusion proposed surrogate-marker screening and an increase of funds for the study of AIDS and the care of patients. Most critically, the statement stressed the importance of individual self-screening based upon moral recognition "that in giving the 'gift of life' there is the responsibility to give the safest gift possible."

Considerable stress was placed by gay groups on the public health dangers of explicit efforts to bar those at risk for AIDS from blood donation. Those whose sexual orientation was still secret might feel pressured into donation in group- and especially workplace-based blood drives. Such pragmatic concerns were, of course, vital from the perspective of public health. Measures that ostensibly reflected a commitment to public health but undermined the public safety were irrational. But more was at stake. Blood bankers had embraced the language of privacy to buttress their concerns about the viability of the blood banking system. Gay leaders had highlighted the potential public health costs of donor exclusion to buttress their concerns about threats to privacy. It was, however, the constricting conception of privacy endorsed by many gay leaders at that time that was so striking. It was a conception of the rights of privacy that made the public expression even of norms of personal responsibility and duty anathema.

Individuals had to consider the risk to others as they decided whether or not to donate blood. Socially imposed exclusionary standards would necessitate unacceptable invasions of privacy and would entail mass stigmatization. Furthermore, exclusion from the donor pool could not be viewed as a self-contained measure, since it would open the way for the identification of gay men who would then be subject to discrimination in other social arenas. Public calls by those who were not gay for the withdrawal of gay men from the donor pool represented a profound threat "reminiscent of miscegenation blood laws that divided black blood from white."[34] In the most extreme case, such calls were equated with the "World War II rounding up of Japanese-Americans in the western half of the country to minimize the possibility of espionage."

Despite the denunciation of either socially or governmentally imposed restrictions, gay physicians and medical groups began a tortured process of attempting to articulate a standard of social responsibility for protecting the blood supply that at the same time placed enormous emphasis on the importance of personal decisions by potential blood donors. Writing in the January 1983 issue of the *BAPHRON*, the newsletter of the Bay Area Physicians for Human Rights, Robert Bolan suggested that in addition to surrogate screening, some donor questions "drawn from current epidemiological data covering the chief apparent risks such as number of different sexual partners, *but excluding specific sexual activities and sexual orientation*," might be appropriate. As an alternative, Bolan asserted that the posting of such sexual orientation-neutral advisories at blood centers could be effective, "rely[ing] on the altruism of those who donate blood to exclude themselves if appropriate." More global in its rejection of even carefully framed screening was the counterpoint proposal of W. L. Warner appearing in the same issue of *BAPHRON*. "To pose questions to a prospective donor about the number of sexual partners he has had . . . is patently ridiculous and viciously invasive . . . even if the response could be considered reliable. Some would consider the questions homophobic in themselves. Any inquiries of that nature carry with them moral attitudes of the questioner. And since morals are internal factors, any application along those lines should be from within." Nevertheless, Warner recognized the important role that gay medical leaders had to play in structuring the personal decisions of gay men, and facilitating the emergence of a culture of restraint and responsibility in the face of a threat to the nation's blood supply. Each individual had to question himself, paying heed to the advice of gay physicians. Gay physicians had the obligation to urge all gay men to avoid blood donation until more was known about the etiology of AIDS. "Gay men cannot, even with the best of intentions, add to the morbidity and mortality of AIDS even if it becomes embarrassing to be the odd man out when the rest of the office troops down to the blood bank to donate." Warner concluded that unless gay physicians took on the responsibility of issuing such warnings, their morality could be questioned and "the homophobes will have a field day."[35]

In New York, the New York Physicians for Human Rights urged those with AIDS or at the risk of exposure, "in particular individuals who have had intimate contact with many different sexual partners," not to give blood. Those in doubt were called upon to consult their physicians.[36] At the same time, private discussions between the New York Blood Center and the medical leadership of the local gay community were begun to develop a method of self-exclusion that would permit those who, though subject to social pressure to donate, believed themselves at risk. The option of completing a confidential form would permit them to indicate that the blood they had given should be used "only for studies" rather than for transfusion.[37] Finally, in February, the American Association of Physicians for Human Rights adopted a statement advising those at risk for AIDS not to donate.[38] But even that decision entailed a deep contradiction. Gay medical leaders acknowledged that the protection of the blood supply required exclusion of those at risk. But even the definition of the at-risk class was to remain beyond the reach of public institutions. In the allocation of the burden of uncertainty, donors were to be guided by gay medical leaders. Public agencies—viewed as they were with deep suspicion—were to remain mute before this critical social challenge, denied the opportunity to establish a communal standard for donor behavior.

The effort of gay leaders to prevent a governmental pronouncement on the exclusion of high-risk individuals from the blood donor pool was ultimately untenable, given the increasing frequency with which they themselves had sought to educate those at increased risk about the dangers of donation. On March 4, 1983, two months after the acrimonious CDC meeting on the risks of transfusion-associated AIDS, the Public Health Service issued its recommendations on the "Prevention of Acquired Immune Deficiency Syndrome (AIDS)."[39] Given the available evidence, the Centers for Disease Control, the Food and Drug Administration, and the National Institutes of Health, which had collaborated in preparing the new recommendations, declared that it appeared that "the pool of persons potentially capable of transmitting an AIDS agent may be considerably larger than the presently known number of cases."[40] In fact, since there was evidence that a latency period existed between exposure and the onset of illness, "physical examinations alone [would] not identify all persons capable of transmitting AIDS."[41] There was, therefore, no alternative but to treat all members of groups at increased risk for AIDS as posing a threat of transmission. Included were homosexual and bisexual men with multiple sex partners, as well as those who had sexual relations with such individuals. In carefully measured language and with full recognition that the blood banking community had expressly rejected the explicit screening of potential donors for sexual orientation, the Public Health Service put forth its "prudent" proposals. "As a temporary measure members of groups at increased risk should refrain from donating plasma and/or blood. This recommendation includes all individuals belonging to such groups even though many such individuals are at little risk for AIDS."[42] The precise method to be adopted to enforce such self-exclusion was not stipulated, and indeed the Public Health Service recommended that "studies . . . be conducted to evaluate screening procedures for their effectiveness in identifying and excluding plasma and blood with a high probability of transmitting AIDS."[43] Though specifying that laboratory tests, careful histories, and physical examinations be included among the approaches to be investigated, the recommendations carefully avoided any reference to the explicit use of questions about sexual orientation, the method proposed by the National Hemophilia Foundation but so opposed by gay leaders.

Despite the very cautious manner in which the Public Health Service recommendations had been framed, the decision to proceed with donor exclusion aroused protests from gay leaders and their political allies. The National Gay Task Force and Congressman Henry Waxman, who had begun to emerge as a vocal antagonist of the federal government's failure to move aggressively to fund research into the causes and possible prevention of AIDS, challenged the very flexibility of the PHS recommendations. Writing to Edward M. Brandt, Jr., the assistant secretary of health, Virginia Apuzzo, executive director of the National Gay Task Force, acknowledged "with some relief" that pressure to identify all gay men as unsuitable for blood donations had been resisted.[44] Nevertheless, she reiterated the arguments put forth by other representatives of the gay community about the preferability of screening blood rather than donors and called for the use of surrogate testing and the rapid development of a test for AIDS. "The medical problem presented by the possible transmittion of AIDS can only be resolved through the implementation of objective blood tests. Solutions dependent on excluding certain classes of blood donors no matter what form the screening assumes and whether driven by medical or political considerations, are inherently unsatisfactory." But most disturbing to Apuzzo was the flexibility of the March 4 recommendations on how donor exclusion was to be accomplished. The failure to reject the option of explicit questioning about sexual orientation was viewed as providing a warrant for such screening. "Such questioning, which has already been implemented in some locations, constitutes an invasion of privacy and carries with it the danger of unfairly and needlessly stigmatizing an entire community. Because of the climate of discrimination that prevails in this country, such questions may have a paradoxical effect. . . . Some men fearful of losing their jobs or suffering other persecution may feel pressured to donate blood." To preclude such "interrogation" the National Gay Task Force called upon Brandt to prohibit it. Henry Waxman echoed much of what Virginia Apuzzo had said, claiming that screening "by group" would be ineffective and probably counterproductive.[45] Furthermore, he noted that the new policy would needlessly restrict donations, thus imperiling the adequacy of the nation's blood supply. On the other hand, because he appreciated the extent to which pressures had been mounted for federally mandated explicit screening for sexual orientation, Bruce Voeller, who had argued so forcefully against donor exclusion at the January 4 CDC meeting, declared that, though he was not pleased with the recommendations, he could live with them.[46]

Three weeks after the Public Health Service issued its statement, the Food and Drug Administration issued its implementation recommendations to those establishments involved in the collection of blood for transfusion and source plasma, as well as to manufacturers of plasma derivatives.[47] Though stipulating that medical histories include specific questions to detect possible symptoms of AIDS, they clearly avoided the suggestion that explicit questions about sexual orientation be employed. Rather, it was proposed that individual donors be informed about those who were considered to be at increased risk for AIDS and about the recommendation that such individuals refrain from blood donations.

With extraordinary sensitivity to the concerns voiced by gay leaders, the American Red Cross moved to implement the FDA recommendations in a manner that was "intended to assist potential donors at risk for AIDS to refrain from donating blood without revealing confidential personal information."[48] Supplemental information was to be added to the pamphlet *What You Should Know About Giving Blood,* read by all potential donors. The new material concluded with advice on how to withdraw from the donor process without undue embarrassment. "If you believe that you are in a group at increased risk for developing AIDS, we ask that you refrain from donating blood at this time. You may leave now without providing an explanation. Or, if you prefer, you may proceed to be deferred confidentially without further questioning by the health history interviewer."

However reluctantly, gay political leaders came tacitly to accept as a temporary measure the Public Health Service recommendations on exclusion. Ultimately, they believed, the development of a specific blood test would obviate the need for screening procedures—no matter how carefully designed—based upon sexual orientation. Thus, when James Curran of the CDC suggested in mid-1983 that some surrogate test might be used *in addition to* the exclusion of gay men with multiple partners, it provoked a sharp reaction by the National Gay Task Force. "The gay and lesbian community will not gladly suffer the stigmatization that inevitably results from the current policy after the point at which a blood test for determining high risk of AIDS has been mandated."[49] But talk of such tests was at that point still quite theoretical. Indeed, as concern about transfusion-associated AIDS persisted and as the epidemiological pattern of AIDS among gay men suggested the epidemic's ever-wider scope, it became increasingly clear that the Public Health Service language of March 4 was insufficiently protective. And so despite the discomfort associated with exclusionary practices based even on subclasses of gay men, the American Association of Physicians for Human Rights recommended at the end of 1983 that only men who had been involved in mutually monogamous relationships for the past three years consider themselves appropriate blood donors.[50]

Deepening anxiety about the blood supply accompanied the publication in the *New England Journal of Medicine* in January 1984 of a major study of transfusion-associated cases of AIDS.[51] With the CDC's James Curran as lead author, the article was bound to affect the social climate. The completed investigations of donors whose blood appeared linked to the development of AIDS in recipients without known risk factors provided "circumstantial evidence that exposure to as little as one unit may result in transmission."[52] But it was the clinical picture of these donors that was most disturbing. "The failure to identify definite cases of AIDS or even severe symptoms among donors examined suggests that affected donors with only mild or inapparent illness account for the majority of cases of transfusion-associated AIDS."[53] Thus it was the asymptomatic carriers of the as-yet-to-be-identified infectious agent that posed the greatest risk. The significance of these findings went beyond the critical issue of protecting the blood supply. The existence of the asymptomatic carrier state had profound implications for the threat of sexual and maternal-fetal transmission of AIDS. How many heterosexual blood recipients were infected? Who posed a risk? Who was endangered?

Though Curran and his colleagues sought to provide some reassurance on the basis of the exclusionary recommendations made on March 4, 1983, the prospects for a marked rise in the number of transfusion-associated AIDS cases was acknowledged: "The current number of cases of AIDS associated with transfusion is small, representing about 1% of the reported cases in the United States. . . . However, most of these patients received their transfusions between 1979 and early 1982, a time when the prevalence of AIDS—and presumably of donors affected by the putative AIDS agent—was much lower than during 1982 to early 1983."[54] In an accompanying editorial, Joseph Bove, who had so forcefully sought to oppose the effort to link blood and AIDS just a year earlier at the CDC's special meeting, noted that "Curran's data provides substantial evidence that transfusion-related AIDS does occur."[55]

The blood banking community, which had been alerted to the impending publication of Curran's findings, sought to blunt an anticipated public response by issuing a statement nine days prior to the article's appearance. Cautiously framed so as to limit the prospect of alarm, the statement suggested that though the number of transfusion-related cases might continue to mount because of the "incubation" period associated with AIDS "[after a few years] we should see a reduction resulting from donor screening measures instituted in March 1983."[56] The statement placed particular emphasis on the implementation of screening strategies designed to make it possible for donors in high-risk groups to refrain from donation voluntarily and confidentially. Furthermore, the blood banking community recommended that especially in those regions with a high incidence of AIDS, mechanisms be available to permit donors to notify collection agencies that blood already provided should not be used for transfusion. It was, said the statement, "important to maintain the right to privacy of all donors."

Despite the emphasis by both the Public Health Service and the blood banking community on confidential self-deferral, it was inevitable that some would seek to guarantee the safety of the blood supply by the threat of the criminal sanction against members of excluded groups who persisted in donating. In what was thought to be the first such legislative proposal, a Republican state legislator in Florida introduced a bill that would have made it a crime for any member of a "high-risk group" to donate blood. "My reason . . . is not to discriminate against anybody or any group . . . it is simply to keep innocent people who need blood from getting a deadly disease."[57] More remarkable than the submission of the proposed legislation was the failure of such measures, even when anxiety about contaminated blood was at its peak, to obtain much by way of legislative support.

Even in the context of transfusion-associated AIDS, where the sense of vulnerability extended beyond those defined as being at high risk and where the public health was so utterly dependent on the withdrawal from the donor pool of those who posed a threat, there was a striking reluctance in the first years of the epidemic to make use of the state's coercive powers. The nascent public health strategy—at times explicitly, at times implicitly—was so focused on eliciting the cooperation of those at risk for AIDS that any potentially insulting or disruptive gesture was viewed as a threat to rational policy. The calculus of public health, here as in the case of the bathhouses, required policy determinations that at times appeared to contradict the dictates of reason. Why not threaten the punishment of irresponsible, at-risk donors as a way of bolstering the purely moral message of self-deferral? Why not enact sanctions as a way of underscoring, if only symbolically, the importance of protecting vulnerable blood transfusion recipients from those who failed to conform their behaviors to the dictates of public health? To those who dismissed legislative proposals for the application of the criminal law, the answer was clear. Criminalization would be a hollow gesture. It might protect a few but subvert the public health. Restraint by public health officials, even symbolic restraint, was critical to the encouragement of restraint on the part of the groups most at risk for transmitting the AIDS virus.

But such conclusions were by no means inevitable. Too frequently those who embraced them were unwilling to confront the difficult question of the appropriate role, as well as the limits, of law, especially criminal law, in the face of the AIDS epidemic. Within the liberal political tradition the exercise of government power as a sanction against those who threatened to inflict harm on others was not only tolerated but expected. Whatever the empirical merits of the policy of legislative restraint in the case of blood-donor behavior, and of the fears about how the application of criminal sanctions would entail the risk of episodic and invidious enforcement, whatever the legitimacy of the concerns about the extraordinary problems of proof that would arise in criminal proceedings (how would evidence of membership in a high-risk group be ascertained and corroborated?), there can be no doubt that the refusal to engage publicly the complex issues involved represented a failure of nerve. At the most fundamental level it was a failure to recognize how public health officials could shape a culture of responsibility by focusing sharply and openly on the social consequences of personal moral irresponsibility, even when more direct and coercive interventions might be deemed impractical and counterproductive.

Screening Blood

A little more than a year after the Public Health Service announced its donor exclusion recommendations, Secretary of Health and Human Services Margaret Heckler announced at a national press conference that HTLV-III, a retrovirus, had been identified as the agent responsible for AIDS.[58] A scientific finding that built upon work of French and American researchers, the discovery would fundamentally affect all future efforts to understand AIDS. It also had immediate implications for protection of the blood supply. Government officials were quick to announce that a blood test for the antibody to the virus would be commercially available within six months. At last a test to protect the blood supply was on the horizon. Within a month of the announcement, the American Red

Cross made public its plans to begin widescale trial testing of blood donations for antibody to HTLV-III.[59]

But no sooner had the prospect of the availability of such a long-awaited test been made public than concern about how it would be applied began to surface. Such anxieties were compounded by uncertainty about the clinical significance of the presence of antibody. In a letter to Edward Brandt, Jr., Neil Schram of the American Association of Physicians for Human Rights posed questions about the ethics of the anticipated research and the course of future public policy. "Clearly," he wrote, "studies of gay males, health care workers, and transfusion recipients among others are needed. But what would a positive antibody result signify? Does that mean the individual is immune (if a state of immunity exists with this disease), is going to develop AIDS, or is a 'carrier' either infectious or non-infectious?"[60] With so many critical uncertainties, how would test results be used? Would health care workers with the antibody be permitted to stay in their jobs? Would research subjects want or have a right to examine the results of their antibody tests? Would physicians have an obligation to inform them? Given these critical questions, Schram proposed that the ethical and practical problems associated with giving informed consent to participation in the proposed research studies of HTLV-III antibody be considered by a special interagency panel that would include representation from those at risk for AIDS—gay men. His goal: the rapid development of knowledge "without causing undue concern."

Very quickly concerns within the gay community extended beyond the conditions under which research on the antibody to the AIDS virus would be conducted, to matters involving the ultimate uses of the test. What in mid-1984 might have appeared to be the alarmist response of those schooled in suspicion about the intentions of government would within two years seem prescient. Thus in early July, Jeff Levi of the National Gay Task Force asked a broad constituency of gay groups to consider a range of issues, including the responsibility of blood bankers to inform donors of test results and to maintain confidentiality. Levi was also concerned about how the test would be used more generally. He urged those to whom he wrote to consider the possibility that the antibody test would be used by insurers to make underwriting decisions, by employers to screen out workers and job applicants, by health care workers to identify those they would not treat, by the military to bar recruitment, and by the immigration and naturalization authorities as a barrier to entry into the United States.[61]

Such anxieties were fueled by every move that suggested that public health authorities might require lists of those who were positive. Lists were but a prelude to surveillance and a threatening breach of the privacy so critical to the protection of gay men from discrimination. Thus, for example, when James Curran of the CDC asked the chief epidemiologist of each state to consider the potential utility of an interstate blood donor deferral registry—a list of those found ineligible for donation—for those who tested positive, he provoked a sharp protest despite his explicit concern about whether such an effort would be compatible with the maintenance of the "right to privacy of persons with AIDS-related disorders or persons who are asymptomatic but antibody positive."[62] Neil Schram wrote to the director of the Centers for Disease Control of his "shock" and "outrage." "The risks," he wrote, "of a national list of people positive for antibody to HTLV-III/LAV are tremendous. If the list follows the same characteristics as the people with AIDS, then the list will be a national list of gay and bisexual men and IV drug users. Since homosexuality is still illegal in over 20 states and IV drug use presumably in all states, the potential of that list falling into police hands is tremendous."[63] In a letter to the members of the American Association of Physicians for Human Rights, Schram made clear the need to mobilize political opposition to proposals that even hinted at the prospect of creating a registry of those exposed to the AIDS virus. "I believe the Curran letter is the first attempt to develop a national list . . . of people positive for HTLV-III antibody. In order for that to be effective, the test would have to be a mandatory reported test in all states. This must be fought early and strongly."[64]

So alarmed had gay groups become about the imminent licensing of the antibody test that early opposition to donor exclusion on the basis of sexual orientation and practices virtually vanished. Thus, in mid-December 1984, when the Food and Drug Administration redefined the class of at-risk men to include "males who have had sex with more than one male since 1979, and males whose male partners have had more than one male partner since 1979"—an exclusionary classification that involved virtually every sexually active gay and bisexual male—there was no sign of protest.[65] That the FDA had demonstrated extraordinary sensitivity by stressing in its recommendations the importance of increasing the effectiveness of confidential "voluntary self-exclusion procedures" certainly contributed to the reception accorded these new exclusionary standards.

As part of the strategy designed to slow the rapid movement toward licensing of the antibody test, an effort was begun by gay political groups to argue that the test in preparation was inaccurate and might actually decrease the safety of the blood supply by inadvertently undercutting the force of voluntary deferral guidelines. In a remarkable about-face, the long-sought objective blood test was cast as the threat and exclusion on the basis of risk group membership was portrayed as the more appropriate strategy. "Few people," said Jeff Levi, "want to consider themselves to be at high risk to AIDS; with the government saying there is now a blood test that will screen out those who are truly at high risk, people will be more likely to donate—thinking the blood test will be their insurance against giving infected blood."[66]

But gay groups were not alone in their concern about how the implementation of the new test would affect the safety and adequacy of the blood supply, especially if, as was anticipated, blood collection agencies would be required by federal officials to notify donors of their test results. Blood bankers were also disturbed about the burden—in time, resources, and professional staff requirements—that the anticipated requirement for notification would place on them. Indeed, there was considerable resistance to the very notion that blood bankers had an obligation to assume such a role.[67]

Finally, there was concern during the prelicensing period about the fact that the planned ELISA test (enzyme linked immunosorbent assay) would produce an unacceptably high level of false positive findings in low-risk populations. Designed to be especially sensitive, as a precaution against the possibility of contaminated blood passing through the screening procedure, the ELISA would, if used without a confirmatory test with a capacity for greater specificity, require the discarding of blood that was in fact untainted. False positive test findings would also result in the identification and potential stigmatization of donors never exposed to the AIDS virus. James Allen of the Centers for Disease Control was not even certain that the most widely used confirmatory test—the Western Blot—would preclude such untoward consequences for healthy donors. "Before I tell a person with no risk factors that he's positive, I'd want to want to know a lot more than I know now."[68]

But to the Food and Drug Administration, licensing of the blood test was a matter of the highest priority despite the uncertainties associated with its implementation. "All we know," said Dennis Donohue, special assistant to the FDA's director of the Division of Blood and Biologics, "at this moment is that an individual whose [blood result] is positive for antibody to HTLV-III has been exposed to the virus. . . . We also know that blood from such an individual should not be used for transfusion."[69] If there were to be errors, the dictates of public health required that they be on the side of safety.

On January 11, 1985, the Public Health Service issued its "provisional" recommendations for the screening of blood.[70] All blood donors were to be told that their blood would be tested for antibody to HTLV-III, that if positive, they would be notified in a confidential manner of the test results, and that their names would be placed on the blood collection agency's donor deferral list along with others deemed unacceptable as donors. Blood that was initially reactive to the antibody test was not to be used for transfusion or the manufacture of other blood products, even though it was admitted that the proportion of false positives among the general donor population on an initial ELISA would be high. It was therefore recommended that no notification occur before at least a second test was done—either a second ELISA or an alternative supplemental procedure. Finally, the FDA made clear that the antibody test was to serve in addition to, rather than as a replacement for, donor self-deferral. Such an approach was necessitated by the small possibility of false negative test results among those who had been infected by the AIDS virus, but had not yet developed sufficiently detectable levels of antibody.

Most remarkable in these recommendations was the insistence upon donor notification. Blood bankers could not avoid the responsibility; donors could not waive the right to such information. So forceful a stance went beyond the patient's "right to know" so central to medical ethics. Typically that right entailed the right not to know the result of medical examinations and tests. Autonomy included the right to shield oneself from the burden of a grim diagnosis. But here the calculus of public health and not clinical ethics was involved. Those who were antibody positive had to know that fact, even if they preferred otherwise, if others were to be protected from exposure through sexual relations or as a result of subsequent blood donations. Restraint and responsibility were predicated on such knowledge.

The insistence upon notification was all the more remarkable since the Public Health Service conceded that the "proportion of these seropositive donors who had been infected with HTLV-III is not known. It is therefore important to emphasize to the donor that a positive result is a preliminary finding that may not represent true infection."[71] Further evaluation by a physician was called for under such circumstances. But whatever the ultimate significance of the test results for any individual, the Public Health Service, having been pressed by representatives of the gay community, underscored the importance of conveying positive findings in a manner designed to protect confidentiality.

Three days after the publication of these recommendations, the Public Health Service's Executive Task Force on AIDS conducted a series of meetings with gay leaders, blood bankers, and public health officials to elicit their reactions.[72] At each session concern was voiced about the conditions under which blood testing would be undertaken, the potential impact on donors, and the consequences for the safety and adequacy of the blood supply. Though a broad coalition of gay organizations had at last acknowledged just days earlier that the testing of blood was an appropriate social intervention, concern about how the blood test might easily be misused in other settings—a long-standing fear—was reiterated. Blood bankers were worried primarily about how the onset of testing might negatively affect the blood supply and stressed the importance of developing a system of alternative test sites that could be used by those seeking to know their antibody status. Some went further and warned that the requirement of donor notification would have serious implications for the safety of the blood supply—even if alternative test sites were available. Inevitably, some high-risk individuals seeking to know their antibody status would use the blood banking system as a source for testing. Speaking for the Conference of Local Health Officials, Mervyn Silverman called on the federal government to fund alternative testing centers where free confidential screening could be done. He warned that a survey in his own city of San Francisco had found that 75 percent of high-risk individuals had stated that they would turn to blood centers for testing unless alternatives were available. Since false negatives could slip through the system, the results could be disastrous. Concerned, as well, about the capacity of local health departments to meet the needs of those who tested positive, Silverman called for a delay in the implementation of testing until an adequate local infrastructure to provide social, psychological, and medical supports was developed.

In the face of the impending licensure of a test designed to protect the blood supply, a broad consensus had thus developed around the need to provide individuals seeking knowledge of their antibody status—no matter how ambiguous the meaning of the test in early 1985—with a network of alternative sites to which they might turn. But at the very moment when this consensus was developing, it masked a profound disagreement that was to have important implications for the evolution of the debate over testing and public health policy in the next two years. Some advocates of testing outside of blood centers anticipated that the ELISA, when subject to adequate confirmation, could be a potentially valuable tool in the effort to meet the challenge posed by AIDS; others saw in the move toward alternative test sites an unfortunate compromise with the demands being made by anxious individuals who, in fact, would learn nothing from the test, whether the results were positive or negative. The January 11, 1985, "Public Health Service Provisional Recommendations" noted that "testing for HTLV-III antibody should be offered to persons who may have been infected as a result of their contact with seropositive individuals, e.g., sexual partners, persons with whom needles have been shared, infants of seropositive mothers."[73] In sharp contrast, Virginia Apuzzo of the National Gay Task Force stated, "[In the alternative test site] it will be essential to provide counseling before and after testing: before testing to *dissuade* the individual from taking the test, so he/she is aware of the potential risks and the fact that there is no clinical value to the test results; after, to try to explain the meaning of the test results—both positive and negative."[74] Even the Association of State and Territorial Health Officials, which was ultimately to become a strong advocate of testing, warned in early February 1985 that it would be inadvisable, given the limitations of the ELISA test, to expand screening beyond blood centers and alternative test sites operated under research protocols.[75]

Though the concern of blood bankers, public health officials, and gay political leaders did not delay the commercial licensing of the ELISA test, the Food and Drug Administration did respond to the challenges raised during the preceding months of public and private negotiation. Most important, it recognized that donor notification had to be delayed pending the achievement of a level of testing proficiency—though even during the start-up period blood donations that tested positive would have to be discarded. In addition, the FDA recommended that the mandated blood testing be preceded by the development of alternative sites to which those seeking to know their antibody status could be referred.[76] Finally, in a "Dear Doctor" letter, Frank Young, commissioner of the FDA, underscored a point repeatedly made by those concerned about the prospects of the widespread misapplication of the ELISA, and the ensuing threat of stigmatization and discrimination. "The test," he wrote, was "not a test for AIDS."[77]

Blood bank testing began in April 1985. As blood collection agencies gained experience with the ELISA test, the importance of performing a Western Blot confirmatory analysis on repeatedly reactive ELISA's became ever more apparent. The American Red Cross reported that of 10,000 initially reactive blood donations, 1,700 were reactive on a second ELISA, and only 333 positive on the Western Blot test.[78] The Red Cross thus determined that no notification of donors would occur until the more expensive and more difficult Western Blot confirmatory test could be done on all repeatedly reactive donations.

In the wake of the implementation of blood bank testing, some states expressly forbade the notification of donors during the phase-in period. In New York David Axelrod, the commissioner of health, wrote to the state's physicians that "individual results will not be provided until a confirmation test has been carried out to avoid the added trauma of false positive results."[79] Furthermore, reflecting the influence of the political and scientific perspective of gay leaders, he actively sought to discourage the use of the test in settings other than blood banks. "The result can provide no definitive medical information and [can] lead to a false sense of security or anxiety. The available data on both the sensitivity and specificity of the test leave the potential for a wide margin of error in an individual test."

By July, three months after the initiation of screening, blood bankers felt prepared to undertake the task of notification. Some collection agencies merely informed donors of their test results and suggested that they seek appropriate medical follow-up. In New York, however, a decision was made by the New York Blood Center to undertake the initial task of counseling those who tested positive. A special task force was convened to review carefully the content of the educational material that was to accompany the process of informing those with confirmed antibody-positive results. Though both the written and video messages sought to avoid an alarmist tone by stressing that "the evidence . . . thus far seems to indicate that the majority of healthy people who are found to have this antibody will remain in good health," the warnings about the risks of transmission were uncompromising. "When you have sexual relations, use condoms. . . . It may be wise to avoid [the] transfer of saliva . . . in French kissing. . . . If you are a woman . . . don't become pregnant. . . . If you are a man . . . do not impregnate a woman."[80]

At a special July conference sponsored by the National Institutes of Health and the Food and Drug Administration, the first months of blood donor testing were evaluated. The conclusion: testing had been a success. The director of the Center for Drugs and Biologics of the FDA reported that "these tests are doing an extremely good job of screening potentially AIDS infectious blood units out of the blood supply."[81] But despite this sense of accomplishment, James Curran warned that there would be no immediate drop in transfusion-associated cases of AIDS. "Most of these will occur in those who received blood prior to the antibody test being introduced."[82]

Studies presented at the meeting dispelled whatever ambiguity remained about the significance of the presence of antibody in a donor's blood. Even given the technical limitations of viral recovery efforts, close to 60 percent of those with "strongly positive" antibody results were found to harbor the AIDS virus, a result that James Allen of the CDC termed "very high."[83] And so a test was now available that could, in fact, identify the asymptomatic carriers of the AIDS virus. The implications were clear for both those concerned with intercepting the spread of the virus and those fearful about how the desire to identify such individuals could lead to the enactment of compulsory broad-scale screening programs.

Seeking to reassure the American people about the safety of the blood supply achieved by virtue of both deferral recommendations and antibody screening, the Public Health Service was quick to respond to suggestions that there remained risks from contaminated blood that had nevertheless tested negative.[84] Indeed, repeated efforts were made to limit anxiety about the remaining statistical risk. It was, however, inevitable that transmission by blood transfusion, though essentially blocked, would still occur, and indeed within the year, the CDC reported the first such case.[85]

That contaminated donations continued to reach the blood banking system suggested that individuals at increased risk for AIDS continued to give blood. Some knew themselves to be at risk. Others did not. Data from one study indicated that of 61 antibody-positive donors 80 percent acknowledged during careful interviews that they were gay.[86] How such individuals could be dissuaded from such reckless behavior would remain a problem for public health officials. Understandably, both legislators and law enforcement officials would be driven—as some had been before the availability of the antibody test—to consider whether the criminal law had a role to play. Of those who unknowingly posed a threat, some had been infected during sexual relations, others as a result of contaminated transfusions in the period before screening was initiated.

It was to assist in the identification and location of those who had been infected by blood transfusions and who thus posed a threat to their sexual partners and potential fetuses, as well as to the blood supply, that the "look-back" program was launched. Designed to locate the recipients of blood from donors who were found to be positive subsequent to the initiation of blood testing, this effort was initially opposed by the blood banking community. On June 7, 1985, a joint statement by the American Association of Blood Banks, the American Red Cross, and the Council of Community Blood Centers declared, "Because we do not know whether an individual with HTLV-III antibodies at a current donation had such antibodies previously, an adequate basis for notification of recipients . . . from previous donations does not exist. The injury to prior recipients which may be caused by such notification is disproportionate to the benefits, which are tenuous and ill-defined."[87] Needless to say, such an effort would have posed yet another administrative burden that blood bankers were not anxious to assume. Within a year, however, there had been a turnabout, as the major blood collection agencies agreed upon the desirability of conducting such a program.[88] In some locales the look-back program was undertaken with alacrity, in other regions with greater caution; and in New York State, the commissioner of health chose to allow each hospital to determine whether to convey to each physician and/or patient information produced by the "look back." "No state statute or regulation requires hospitals or physicians to inform transfusion recipients of a possibility that the blood they received might have been contaminated. Hospitals and physicians may decide independently, based on the best interests of the patients and individual circumstances to inform patients of the potential for HIV infection."[89] This position, so consonant with the excessive restraint of New York State in the first years of the AIDS epidemic, provoked an angry response from a New York Blood Center task force that had, for more than a year, struggled with the ethical and social issues raised by blood screening. This group accused the commissioner of failing to take full account of the right of the potentially infected to be informed of their situation. He had failed to appreciate the full public health implications of not notifying those who inadvertently could be transmitting the virus to others.[90] Called upon to mandate the notification already undertaken in other states, Commissioner David Axelrod made no response.

With the initiation of the look-back program, the final element in a broad public effort to protect the blood supply had been put in place. Donor deferral, blood screening, and finally, the location of those who might have been inadvertently infected by past donations, were all critical features of this effort. But the unassailable goal of protecting the blood supply was inextricably linked to the identification of those capable of or at increased risk for transmitting a lethal infection. It was this dimension of the blood safety program that had from the beginning provoked the most serious of political conflicts. Fears of how identification could subject the infected or possibly infected to stigmatization, limitations on economic and social well-being, and perhaps most threatening, the loss of liberty itself, had motivated the reactions of those alarmed by policies that, from the perspective of public health, could only have been lauded.

What the controversy surrounding the blood supply had demonstrated was that there could be no public health interventions that were merely technical in nature. All entailed political judgments, judgments about the distribution of burdens and benefits. A failure to take steps to retard the spread of HIV infection carried with it serious implications for communal health and, more critically, subverted the prospects for the emergence of a public culture of restraint and responsibility that would reinforce private decisions to behave with due regard for the vulnerability of others. Yet those very same measures, if unwisely crafted, could hinder the emergence of such a culture by fostering an antagonistic climate within which those most at risk for transmitting the AIDS virus would view themselves as under siege.

The capacity of gay political, legal, and medical organizations to articulate the fears of those whose social vulnerability was intensified by the AIDS epidemic had shaped the debate over the directions of public health policy in the first years of the epidemic. The controversies that had first surfaced in the clash over the screening of blood were to be replayed again and again as the role of antibody testing in the public health response to AIDS became the subject of often bitter debate.

Chapter 4

Testing, Reporting, and Notifying

The Politics of Identification

From the outset the test developed to detect antibody to the AIDS virus—and first used on a broad scale in blood banking—was mired in controversy. Uncertainty about the significance of the test's findings and about its quality and accuracy provided the technical substrate of disputes that inevitably took on a political character, since issues of privacy, communal health, social and economic discrimination, coercion, and liberty were always involved. For those who feared that public anxiety about AIDS would turn individuals identified as infected with the AIDS virus into targets of irrational social policy and practice, the antibody test became emblematic of the most threatening prospect in the community's response to AIDS. They believed that the ELISA test would inevitably be extended beyond blood banking. Vigorous encouragement of testing would ineluctably lead to mandatory approaches as the impatient appealed to the authoritarian history of public health. Since confidentiality would not be preserved, the consequences would be stigmatization and deprivation of the right to work, go to school, and obtain insurance. Most ominously, the identification of the infected could threaten freedom itself. No marginal advance of the public health, those who argued against wide-scale testing asserted, could warrant such a catastrophic array of personal burdens.

Those who believed that the identification of the infected or potentially infected—through testing or other public health efforts—provided an opportunity for strategically targeted measures viewed the availability of the antibody tests as a great opportunity. Some advocates of testing, opposed to the use of coercion and attentive to matters of privacy so forcefully articulated by gay groups, would stress the importance of preserving the right of each individual to determine whether to be tested, protecting the confidentiality of test results, and guaranteeing the social and economic rights of those whose test results revealed infection with HIV. Theirs was a posture that sought to demonstrate the compatibility of an aggressive defense of the public health with a commitment to the privacy and social interests of the infected and those at risk of infection.

Others asserted that the defense of the public health required coercion and limitations on the liberty of the infected. For them screening on a compulsory basis was both necessary and inevitable. Assertions that the public health would not require such efforts merely masked, they argued, the willingness to sacrifice the communal welfare to private interests. The specter of such coercion haunted the discussion of all public health efforts, even the apparently voluntary attempts to facilitate identification of the infected.

Ultimately, the debate over testing and other public health measures designed to identify the infected would force a confrontation over which proposed interventions could most effectively contribute to the transformation of the private behaviors linked to the spread of HIV infection and the development of a public culture that would encourage and reinforce such changes. Bold moves might advance the cause of public health in the face of the AIDS epidemic, or they might subvert that very cause. Caution might represent wisdom or a failure to grasp the opportunity to affect the pattern of HIV transmission. Appeals to the history of public health would inform the perspectives of those who encountered each other as antagonists; so too would profound differences over the weight to be given to communal well-being and personal liberty. Empirical considerations, historical perspectives, and philosophical commitments each thus helped to shape the fractious struggles that characterized the politics of identification.

Testing for Antibody to the AIDS Virus

Months before the AIDS virus antibody test was licensed by the Food and Drug Administration for use in blood banks, anxiety had already surfaced in the discussions of gay leaders. "Don't take the test" became the rallying cry. In an editorial, the *New York Native* wrote, "No gay or bisexual man should allow his blood to be tested. . . . The meaning of the test remains completely unknown, beyond indicating exposure to the virus. The meaning of exposure to the virus is completely unknown. Scientists and physicians agree that a positive test result cannot be used to diagnose anything." What was far from uncertain, however, was the "personal anxiety and socioeconomic oppression that [would] result from the existence of a record of a blood test result. . . . Will test results be used to identify the sexual orientation of millions of Americans? Will a list of names be made? How can such information be kept confidential? Who will be able to keep this list out of the hands of insurance companies, employers, landlords, and the government itself?" What was critical was for gay and bisexual men to modify their behaviors in order to protect their own health and that of their sexual partners. For those purposes, what role could such an ambiguous and potentially dangerous test play? "If you test positive, will you act with any more wisdom or concern than if you test negative? Will you be less or more conscious of following safe and healthy sexual guidelines?"[1]

In the same issue of the *Native* Stephen Caiazza, president of the New York Physicians for Human Rights, warned his readers that the test was "pernicious" and would cause great harm. "We have reached the point in medical technology where we can accumulate data upon data without knowing what they mean. Unfortunately, there are times when the information collected can hurt the individual. This is at present the case with AIDS."[2] Here then, before the test was available, were the elements of what would harden into an orthodoxy among gay leaders: the test was technically limited; the findings it produced would be of no benefit to the individuals tested or to their sexual partners; those who were antagonistic to gay interests would seize upon the test to foster irrational discrimination wrapped in the mantle of public health.

But despite such opposition, gay leaders were driven by the imminence of blood bank screening in early 1985 and the FDA requirement that individuals whose blood was found to contain antibody to the AIDS virus be so notified to support, along with some public health officials, the creation of alternative test sites. Only such testing centers could protect the blood supply from the hazard that those at increased risk for AIDS might turn to blood banks for testing. Thus the American Association of Physicians for Human Rights declared that while "current uncertainties about the accuracy or prognostic significance of the available antibody test mitigate against [its] widespread use . . . in screening individuals . . . some individuals will ultimately fail to be dissuaded from seeking testing."[3] Confronted by the realization that an undetermined number of gay men would seek testing, AAPHR was compelled to advance protective guidelines for the governance of alternative test sites while opposing the use of tests for such extra–blood-banking purposes.

Opposition to the use of the antibody test outside the context of blood banking and research protocols was not, however, restricted to gay groups. A number of health departments, sometimes strongly influenced by concerns of gay medical and political leaders, also expressed alarm. The Philadelphia Health Department petitioned Secretary of Health and Human Services Margaret Heckler to revise her decision to provide federal funds for the creation of alternative test sites. "We believe that the Public Health Service loses credibility when it tells Americans that they should not have the test, but then makes it generally available anyway. . . . If we expect the public to believe us on complicated and sensitive issues, we should be consistent and credible in our scientific and public position."[4] The insistence of the Public Health Service on the notification of blood donors about their test findings had *created* the need for the new sites. Eliminating that requirement would also eliminate the need for special settings where testing could be done. Chicago joined Philadelphia in challenging the public health grounds for creating the alternative sites.[5] And in New York City the health commissioner not only refused to establish alternative sites but sought by every means at his disposal to create impediments to the use of the test outside of blood banking. New York, the epicenter of the American AIDS epidemic, thus became the only major American city where testing would not be readily available.

Perhaps most striking, the Association of State and Territorial Health Officials, which ultimately was to become a strong proponent of broad-scale voluntary testing, expressed doubts about the use of the test. In early February 1985 ASTHO noted that the ELISA test would simply generate too many false positive results, and the association, like others, stressed the unknown prognostic significance of the results that were truly positive.[6] In all, the test was not appropriate for public health screening purposes. One month later, on the eve of the licensing of the antibody test, ASTHO convened a national consensus conference designed to provide guidance to public health officials. The final report of the meeting asserted that beyond the screening of blood and in research protocols the test was of "extremely limited utility."[7]

Despite the award of $9.7 million by the Centers for Disease Control to more than fifty localities to facilitate the establishment of alternative test sites, it took many months for such centers to become operational. Even in California, where the legislature moved aggressively to provide funding for such sites, where testing could be conducted under conditions of anonymity, and where the nation's most stringent confidentiality legislation was enacted to protect those who took the test, it was not until July that testing was begun.[8] During this period, gay groups intensified their efforts to discourage use of the test. In New York City, the Gay Men's Health Crisis—the city's largest AIDS service organization—warned in a paid advertisement, "The test can be almost as devastating as the disease."[9] In Washington the AIDS Action Council, speaking for a coalition of gay political and health organizations, urged, "If you are a member of a group at risk for AIDS, you have it within your power to short circuit the dangers that this test poses for you and millions of others. How? By refusing to be tested yourself and by refusing to let any of your friends be tested. Don't donate blood and don't ask your physician, clinician, or public health service to give you the test. It's that simple."[10] This perspective was extended to those responsible for the treatment of drug users, as typically more sophisticated gay leaders counseled them about how testing could have only deleterious effects upon those who were in their care. And so such treatment personnel began to articulate positions indistinguishable from their gay tutors, despite the grave implications for the heterosexual transmission of the AIDS virus and the transmission of HIV to fetuses as a result of maternal infection.

At the same time that gay leaders were denouncing the antibody test, a countercurrent began to emerge that perceived in the test, especially when the ELISA was done in conjunction with the technically more difficult and more expensive Western Blot confirmatory test, a potentially invaluable adjunct in the struggle against AIDS. The proponents of testing did not deny that there were lingering technical problems with the test and especially with the standardization of the Western Blot procedure, but they asserted that similar problems were associated with virtually every test done in medicine. They did not view the test as a substitute for individual counseling and mass education but as a potent tool for fostering the behavioral modifications that everyone understood to be essential to any AIDS control program. They did not discount the risks posed by threats to confidentiality but sought to protect the privacy of those who needed testing, frequently by arguing that the option of anonymity be available. Finally, and most critically, those who supported the use of the test believed that the emerging understanding of the significance of confirmed positive findings was of great personal and public health relevance. Unlike those who persisted in asserting that the test demonstrated little about current infectivity, the test's proponents relied on studies revealing that the presence of the antibody was indicative of current infection with the AIDS virus and of a presumed capacity to transmit infection to others. In sum, at each juncture where uncertainty and ambiguity led opponents of the test to stress the threats to privacy and civil liberties and the absence of compensating public health benefits, proponents of testing underscored the potential for a contribution to the struggle against AIDS.

Thus in March 1985, when many public health officials were still counseling caution and when the precise significance of antibody test results remained very uncertain, Franklin Judson, an aggressive Colorado public health official and president of the American Venereal Disease Association, wrote to the association's membership, "I am concerned about the lack of movement towards an organized HTLV-III control program."[11] AIDS, Judson asserted, was "the most deadly" sexually transmitted disease in recent history, and yet the antibody test was being conceived of only as a way of preventing transfusion-associated cases—less than 1 percent of all cases. Neither technical limitations of the test nor fears about how results could be abused provided a warrant for inaction. "The realities of imperfect diagnostic tests and fear about confidentiality should not drive us to the sidelines to observe the natural history of this epidemic. In my mind the consequences to gay men and other high risk groups of doing nothing are far worse than the consequences of an active program that at least considers the use of traditional public health disease control measures." Among such measures would be the screening of high-risk group members, the reporting of the names of those found positive to well-guarded public health registries, contact tracing—a method commonly used in venereal disease control programs—and "legal restrictions on the sexual activities of seropositive individuals."

It was precisely the threat of such a broad-gauged public health program and the ominous implications of establishing registries as well as legal restrictions on sexual activities that provoked the reaction of gay leaders as they heard Donald Francis, a virologist on the staff of the Centers for Disease Control, address a meeting in the spring of 1985, just before the commencement of the First International AIDS Conference in Atlanta. Francis called upon gay men to seek out testing voluntarily in order to limit the transmission of AIDS. There was no question but that those who were positive for the antibody to the AIDS virus were infected. There was no question but that they could transmit the virus to others. They had to know those facts.[12] Though Francis stressed that he was speaking in an unofficial capacity, to those who heard him the imprint of the government marked his words. Some in his fearful and outraged audience termed his proposal "unworkable," others "diabolical."[13]

But it was not simply those officially involved with public health who had begun to argue that testing for the antibody to the AIDS virus was important. A few gay leaders, most often physicians or scientists, began to break ranks on the issue. In April 1985 Bruce Voeller, former executive director of the National Gay Task Force, a member of a number of federal scientific advisory panels and an active participant in the early controversy over blood safety, published bold appeals for testing in the Los Angeles–based *Advocate*[14] and in the *New York Native*.[15] "Gay leaders have warned that lists of test-takers could fall into the wrong hands. Maybe so, but I'd rather be alive and on a list than dead because I'd been misled into believing I could get no value from knowing my test results. Lives are more important than lists." Unlike those who argued that the test produced no clinically or socially relevant information, Voeller argued that knowledge of one's own antibody status was necessary, not only to protect oneself, but to protect one's lovers.

In time, on both the East and West coasts, gay physicians began to question the rigid rejection of testing. In New York Stephen Caiazza, who as president of the New York Physicians for Human Rights had written in October 1984 with such passion about the dangers of testing, began by October 1985 to challenge the policy of the New York City Health Department that attempted to restrict the test's availability.[16] In California, Robert Bolan, president of the San Francisco AIDS Foundation (which had played so critical a role in providing education about AIDS to the gay community), who had sounded the alarm about the direct questioning of blood donors about sexual orientation, charged that many of his colleagues had permitted their anxiety about the potential misuse of the test to cloud their vision. Writing in the *Newsletter* of the American Association of Physicians for Human Rights, he asserted that any gay or bisexual man who was sexually active outside of a monogamous relationship and who did not "consistently and regularly" follow safe sexual practices had to be encouraged to be tested.[17] Rather than warning gay men about how testing itself could threaten the gay community, gay physicians had to sound a tocsin about the threat to survival posed by AIDS. "We must abandon our reluctance to encourage testing in persons for whom a positive test may result in a significant adverse psychological effect. With antibody prevalence now being estimated at close to 50 percent of our community in San Francisco, we are fast reaching saturation kinetics and will lose our community if we do not abandon our timid approach to this antibody test. Legitimate issues like civil rights can create a smokescreen and excuses for not being as fully informed about one's risks as possible." Gay physicians had a public health duty to dispel denial about the grim significance of the test's results and challenge the prevailing misinformation about the test's accuracy. "I think the position 'don't take the test' was erroneous, especially after the alternate test sites were secured. We have been able to deal effectively, if not immediately, with panic, repression, abrogation of personal rights." There would be no "AIDS Dachau." What the gay community had not done well was to confront the "real enemies: personal denial and the AIDS virus."

Not surprisingly, Bolan was sharply attacked for his position. In an essay that ran as a companion piece in the *AAPHR Newsletter*, Bolan's science and politics were challenged. "Even if the test were foolproof (which it clearly is not) would this information be worth the inherent dangers of a freely available AIDS antibody test?" Though there were confidentiality protections in California, the legislature that enacted them could just as easily rescind them. And beyond California there were no such protections. With allusions to the history of American racism and the experience of Japanese-Americans during World War II, the dangers of identification were stressed. "It is a fact that the AIDS antibody test is being used now and will be used increasingly in the future to identify a minority and deprive that minority of rights not consistent with the significance of that test but consistent with hysteria and homophobia." Those who advocated testing were guilty of denial. An "AIDS Dachau" was a possibility. "Loss of civil liberties [is] our real enemy."

Despite such attacks there clearly was, by the end of 1985, a more nuanced perception of the test on the part of an increasing number of gay leaders. No longer was testing viewed simply as a threat. Some of those who continued to attack the accuracy of the test publicly, acknowledged privately that technical matters were being used for political reasons, as a way of forestalling what they saw as the true danger: a politically inspired rush to mass screening. In November 1985, nine months after the test was licensed, AAPHR urged gay and bisexual men to take the test if they needed it "to practice low risk sexual behavior all the time."[18] In justifying the position of the association, Neil Schram, chair of its AIDS Task Force and its past president, acknowledged that his deepening realization that AIDS posed the "most serious threat of our lifetime" had impelled him and the gay and lesbian physicians' group to a change of mind.[19] Like others, he had strongly opposed the use of the test outside of blood banking. From the vantage of early 1986 he believed that he had been mistaken. "In 1984 . . . I saw the test as the greatest threat to the gay community and advised loudly 'don't take the test.' I was wrong . . . the greatest threat to gay and bisexual men is not the test (at least where it is anonymous), it is infection with HTLV-III." Expecting to be denounced by those who held rigidly to the earlier position, Schram declared, "Our frustration at seeing the denial that exists in the gay community, contributed to by the gay media, forces me to respond. AAPHR is certainly not antigay. . . . We are fighting for our survival both as individuals and as a community."[20]

While increasing numbers of gay leaders were beginning to accept the need for testing under carefully defined circumstances, many within the public health community were beginning to place ever greater stress on the potential benefits that would result from the broad-scale voluntary testing of those at increased risk for HIV infection. Not a substitute for counseling, the test, they held, could act as a potent reinforcement for behavioral change. In August 1985 the Association of State and Territorial Health Officials once again convened a national consensus conference devoted to the antibody test. On this occasion, doubts about the test, its use, and the recommendations to be made to those who tested positive had all but gone. "With less than six months' experience, it is clear that [the tests] are more than simply measures to screen donated blood. Their high sensitivity, specificity, and in higher prevalence groups, their predictive powers for exposure to HTLV-III will substantially assist the disease prevention effort. When properly used, test information may also enhance the education efforts which remain for now the principal intervention to prevent HTLV-III transmission."[21] But an increased reliance on voluntary testing was predicated on the capacity to protect the confidentiality of test results. Acknowledging the skepticism of the gay community, the ASTHO report stressed the importance of convincing those at risk that all measures would be taken to preclude the unwarranted disclosure of test findings.[22] The defense of confidentiality was not antithetical to the protection of public health; it provided the condition for the required interventions.

The move toward wider testing was further reflected in December 1985 when *Morbidity and Mortality Weekly Report* published recommendations on the prevention of transmission of the AIDS virus by infected women to their fetuses.[23] These recommendations underscored the importance of testing women at increased risk for AIDS so that they could know and understand the implications of their antibody status. Such information would provide the basis for "informed decisions to help prevent perinatally acquired HTLV-III/LAV."[24] Though carefully worded, the recommendations clearly suggested that given the prevailing understanding of the risk of mother-to-fetus transmission infected women would be best advised to delay pregnancy. The recommendations were more circumspect about the function of testing in pregnant women. Unable—for political reasons—to utter the word "abortion," federal health officials could only note the potential need for "additional medical and social support services."[25] Finally, given the risks of social isolation, the importance of preserving the confidentiality of test results was noted.

How sensitive the issue of broad-scale testing for identification of those who were infected remained was made clear from the response to these recommendations by the New York City Health Department's Bureau of Maternity Services and Family Planning. Alarmed by the breadth of the federal initiative on perinatal transmission and particularly concerned about how such screening might impinge on the reproductive rights of black and Hispanic women, who comprised the largest number of women at risk, the bureau convened a special committee and charged it with the task of reviewing the federal guidelines.[26] Like those who were involved with protecting gay men from the potential abuses of testing, this committee, which was clearly influenced by feminist concerns about the reproductive rights of women and which included departmental as well as nondepartmental representatives, sought to circumscribe carefully the conditions under which testing would be deemed appropriate. At stake were the rights of women and the dangers of stigmatization. To prevent the subversion of those rights and to preclude stigmatization, the committee rejected as overbroad the definition of those at risk. Thus setting aside the biological logic of male to female HIV transmission, the committee was willing to class as at risk the female partners of male intravenous drug users but not the female partners of bisexual men. The still-limited evidence provided by epidemiology was allowed to justify an untenable conclusion. Reflecting the antitesting perspective of the New York City Health Department and the hegemony of the perspective articulated by gay political leaders, the committee asserted that it was counseling and education rather than testing that should be the focus of the city's effort to protect women. Indeed, the recommended pretest consent procedures, in warning about the potentially negative consequences of the test, did all but suggest to those seeking to know their antibody status that they not do so. Finally, the committee sought to protect women who chose to be tested from the threat of coercion by their own physicians. "At this time, there is little clinical benefit to a patient of informing her physician of her HTLV-III test results."

The report was never released, in part because of a change in the leadership of the Health Department, and in part because of the furor it created among some obstetricians and gynecologists who were appalled by its posture toward physicians. For those who believed that testing was necessary for at-risk women and that knowledge of antibody status would permit women to make informed choices about pregnancy and abortion, the cautions of the committee were a tragic parody. Some simply termed the report a recipe for public health malpractice.[27]

How different were the recommendations regarding women at risk for AIDS prepared by James Chin, chief of the Infectious Disease Branch of the California Department of Health.[28] Distributed to California's local health officials months before the CDC had issued the December guidelines, the recommendations stressed "the potentially disastrous result for the fetus when an expectant mother is infected with the AIDS virus." Women at increased risk had to be identified "and followed by serologic examination and educated about AIDS." Though acknowledging that the task of identifying, counseling, and testing women at risk would be difficult and would involve matters of great sensitivity, Chin declared such interventions "medically and legally appropriate."

Chin's aggressive posture on testing reflected the changing perspective of many health officials and, given his prominence, helped to shape the shifting outlook as well. That shift was crystallized in March 1986 when, after months of deliberation, the CDC published recommendations placing federal health authorities behind proposals that would involve the voluntary testing of all Americans at risk.[29] Among those included were homosexual and bisexual men, present or past intravenous drug abusers, persons with clinical laboratory evidence of HIV infection, persons born in countries where heterosexual transmission was believed to play a major role in the spread of AIDS, male and female prostitutes, sex partners of infected persons or persons at increased risk, all persons with hemophilia who had received clotting factor products, and newborn infants of high-risk or infected mothers. In short, millions of Americans were brought within the scope of the CDC proposals. Such testing was necessary to "facilitate the identification of seropositive asymptomatic individuals" so that they might be counseled about risk reduction and the importance of ongoing clinical evaluation.[30] Broad-scale testing and counseling would, in turn, necessitate a vast expansion of the settings within which efforts would be made to reach those at increased risk. No longer were the alternative test sites adequate to the task. Instead, counseling and voluntary testing had to be routinely offered to individuals at increased risk wherever they received medical care—clinics for the treatment of those with sexually transmitted diseases and drug abusers were singled out. The CDC used the occasion to underscore the importance of confidentiality protections to the new strategy of public health intervention. Only if those at risk believed their privacy was protected would efforts to increase the numbers seeking testing succeed. So important was such confidence-building that the CDC supported testing under conditions of anonymity if confidentiality could not be assured.[31]

Antagonism on the part of gay groups to the CDC recommendations had surfaced well before they were formally published in March. Given an opportunity to comment on a preliminary draft, gay leaders expressed their alarm about the sweeping nature of the proposals. Voluntary mass testing was but one part of an intensified public health program that included an endorsement of measures like sexual-contact tracing and a call for the closing or regulation of gay bathhouses. For gay leaders it was clear that a serious threat to privacy rights was in the offing. Writing to James Mason, director of the CDC, Jeff Levi of the National Gay Task Force charged that the federal agency's commitment to testing was without scientific merit. There were no empirical grounds to substantiate the assumption that mass testing would contribute to the goal of behavioral modification. Furthermore, despite the available research indicating that those who were antibody positive also carried the AIDS virus, Levi questioned the assumption that "such tests have value in predicting which individuals are infected." In short, testing would expose the individuals so identified to social hazards without a measurable advance of the public health.[32]

When the CDC recommendations appeared in mid-March, they not unexpectedly became the target of sharp denunciation. Neil

Schram, who had so recently defended the voluntary testing of those gay men who needed it to foster behavioral change, was particularly appalled by the emphasis placed by the CDC on the importance of the test for *identifying* those who were infected but asymptomatic. Mass testing for the purpose of identification was far different from more circumscribed efforts and would lead to a disastrous outcome. Schram urged that "the gay community . . . resist such efforts since [they] will surely lead to calls for universal mandatory testing."[33] Because of the history of homophobia in America, many gay leaders were so deeply suspicious of the intentions of government officials that they easily conceived of apocalyptic scenarios. Thus the American Association of Physicians for Human Rights argued, "Since gay and bisexual men cannot be identified to get them to voluntarily take the test, it is clear that calls for massive voluntary testing will fail. . . . Therefore, there is only one logical explanation for such a recommendation . . . the CDC is laying the groundwork for universal mandatory testing." Perhaps more ominously, such testing and identification would provide the conditions for adopting the "classic public health strategy [of] separating [the] infected from [the] uninfected," for mass quarantine.[34] Not informed by the diction of politics, a statement of the National Hemophilia Foundation also rejected the call for wide-scale testing, stating that "there is no substitute for an effectively designed and targeted education strategy directed at modifying behavior in order to reduce the transmission of HTLV-III virus."[35] It would be another year before the foundation would change its stance.[36]

In the next months, a broad coalition of gay groups collaborated in the framing of a consensus statement that sought to define sharply a limited role for testing, thus further distancing these groups from the public health officers who, with increasing confidence, were pressing for wide-scale voluntary testing. Ultimately signed by more than fifty gay political, medical, and community organizations from across the nation, the statement opposed the course outlined by federal health officials. Stress on mass testing was denounced as an assault on the principle that "taking the test must be a very individual decision." The spirit of mass testing, with its commitment to the identification of the infected, thus was perceived as subverting the possibility of voluntary choice. In the face of an epidemic with profound communal implications, many gay leaders remained committed to a perspective within which individuals would choose independently and privately the appropriate course of action. But wide-scale testing—even if superficially voluntary—was a grave threat not only to privacy but to the rational social allocation of resources. It would involve a massive and wasteful diversion of resources from education and counseling "that have proven successful in reducing transmission of HTLV-III to a program of unproven value."[37]

Fear, rooted in the social experience of American homosexuals, of how mass voluntary testing and counseling could produce a disastrous train of events for those identified as infected had thus compelled the mainstream of gay political and medical organizations to assume a defensive posture. Dismissive of those who claimed that testing could serve a vital role in fostering behavioral change and suspicious of the intentions of those who would devote considerable resources to a counseling program linked to testing, gay leaders responded with a rigidity for which only time and the ever-growing impact of the epidemic would serve as an antidote. Anxieties about the threat of AIDS and irrational discrimination made consternation about the impact of testing wholly understandable. But, however understandable, the result was an impediment in the struggle against AIDS.

Fear of the consequences of exposure also framed the response to other proposed public health measures that would entail the identification of the infected: the required reporting of the names of those who tested positive on the AIDS antibody test to public health departments and the effort to locate the sexual partners of those found to be infected, so that they too might be tested and counseled. In both cases officials who advocated the extension of these traditional public health measures to AIDS argued that the full panoply of interventions had to be brought to bear if the epidemic was to be limited, that AIDS should be treated no differently from any serious public health threat. Those who opposed such a strategy warned that the identification of the infected by public health interventions would not only threaten privacy but prove counterproductive, undermining the cooperation of the gay community that was so critical in the struggle against AIDS. AIDS was different, they asserted, because of those who bore the burden of disease in America. AIDS was the illness of the vulnerable. That difference, they argued, required radical modifications in the practice of public health if the epidemic was to be brought under control.

Public Health Reporting

As the dimensions of the threat posed by AIDS became increasingly apparent soon after the recognition of the disorder by the CDC, state and local health departments moved to require that physicians and hospitals report by name those diagnosed with the new syndrome. Only such reporting would permit health officials to have an accurate epidemiological picture of the disease with which they were confronted. Only such reporting would permit the application of other appropriate public health measures to the sick. The public health required this abrogation of the principle of confidentiality, as had always been the case when epidemic threats were involved.

The history of public health regulations requiring such reporting, with their obvious intrusions into the privacy of the physician-patient relationship, has been fraught with conflict.[38] Disagreements over what the public interest required, over professional prerogatives, and over the rights of privacy have been as critical in these controversies as matters of science and therapeutics. However such conflicts were formally resolved, private physicians, in fact, dictated the ultimate pattern of reporting. Sheer resistance, especially when sexually transmitted diseases were involved, often limited dramatically the extent to which public health officials had before them a true picture of the pattern of disease in their communities. Promises, enshrined in legislation and regulation, that the identity of those reported would be shielded from the scrutiny of those with no public health interest, often did little to affect the willingness to report, especially when private patients were involved. It was in recognition of the capacity of private physicians to exercise a de facto nullification of public health regulations that in 1937 the Conference of State and Territorial Health Officials declared that "qualified physicians—with the approval of local health authorities—should be given the option of reporting their cooperative patients by initials, date of birth, and community of residence, rather than by name.[39]

It is thus remarkable, given the salience of concerns about the privacy of individuals with AIDS, that there was little resistance to efforts to mandate case reporting by name. Indeed, an appreciation that only accurate epidemiological information could unlock the mysteries associated with the transmission of the new disease led the Board of the American Association of Physicians for Human Rights in 1983 to call upon local health authorities to make the names of AIDS cases reportable.[40] Controversy did emerge, however, when the CDC called upon local health departments to forward to Atlanta full case reports, including the names of those about whom they had been informed. For the CDC such identified reports were essential if an accurate, unduplicated record of cases was to be developed for the nation as a whole. Distrust of the intentions of the federal authorities and anxieties about how such a national list might be abused led gay leaders to oppose such efforts. As a result, some treating physicians and local health departments began to resist the requests by federal health officials for case reports.[41] Ultimately the CDC was compelled to agree, albeit reluctantly, to reporting by a unique coding mechanism—called Soundex—that would preclude duplicate reporting without the use of names or other personal identifiers such as social security numbers. James Allen—then chief of the Surveillance Section of the CDC AIDS Activities Branch—acknoledged that the compromise would complicate his efforts, but noted, "It's better than the alternative: persons refusing to cooperate by giving inaccurate information. That would make the situation worse. By agreeing to this compromise we can reassure them that we are acting in good faith and won't jeopardize their privacy."[42] Others within the CDC expressed exasperation. "They say the government isn't doing anything, then they accuse us of breaching confidentiality when we try to carry out responsible studies."[43]

The relative ease with which AIDS was incorporated under state and local health requirements governing the reporting of communicable diseases did not extend to efforts to make results of the antibody tests reportable. The first encounter over a proposal for such reporting occurred in New Jersey just a month after the testing of blood donations began in April 1985.[44] Drawing a sharp distinction between reporting cases of AIDS and the results of the new antibody test with its ambiguous clinical implications, the local gay community denounced the proposal. Opposition came also from the national Federation of AIDS-Related Organizations and the United States Conference of Local Health Officers.[45] Confronted with so determined an opposition, the New Jersey Public Health Council decided to defer to the legislature rather than act through administrative determination.[46]

For those who had viewed New Jersey's effort as medically unwarranted and as a potential threat to the privacy of those whose names would be reported, the decision was an "important victory."[47] But there was also some trepidation about whether other states would succeed where New Jersey had failed. "We are in the first skirmish," said Timothy Sweeney of the Lambda Legal Defense and Education Fund, a national gay civil rights organization. "This does not mean they will not come back and try again or [that] other states will not try this."[48] Such fears were confirmed just days after New Jersey had held its hearings on reporting, when CDC director James Mason declared in a May 1985 radio interview that public health departments might seek to keep records of those who were antibody positive. Linking the reporting of such test results to standard public health practice in venereal disease control, he asserted, "The same sensitive confidential system that has served this nation so well in the past for a series of other sexually transmitted diseases . . . doesn't have to be rearranged or reworked to serve equally well in the control of AIDS."[49]

The National Gay Task Force responded forcefully to Mason's remarks.[50] Centering its objections on what it perceived to be a threatened invasion of privacy that would not be balanced by any public health benefit, the NGTF sought to draw a sharp distinction between mandatory reporting for communicable diseases where treatment or appropriate public health interventions were available and the reporting of positive results on the antibody tests. "What will public health authorities be able to do with this information to prevent the spread of the disease? . . . This is not a test for AIDS; it is simply a test for the presence of antibodies to HTLV-III, the virus associated with AIDS. While this is not a test for the virus itself, even if one conceded that the presence of antibody indicated continued presence of virus—a matter under debate by the scientific community—the data is even more inconclusive regarding infectiousness at this time. Unfortunately there is no intervention for those who test positive." Furthermore, reporting would subvert the viability of the alternative test sites just being established across the nation. Such centers were pledged to provide completely confidential, and frequently anonymous, testing. Reporting would make a shambles of those efforts.

The first successful attempt to mandate public health reporting of HIV antibody test results came in Colorado. There, in August

1985, Thomas Vernon, the executive director of the Department of Health, proposed that the state require such reporting.[51] Drawing upon the evolving scientific understanding of the significance of the test—federal health official had just reported very high rates of viral recovery from those who were "strongly reactive" to the ELISA test—he noted that positive findings were "a highly reliable marker" for infection with HTLV-III and "probably for infectiousness as well."[52] As a result, he argued, reporting could alert responsible health agencies to the presence of persons likely to be infected with a dangerous virus; allow such agencies to insure that such persons were properly counseled about the significance of their laboratory tests and about what they needed to do to prevent further transmission of the virus; permit those charged with monitoring the prevalence of infection with the AIDS virus to better accomplish their tasks; and create the possibility of expeditiously notifying the infected when effective antiviral therapeutic agents became available. Every traditional public health justification for reporting applied, according to Vernon, to infection with the AIDS virus. A failure to extend reporting to this situation would thus represent a dereliction of professional responsibility in the face of a new deadly disease. Responding to concerns about breaches in confidentiality that could result in social ostracism, loss of insurability, and loss of employment, Vernon and his deputy for sexually transmitted diseases asserted that the system for protecting such public health records had been effective for decades. There was no reason to believe that in the case of infection with the AIDS virus the department's record would be tarnished.

Despite Vernon's vigorous defense and his belief that his proposal was in the grand tradition of public health measures, his effort to make Colorado the first state requiring reporting provoked a sharp response from his opponents in a hearing before the state's Board of Health.[53] The director of public health for Denver warned that reporting would have the counterproductive impact of driving high-risk individuals away from testing, regardless of the health department's pledges to preserve the confidentiality of test results. Julian Rush, director of the gay community-based Colorado AIDS Project, asserted that his organization would not encourage testing if Vernon's proposal were adopted. The president of the board of Colorado's Civil Liberties Union joined the challenge. In each case, Vernon's opponents underscored their fear that regardless of the historical and prevailing standards of confidentiality, a repressive turn caused by the hysteria associated with AIDS could well result in social policies that Vernon and his associates would consider anathema. To these concerns Vernon responded with a claim that he was to make repeatedly in the next months: widespread perception that public health officials had failed to do "everything possible" to control AIDS could foster social anxiety and thus produce the very repression so feared by those concerned with the rights of the infected.

Despite the bitter protests by gay and civil liberties groups, as well as the concern of some health officials, one month after Vernon made his proposal the Board of Health unanimously adopted a resolution making Colorado the first state to require the reporting by name of those with positive antibody test results.[54] To those who continued to stress the possibility that the health department's list of seropositive individuals could be put to ill use, Vernon responded, "The issue before us is the reality of a tragic epidemic of AIDS, not the theoretical risks [that] our confidentiality system will be breached."[55]

In the aftermath of the imposition of mandatory reporting, there was, in fact, a marked downturn in the number of individuals seeking testing in Colorado. To those who had warned of such an outcome, the result only proved how an apparently aggressive public health posture could have counterproductive consequences.[56] To those who defended the new course, the downturn was explained as largely coincidental, paralleling the experience of states that had not adopted a policy of reporting.[57]

To limit the extent to which fears of reporting would, in fact, deter individuals from seeking testing, a tacit and remarkable compromise was struck that suggested to opponents of reporting how ludicrous were the public health claims made on its behalf. Individuals who appeared at Colorado's test sites would not be asked for proof of identity, thus making available the option of using pseudonyms. Months later Vernon was to defend this policy publicly: "Would we ask for or require personal identification of those infected? No! The option of not using one's own name has always been available in disease control programs. HIV testing is not different."[58] Some of Vernon's opponents reported that perhaps as many as one third of those seeking testing used this option.[59]

In the wake of the Colorado decision and of efforts by other state officials clearly identified with an aggressive public health posture to require the reporting by name of those infected with the AIDS virus, James Mason, director of the Centers for Disease Control, wrote to state health officials asking them to consider the possibility of requiring "some kind of reporting."[60] Such a move, Mason stressed, would necessitate the existence of confidentiality protections, including legislative shields for health department records against disclosure. But while noting the public health benefits that might follow from the adoption of mandatory reporting, Mason warned that such a move had to be "weighed against the possibility that such a requirement might discourage persons from agreeing to nonanonymous testing."

Gay political groups responded to Mason's letter in an expected manner. The AIDS Action Council warned that "even where statutes to protect confidentiality are in force, anonymous testing is the best means of insuring voluntary compliance in high risk groups."[61] The National Gay Task Force argued that reporting would be counterproductive from a public health perspective. "Individuals will be legitimately frightened about what will be done with that information, in a fairly hysterical climate surrounding AIDS." As a consequence they would avoid testing.[62]

When the CDC finally published its recommendations for broadscale voluntary testing in March 1986, Mason's initial suggestion had been considerably softened.[63] State and local officials were simply urged to "evaluate the implications of required reporting." But it wasn't only civil liberties organizations and gay political groups that had opposed reporting. Many local and state health officials were concerned about the potential impact of Mason's proposed move. In January 1986 the United States Conference of Local Health Officials debated the issue of whether testing under conditions of anonymity—the standard at many alternative test sites—was preferable to confidential testing.[64] Anonymous testing would preclude reporting. Confidentiality would make it possible. Slightly more than half of the officials rejected efforts to encourage the substitution of confidentiality for anonymity. Most remarkable was what the vote revealed about the politics of public health. Officials from cities with relatively few AIDS cases supported a more aggressive posture. Those from cities with many cases tended to favor a policy that would thwart the prospect of reporting. Constrained by the necessity of having to preserve collaborative working relationships with relatively large and well-organized gay communities and concerned about how reporting would affect the willingness of individuals to be tested, they could not support a measure that would almost certainly produce alienation with no assured contribution to the public health. Less constrained by such factors, those from cities with few AIDS cases could favor policies that represented the application of traditional public health practice to HIV infection.

This pattern was repeated as the Association of State and Territorial Health Officials sought to formulate a policy on reporting in 1986. But in this instance the advocates of reporting prevailed. The ASTHO position was particularly distressing to gay leaders who had worked so diligently to win the support of public health officials in cities like New York and San Francisco. Christopher Collins, who had represented the Lambda Legal Defense and Education Fund at the consensus conference from which these recommendations had emerged, thus wrote in protest, "I believe credence should be given to the views of those whose states are most affected by the disease. They have had the most experience . . . and should not be 'horse whipped' into having to go along with the views of those health commissioners from states where the disease has not yet reached the extent that it has in New York and California." For Collins, health officials from regions with large numbers of AIDS cases had come to appreciate the misgivings of the gay community and share its concerns about how antibody testing could threaten the privacy of those at increased risk for AIDS. They understood that "until such time as the fear, stigma, and politicization of this disease has diminished, you cannot continue to treat [it] as just any other sexually transmitted disease."[65]

Those who rejected anonymity and who believed that reporting by name to state health departments had a potentially important role to play in the public health strategy against AIDS, provided a different analysis. In their view, the stance of health officials from areas with large numbers of AIDS cases was not a matter of greater experience. Rather, it entailed an unwise accommodation to the immediate and narrow political interests of those whose primary concern was the defense of "gay rights" and the advance of a "civil liberties agenda." The demands of the public health, they felt, had been ignored in this process. Dominated by the desire to avoid a breach with the organized gay community, some officials had lost the ability to articulate a defense of the public health. Kristine Gebbie, administrator of the Oregon Department of Health, a former president of ASTHO and a moving force for the vigorous application of standard public health practices to the AIDS epidemic, characterized the collaboration of some health officials and gay political groups as "a public health equivalent of the Stockholm syndrome," the identification of hostages with their captors.[66]

Remarkably, however, Gebbie could not get her own state to adopt a standard public health reporting policy for those who were antibody positive. Instead, in a compromise move that she described as "devilishly clever,"[67] and which replicated the ASTHO position adopted forty years earlier, Oregon's AIDS task force recommended that each physician be required to report by initials only those who had positive test results. Physicians would then be required to attest to having provided appropriate counseling about risk reduction to each reported case.[68] Gebbie herself could not escape the political constraints within which public health policy in her own state was fashioned—nor could those public health officials who sought to identify the infected through the process of sexual contact notification, in order to warn them about the hazard they posed to others.

Sexual Contact Notification

Despite the well-established role of public health departments in identifying and notifying the sexual contacts of those reported to have venereal diseases, this strategy of intervention—designed to break the chain of disease transmission—played no role in the early response to AIDS. Not until the commercial development of the antibody test was it possible to consider contact tracing, since only the test made possible the detection of the asymptomatic carriers of the AIDS virus. But even subsequent to the test's availability, and the realization that virtually all antibody positive individuals were also carriers of HIV, contact notification was almost never undertaken by public health departments. Matters of practicality as well as concerns about privacy were involved. Unwilling to antagonize gay leaders, concerned about the costs of so labor intensive an effort, and unclear about how the absence of a therapeutic intervention for AIDS would alter the justification for notifying the sexual partners of those who had been infected with the AIDS virus, public health officials too often chose to do nothing. The result: a paralysis of imagination and will, a failure to warn those who might inadvertently transmit HIV infection to others.

In mid-1985, as part of an effort to limit the spread of AIDS among heterosexuals, San Francisco launched a pilot program in which bisexual males reported to the health department as having AIDS were asked to provide the names of their female sexual partners so that these women might be notified about the possibility of exposure to the AIDS virus. In an editorial in the *Journal of the American Medical Association,* Dean Echenberg, the city's chief communicable disease officer, asserted that such a program was of critical importance since the mass educational campaign designed to warn about the risks of HIV infection and transmission would inevitably have less impact among heterosexuals than among gay males. Furthermore, the female partners of bisexual men would have no reason to believe that they had been exposed to AIDS and would have little reason to modify their sexual and procreative behaviors. Only by warning them directly and by urging them to be tested would it be possible to avoid the unwitting transmission of the AIDS virus to others. "The foundation of this approach," wrote Echenberg, "rests on the assumption that no individual would want to unknowingly infect others."[69]

Though limited in its scope—the program would not reach the female partners of asymptomatic but infected bisexual males—and committed to the preservation of the confidentiality of the named partner as well as the anonymity of the "index case" (the patient with AIDS who had provided the contact's name), San Francisco's effort was denounced by representatives of gay and civil liberties groups as an "Orwellian nightmare." Thomas Stoddard of the New York Civil Liberties Union declared, "Contact tracing is a euphemism. What they want to do is to keep a list of sexually active people."[70] Though acknowledging that contact notification had been used historically to interdict the spread of other sexually transmitted diseases, he argued that to become part of a list of those exposed to AIDS would have social consequences "far graver than with any other disease."[71]

That so vigorous a response could be provoked by San Francisco's modest and circumscribed program of sexual partner notification was evidence of how intense anxiety about privacy and the power of the state had affected the milieu within which public health policy was being made. The response was all the more striking since contact notification had been a central feature of American venereal disease control programs for almost five decades. Thus, Thomas Parran, the architect of the federal antivenereal program in the 1930s, had stated: "A physician would not consider treating a case of smallpox without investigating fully the source of infection. He would either undertake this himself or report to the health department to make the investigation. On the other hand, one does not feel any such responsibility in the case of early syphillis."[72]

That had to change if syphillis was to be brought under control, and so in 1936 Parran told the National Conference on Venereal Disease Control, "Every early case must be located, reported, its source ascertained and all contacts followed up to find possible infection."[73] Each contact could then be informed about the possibility of infection, provided with a Wasserman test, and if infected, treated. Thus could the disease be cared for early on and the chain of transmission broken. The most ardent advocates of contact tracing and of reliance on "public health sleuths" believed that such interventions could prevent pyramids of infection from developing out of a single source.[74]

Contact tracing, so reliant upon the ability of public health employees to elicit the cooperation of those whom they interviewed, did not begin in earnest until the 1940s, when effective treatments for syphillis became available. In subsequent years, the rise and decline of federal funding for venereal disease control programs did much to affect the resources available for such labor intensive efforts at case finding. But on each occasion when a renewed commitment to the control of such diseases was made, case investigation and contact tracing were viewed as a cornerstone of the public health strategy. This was true for syphillis in 1961, for gonorrhea in 1972, and for chlamydia in 1985.[75]

How effective such efforts have been is difficult to determine. Allan Brandt's history of venereal disease, *No Magic Bullet,* notes the difficulties that have beset such programs—the reluctance of individuals to speak with strangers about their sexual partners and of private physicians to notify public health officials about venereal diseases in their patients.[76] Public health officials have been more enthusiastic, even when they have ruefully acknowledged that limited resources have required the modification of standard approaches, by placing greater emphasis on the role that infected individuals might play in notifying their own sexual partners.[77]

It was only at the end of 1985, as the Centers for Disease Control began to consider a range of proposals designed to intensify AIDS prevention activities, including an increased emphasis on the identification through testing of asymptomatic infected individuals who could transmit HIV infection to others, that the first open discussion of contact tracing by federal health officials took place.[78]

Alarm over the threat to privacy posed by contact notification intensified as federal officials made public their support for the adoption of such efforts. In a letter to the director of the CDC, Jeff Levi of the National Gay Task Force wrote of his organization's opposition to all such proposals and strategically stressed the negative public health consequences that might, inadvertently, be produced. "This, second only to mandatory reporting, has the greatest likelihood of scaring people away from being tested. The possibility that partners might be informed of their exposure (even though the tracing is voluntary) may result in individuals not even entering the . . . clinic in the first place."[79] But Levi went further. Contact notification might actually encourage anonymous sexual encounters by individuals who feared that their partners would "turn their names in to the public health authorities." Gay groups also expressed concern about how costly contact notification programs might divert already limited public resources from broadly targeted programs of risk reduction education. Thus, in an editorial entitled "Contact Tracing Dupes Gay Community," Mark Behar, chair of the National Coalition of Gay STDs [sexually transmitted diseases], stated that such programs were designed to "deceive the public into believing that something is being done. [The strategy] will do little to help the largest percentage of people who are at risk for AIDS because attention and funds are being diverted away from effective public education measures."[80]

Finally, fueling these arguments was a deep concern about how contact notification would inevitably broaden the extent to which the state would have in its possession the names of the infected. Identifying the infected, even for purposes of warning them, would represent but one more step in a threatening chain with consequences that not even the most committed of public health officials could forestall. "We have been reassured by public health authorities that their record of maintaining confidentiality of records of persons testing positive for other [sexually transmitted diseases] is excellent. We have no reason to doubt that claim. However, AIDS is not an ordinary STD. The hysteria associated with it makes more likely breaches of confidentiality, whether by overzealous employees or as a result of efforts by other government agencies wanting to know the status of their employees."[81] Against such anxiety no promise to protect the names of those infected or those named as contacts could suffice.

The response to contact notification that came from civil liberties groups mirrored that of gay political organizations. Though such groups had never opposed contact notification during the decades when it had become a standard feature of efforts to limit the spread of sexually transmitted diseases, the very earliest suggestion that contact notification could play a role in the face of the AIDS epidemic provoked striking opposition. The adoption of this posture reflected deep concern about endangering the privacy of those at increased risk for AIDS, a willingness to challenge the exercise of public health authority in a manner that entailed an important ideological shift, and the direct influence of gay men and lesbians on the formulation of the policies of civil liberties groups.

In San Francisco, the Ad Hoc Committee on AIDS and Civil Liberties of the Northern California Branch of the American Civil Liberties Union denounced the "compulsory tracing" of sexual partners.[82] Seeking to distinguish between the use of contact notification for the control of other venereal diseases and its use with HIV infection, the committee drew upon empirical and philosophical arguments. Despite the abundance of evidence by late 1985 regarding the extent to which antibody-positive individuals were also carriers of the AIDS virus and the universally shared public health assumption that those who were infected were also infectious, the committee declared, "Seropositives have been exposed to the AIDS virus, but there is as yet no way of knowing if the individual is actually infected with the disease or is capable of transmitting it to sexual partners." By insisting upon definitive evidence about infectivity and by rejecting the presumption that those who were antibody positive were also infectious, the committee dismissed the philosophical commitment to erring on the side of safety so central to the practice of public health in the inevitable presence of degrees of uncertainty. The committee also sought to distinguish between contact notification in the case of venereal diseases for which a therapeutic intervention existed and AIDS, for which there was no treatment. In the absence of a cure there was no compensating benefit that could be offered to those whose privacy would be violated by notification. In lieu of notification, the committee counseled the adoption of self-protective measures as the sole strategy for interrupting the transmission of the AIDS virus. The committee elected to remain silent on the question of whether those who had no reason to suspect that they had been exposed to an infected individual had a right to such information. Nor did the committee address the question of whether there was a legitimate public health interest in warning the unknowingly exposed about the potential risks they could pose to their future sexual partners or offspring.

When the Northern California Branch of the ACLU adopted its full policy statement on AIDS, not only did it declare its opposition to measures designed to "compel involuntary disclosure of sexual contacts"—though contact tracing had, in fact, always relied ultimately on the willingness of infected individuals to provide the names of those with whom they had had sexual relations—but it also denounced the "unconsented disclosure or unauthorized use of such information when voluntarily provided."[83] Thus the privacy interests of named contacts were defined in so cramped a manner as to preclude notification and warning, even if an infected individual believed that past or current sexual contacts might have been placed at risk, and even if such an individual sought the assistance of public health agencies in informing those who might be the unwitting source of further infection.

As the Privacy Committee of the national ACLU began to fashion proposed recommendations on AIDS for its Board of Directors, it too confronted the issue of sexual contact notification, and without much difficulty concluded that "compulsory tracing of sexual partners [is] offensive to privacy standards" and would not prove to be an effective strategy of public health intervention.[84] But despite the ease with which the Privacy Committee was able to dispatch the matter, it did provoke a lively debate at the ACLU's national board meeting in the spring of 1986.[85]

Those who questioned the committee's recommendations noted that the Civil Liberties Union had never opposed contact tracing for other venereal diseases, that there was a public health interest in warning individuals who might unknowingly transmit the AIDS virus to their sexual partners, that, in short, the Privacy Committee had given insufficient attention to public health concerns toward which the ACLU had always been "deferential." Opponents of contact notification responded by suggesting that the ACLU might have been in error for failing to oppose such efforts in venereal disease programs "considering . . . the deep intrusion into privacy rights" that was entailed, that compulsory or voluntary notification under the aegis of public health officials would be ineffective, and that broad educational programs were a more desirable strategy for halting the spread of AIDS and HIV infection.

A divided board adopted a far-reaching statement that characterized sexual contact tracing in the case of AIDS as raising "grave civil liberties concerns because major identifiable groups that are most at risk are deeply discriminated against." The very prospect of a government list of the sexual contacts of homosexual and bisexual men was portrayed as "ominous." Though there was little evidence that public health officials planned to rely upon coercion to elicit the names of contacts, notification programs were characterized as "compulsory." In lieu of such intrusive measures "public education and counseling schemes under which the infected person could be urged voluntarily to inform his/her sexual partners" were deemed preferable from the point of view of both public health and civil liberties. Swept aside were the concerns of board members who had argued that some individuals might seek the assistance of public health officials in warning sexual partners. So, too, were the concerns about the rights of those who would remain ignorant about their potentially infective status.

Remarkably, as was true in the case of public health reporting, the earliest and most acrimonious conflict over the role of contact notification took place not in the states with many reported cases of AIDS, or where the incidence of HIV infection among gay and bisexual men was assumed to be substantial, but in Minnesota. There, in January 1986, the state's chief epidemiologist, Michael Osterholm, put before the health commissioner's AIDS Task Force a far-reaching proposal to employ contact notification.[86] Unlike the program in effect in San Francisco, however, notification services were not to be restricted to heterosexual contacts of bisexual men, nor were they to be activated only in the case of clinically diagnosed AIDS. Rather, Osterholm sought to employ notification services in each case of infection with the AIDS virus, whether the partners involved were homosexual, heterosexual, or those who had shared intravenous drug paraphernalia.

To bolster support for his proposals Osterholm invited Willard Cates, director of the Sexually Transmitted Disease Division of the CDC, to address the AIDS task force. Minnesota, Cates said, could serve as a laboratory for evaluating the efficacy of contact notification in combating the AIDS epidemic, precisely because it was a state with few diagnosed cases and with a relatively low level of HIV infection among gay and bisexual men.[87]

Not unexpectedly, the response of Minnesota's gay community was hostile. The two gay members of the AIDS task force warned that contact notification might drive those at risk away from HIV antibody testing sites.[88] Furthermore, they urged that "less intrusive" options be examined. Specifically, they suggested that counselors emphasize to all seropositive individuals the importance of contacting their own sexual partners. Alternatively, they proposed that a nongovernmental body—the gay community-based Minnesota AIDS Project, for example—undertake notification. At base was a deep suspicion of the state and uncertainty about the capacity of public health officials to undertake notification without placing named individuals at considerable social risk.

At a public forum organized for the gay community, Osterholm sought to place contact notification within a broad program of prevention strategies.[89] Warning his audience of the catastrophic consequences of failure, he urged support for a full panoply of efforts. But it was contact notification that had sparked the gay community's alarm, and it was to a defense of that element of the state's overall proposed strategy that Osterholm was compelled to devote his most ardent defense. Most important, he argued, was the role health professionals could play in interrupting the transmission of infection, a goal that could not be achieved by relying on individuals to contact their own partners. Programs that placed primary emphasis upon patient-initiated outreach could never attain the level of consistent follow-up of contacts that could be expected when carefully trained health officers undertook the task. Underscoring the centrality of confidentiality to the entire process, Osterholm sought to disarm those who feared the state's intrusion. In noting the system of protections that shielded the names revealed to health department officials, he attempted to reassure those concerned that contact notification could set the stage for discrimination.

But despite Osterholm's efforts, the audience was not reassured. The first speaker to respond to his presentation evoked the horrors of Nazi Germany. "The road to the gas chambers began with lists in Weimar Germany."[90] Osterholm's attempts to press for contact notification—a program that he acknowledged could not be undertaken without the support of the gay community—had opened a deep fissure and had jeopardized the collaborative relationship so critical to the public health struggle against AIDS.

Writing to the *GLC Voice*, a gay newspaper, Rick Osborne, a gay member of the Minneapolis Civil Rights Commission, asserted, "The fear, anger, and mistrust felt by me and many other gays reflects neither a 'pro-AIDS' nor an 'anti-health department' sentiment. Rather they reflect our profound belief that the threat to our fundamental human rights posed by the existence of AIDS is an evil of equal strength to the disease itself. . . . To ignore our feelings will only further alienate the gay community, thereby imperiling the Department's often legitimate efforts to arrest this serious health problem."[91]

By mid-May 1986, after months of controversy and negotiation, the state's commissioner of health was prepared to announce Minnesota's commitment to a program of contact notification. Scaled back and reconceptualized, the program would place primary emphasis on "client-initiated referral." Third-party notification—involving health department personnel—would be undertaken only as a matter of last resort.[92]

When a final contact notification protocol was promulgated by the state in November—ten months after it was first proposed—the effectiveness of the opposition to "overintrusive government" was apparent.[93] As the state's health commissioner had suggested in May, primary emphasis was given to the role of private notification. "It should be the responsibility of HIV seropositive persons to assure that their partners are notified of their exposure, so they can be given the opportunity to receive appropriate medical and counseling services." Within this scheme, the health department would provide guidance and support to those who were to assume this critical responsibility. Because third-party notification would occur only at the request of individuals who could not—because of fear, shame, or anxiety—undertake the task themselves, threats to privacy would be limited. Finally, in acknowledgment of the doubts of those who believed that the mere existence of lists of sexual contacts would always pose a threat to privacy, an extraordinary gesture was made. Within six months after the completion of contact all forms containing personal identifiers would be destroyed.

If this final program fell short of Osterholm's initial vision of the responsibility of state health officials to identify and warn the potentially infected and infectious, it nevertheless placed Minnesota at the forefront of states seeking to apply standard public health practices to the AIDS epidemic. That modifications had been necessitated by political realities only underscored the point that public health interventions must inevitably bear the mark of the social matrix within which they are forged. They are never simply technical in nature.

The political controversy over contact notification was reenacted in a less public form as the Association of State and Territorial Health Officials attempted to fashion its programmatic recommendations for health departments facing the AIDS epidemic. Like the bitter conflict over reporting of antibody status that had so divided ASTHO, the dispute over contact notification revealed the way profound disagreements over public health policy were shaped by local political and epidemiological considerations.

At the ASTHO consensus conference convened to forge a position on AIDS, the initial proposal on contact notification bore the imprint of Osterholm, who had drafted it. It provided vigorous arguments for contact notification while stressing that any such program would require the voluntary cooperation of infected individuals.[94] Not insensitive to the potential impact of notification on an unsuspecting sexual partner, the proposal nevertheless asserted that there was no alternative but to warn those who had been exposed to infected individuals. "While the potential trauma to the individual must be acknowledged, the primary concern of public health must be to prevent new infections, so that this trauma and the devastation of HTLV-III/LAV can be avoided in the future. If . . . infected persons continue their current high-risk behaviors . . . in effect they are continuing the spread of the epidemic." Though this initial formulation acknowledged that contact notification could follow either a "patient referral" or "third party referral" model, only an approach that involved some direct role for public health officials was considered adequate to the task at hand.

The draft met with a critical response from the National Gay Task

Force.[95] Jeff Levi, who had been an invited participant at the ASTHO consensus conference, rejected any system that involved public health officials in the notification of past sexual partners. "The only form of contact notification that is in the realm of acceptability is that of patient referral." Somewhat more surprising was the reaction of Wendy Wertheimer, director of public and governmental affairs for the American Social Health Association, the national organization that had been so central to the historical evolution of the public response to sexually transmitted diseases in the United States. "No data exists to show that . . . contact tracing will be [an] effective tool to control the disease, given the lack of an effective medical intervention."[96]

In the end, a much revised statement on contact notification was endorsed by ASTHO. Softer in general tone, the position adopted a stance of neutrality between the client referral and third-party notification models.[97] Thus, the major recommendation that "some form of contact notification should be encouraged in every community" entailed nothing more than a willingness to acknowledge that each community would have to achieve its own solution based upon epidemiological, political, fiscal, and professional constraints. Only those who viewed contact notification by public health officials as utterly unacceptable and who would have preferred an outright rejection of such an approach found this compromise wanting. For those who believed that public health departments had a crucial role to play in seeking out infected and infectious individuals, especially when they had no reason to suspect that they had been exposed to HIV, the ASTHO compromise represented yet one more demonstration of the unwillingness or inability of public health officials to stake out a forceful and unambiguous position in the struggle against AIDS.

But despite the inability of ASTHO to give a clear endorsement to third-party notification programs—even under carefully circumscribed conditions—there was, in fact, growing recognition across the country that state and local health departments had some obligation to make such services available when infected individuals sought assistance in warning those whom they might have exposed. Even in New York City, where officials had in 1985 and 1986 adamantly resisted suggestions that contact notification had any role to play in the response to AIDS and where the provision of testing in alternative test sites came so late, the first moves were made in 1987 toward making third-party notification available to those who tested positive and requested assistance in alerting their sexual partners.[98]

Identification of the Infected: The Voluntarist Consensus

The gradual recognition that voluntary contact notification did in fact have a role—albeit limited—to play in the response to AIDS, especially where epidemiological circumstances made such labor intensive measures feasible, was a victory for those who believed that the history of public health interventions provided important lessons that should not be put aside. Contact notification did not represent a deviation from the broad consensus forged by public health officials, in large measure out of intense and often acrimonious confrontations with gay leaders and advocates of civil liberties. Voluntarist at its core, it was a consensus marked by an appreciation of the gravity of the AIDS epidemic and a recognition of the very limited role that coercive public health measures could play in the years ahead. Perhaps most critically, it was a consensus which recognized that some coercive measures could harm the public health by driving those most at risk of infection into defensive postures by subverting the prospects for the broad-scale modification of private behavior so central to any effective campaign against AIDS.

Both the surgeon general of the United States and a special committee established by the Institute of Medicine of the National Academy of Sciences underscored these themes in reports issued in the fall of 1986. Coming just months after the Public Health Service had announced its grim forecast for the next five years—270,000 cases of AIDS by 1991, 179,000 AIDS-related deaths by that year—these recommendations were all the more striking. In his *Report on AIDS*—a pamphlet designed for broad-scale distribution—Surgeon General C. Everett Koop rejected proposals for mass mandatory screening as "unnecessary, unmanageable, and cost prohibitive."[99] Instead, voluntary testing conducted under conditions of confidentiality was recommended for those whose behaviors placed them at risk. Indeed, to foster a social climate of trust between those at risk and the nation's health institutions, Koop—going beyond the CDC's positions—rejected both the reporting of positive antibody test results to public health departments and sexual contact tracing.[100] To mandate such procedures would, he asserted, drive the potentially infected "underground, out of the mainstream of health care and education."

The Committee on a National Strategy for AIDS, created by the Institute of Medicine and the National Academy of Sciences, similarly rejected compulsory testing as a method of identifying the infected. Its report, *Confronting AIDS*, argued forcefully that the history of compulsory health measures revealed not only that they had commonly been applied in an invidious and discriminatory manner but that they had often been ineffective.[101] Its perspective on intervention was thus dictated by philosophical commitments as well as a concern for the efficient use of public health resources. In the case of AIDS, where so much irrational fear had already surfaced and where those at increased risk were socially vulnerable because of their sexual orientation or illicit behavior, the necessity of fashioning policies that would strike an appropriate balance was especially critical. It was thus that the committee sought to put forth proposals that would protect individuals from HIV infection "in a society that values privacy and civil liberties."[102]

It followed that mass mandatory HIV antibody screening of the American people was "impossible to justify on either ethical or practical grounds."[103] Furthermore, proposals for more targeted mandatory screening of at-risk individuals were rejected as impractical and infeasible in an "open society." Instead of such compulsory measures, the committee, albeit with less enthusiasm than the Public Health Service, endorsed the availability of wide-scale "voluntary, confidential testing (but with provision for anonymous testing if desired)."[104] Both a commitment to privacy and concern about creating conditions conducive to voluntary testing led the committee, like the surgeon general, to oppose the reporting of antibody test results to local and state health departments.

But to those who viewed the future with a sense of not only gravity but alarm, the voluntarist consensus as expressed by the surgeon general, the Institute of Medicine, and the National Academy of Sciences represented too timid a response, too much of an accommodation with those who sought to restrain the effective use of the government's authority to intervene forcefully to protect the public's health. It was not the limits imposed by AIDS, its modes of transmission, and the absence of effective medical prophylaxis, but rather the triumph of interests committed to the protection of privacy that accounted for the peculiar disjunction between the gravity of the situation confronting America and the prescriptions that had been put forth. At first this challenge was given articulate expression by those of the sectarian right wing of American politics. Eventually it would find a sympathetic hearing among America's politicians and by the White House itself.

If the fear of how public health authority could be abused had often compelled gay leaders passionately to oppose measures, like voluntary testing and sexual contact notification, that could have contributed to the overall strategy of limiting HIV transmission, those who were frustrated by the complex tasks imposed by the AIDS epidemic turned in a reflexive way to the authoritarian traditions of public health. Fear and frustration thus colluded ironically and inadvertently to weaken the goal of effecting long-term behavioral change: fear by seeking to thwart the implementation of public health policies designed to identify and counsel voluntarily those who could transmit HIV infection, frustration by threatening the infected in ways that would render collaboration with public health officials difficult to attain. Both subverted the prospects for the emergence of a public culture of restraint and responsibility that could affect the course of the epidemic.

Chapter 5

Compulsory Screening

The Politics of Exclusion

Historically, public health officials have sought to identify those who carried infectious diseases as a way of controlling the spread of dangerous pathogens. Identification has served as the prelude to compulsory treatment, as the prelude to exclusion from settings in which infection might be transmitted, as the prelude to isolation and quarantine. Thus the history of mass testing and screening for disease has been linked to a range of public health measures entailing the exercise of coercive authority.

In the context of the AIDS epidemic, where no effective therapy was available during the epidemic's first seven years, proposals for wide-scale voluntary testing and counseling, contact notification, and even public health reporting have been based on the assumption that the identification of individuals infected with the AIDS virus was essential to any social program whose goal was the broad-based modification of behaviors linked to the spread or acquisition of HIV infection. Proposals for mandatory screening have typically sought to serve a very different purpose. There have, on occasion, been proposals to screen all high-risk individuals as they passed through a variety of medical and social institutions, thereby compelling the asymptomatic to know their antibody status. More generally, proposals for mandatory testing have been made in order to permit the identification of the infected so that restrictions and exclusions might be imposed on them.

In a few circumscribed settings mandatory testing for the antibody to the AIDS virus has been adopted without protest because of the virtually universal recognition that an important public health good, not otherwise attainable, would be secured. Screening of blood, organ, and semen donors has provoked little outcry—after the initial uncertainties of 1985 in blood banking—because all parties understood that the exclusion of contaminated body fluids and tissue from the donor pool was essential for the protection of others. In virtually all other settings proposals for mandatory screening have provoked controversy, not only because of the invasion of privacy and application of coercion involved, but because of the restrictive and exclusionary purposes they have been designed to serve. The proponents of mandatory screening have asserted that even the theoretical possibility of transmission warrants the identification and special treatment of the infected. Such moves were opposed by those who characterized them as a response to irrational fears, as scientifically unwarranted discrimination and nothing more than the application of the patina of public health to the invasion of privacy—in short, thinly disguised efforts to identify and then exclude homosexual or bisexual men or those with a history of intravenous drug abuse.

Public Health Officials and the Opposition to Mandatory Screening

Despite repeated reassurances by public health officials about the very restricted ways in which the transmission of the AIDS virus was believed to occur, social anxiety about the epidemic and the unwillingness of scientists to frame their statements about risk in absolute terms created the setting within which the calls for the exclusion of both those with AIDS and the asymptomatic carriers of HIV were to be heard. It is not surprising that schools became an early focal point for such efforts, as parents, terrified by the new disease, acted to protect their children from what they believed was the unacceptable, if remote, threat of a lethal disease. Although no more than a handful of schoolchildren were involved, the ensuing conflict dramatized the more general gulf between those who argued that great care was necessary when exclusionary policies were being considered and others who believed that in the face of a threat like that posed by AIDS no precaution was too great. That it was children who would either suffer the consequences of exclusion—shame, stigma, isolation—or bear the risk of infection only sharpened the conflict.

In the fall of 1985 several school boards yielded to parental anxiety and barred children who had AIDS or were suspected of being HIV-infected from the classroom. Where local boards, acting on the advice of health officials, refused to take such action, parents sometimes organized classroom boycotts. In New York City a bitter controversy pitted two local community school boards against the city's central Board of Education and Department of Health.[1] Parents angered by the insistence of public health officials that pupils with AIDS be permitted to attend class marched with placards that declared: "Our children want grades, not AIDS"; "Better safe than sorry"; and "Stop the lies: We want facts."[2] To the efforts at reassurance parents responded with the disbelief of those who expected manipulation by medical experts and public officials alike. Ultimately the New York State Supreme Court held that given the scientific evidence on the risks of transmission "automatic exclusion of all children with AIDS would violate their rights."[3]

Anticipating such challenges to what it considered rational public health policy and social order, the Centers for Disease Control convened a group of consultants in June 1985 to assist in the preparation of recommendations on the issues that would be raised by the presence in the classroom of children infected with the AIDS virus as well as those clinically diagnosed as having the disease itself. At the end of August, just before the beginning of the school year, the CDC issued its recommendations.[4] Reassuring in tone, the statement reviewed the epidemiological evidence and concluded that "casual person to person contact as would occur among school children appears to pose no risk."[5] Only in the case of very young children and those who were neurologically impaired, where control over bodily secretions was limited, was there even a "theoretical" risk of transmission.[6] Though this formulation left open the question of day care for and the foster placement of infants born to infected mothers—an issue that would haunt later discussions—it was adequate to the immediate task. There were no grounds for excluding most infected children, many of whom would have acquired HIV infection from blood transfusions or the clotting factor used by hemophiliacs, from the classroom. "Mandatory screening as a condition for school entry [is] not warranted," the CDC concluded.[7]

Like the threat of AIDS in school, concern by employers and workers provoked a rash of efforts to bar from the workplace those considered to pose some risk of transmitting AIDS.[8] Although the epidemiological evidence and scientific understanding of the transmission of HIV had by mid-1985 made such acts groundless from a public health perspective, private as well as some public sector employers responded with alarm, at times because of fears of contagion, on other occasions because of pecuniary concerns. Thus the city of Hollywood, Florida, sought to screen all prospective employees in order to prevent the employment of individuals who might develop AIDS, in part because of their potential impact on the city's employee benefit plan, in part because of a belief that any investment in training such workers would be wasted.[9] In neighboring Dade County, despite the advice of its chief health officer that AIDS, like other blood-borne diseases, could not be transmitted through food, the county board announced plans to screen all food-service workers for AIDS.[10] And although the 16th Biennial Conference of the AFL-CIO had voted to oppose the screening of workers,[11] the National Educational Association had already resolved that schools be permitted to screen employees and students if "reasonable cause" existed to believe the individual was infected with the AIDS virus.[12] Similarly, unions representing prison guards began to press for the screening of inmates so that the infected could be subject to special handling and even segregation.[13]

As it had done in the face of the threat of discrimination against schoolchildren, the CDC, committed to an antialarmist course, sought to stanch the tide of AIDS-related anxiety in the workplace. Less than three months after it had issued its recommendations on schools, the federal agency published a comprehensive statement on the prevention of HIV transmission in occupational settings.[14] Juxtaposing the workplace to the close family setting, where epidemiological studies had shown no transmission from infected individuals to those who were neither sexual partners nor the infants of infected mothers, the CDC could assert that the kind of nonsexual person-to-person contact that typically occurred in occupational encounters posed no risk for workers, customers, or clients.[15] There was no reason to restrict the use of telephones, office equipment, toilets, showers, eating facilities, and water fountains by those known to be infected. Nor was there any reason to restrict the employment activity of food-service workers, given the epidemiological and laboratory evidence on the transmission of blood-borne diseases. Finally, the CDC asserted that there was no reason to limit the activity of otherwise competent infected health-care workers.

Because of the theoretically greater risk they posed, the CDC devoted a special set of recommendations to those who performed invasive procedures where blood contact was possible.[16] But there, too, despite the fact that many would continue to argue that HIV-infected clinicians should not perform invasive procedures where there was some risk that blood contact could accidentally occur, the CDC denied the necessity of restricted activity. In sum, there were no grounds for the exclusion of workers otherwise capable of performing their jobs because of AIDS. There were no grounds for routinely screening asymptomatic workers to detect the presence of HIV infection.

But if infected workers posed no risk to clients, customers, and patients, what of the risk posed by infected patients to those who came into contact with them and especially with their blood and other body fluids? Here, too, the CDC provided a voice of reassurance. The adoption of standard infection control precautions in dealing with all patients would be sufficient to protect health-care workers from those who were infected with the AIDS virus.[17] As the model of close interpersonal contact within the family had served to provide the margin of safety in the analysis of the risks associated with nonmedical occupational exposure, the epidemiology of hepatitis-B viral transmission was used to demonstrate how little risk there was for medical workers exposed to infected patients when standard infection control measures were applied. Since hepatitis B was so much more infectious than HIV, it represented a "worst-case" model, and since hospitals had never screened all their patients for hepatitis B, there were no grounds for the routine screening of patients for the AIDS virus. Such screening was "unlikely to reduce the risk of transmission which even with documented needle sticks is extremely low. . . . Moreover results of routine serologic testing would not be available for emergency cases and patients with short lengths of stay."[18]

Anticipating that some would charge it with having become the captive of those committed to the protection of gay interests and with no longer representing the health interests of the community, the CDC was obliged to state that in preparing its recommendations "the paramount consideration had been the public health."[19] To conservative and openly antihomosexual California congressional representative William Dannemyer, who was to emerge as a persistent critic of the CDC and the entire public health establishment, the workplace recommendations were utterly unacceptable. Risks had been minimized and inadequate margins of safety applied. Civil rights, not protection against disease, had provided the yardstick. "The people in the public health service are erring on the side of the victims of AIDS when they should be erring on the side of protecting the public health."[20]

But despite the objections of Dannemyer and of those who believed that mandatory screening had to be undertaken where even the remotest of risks might exist, by 1985 the broad spectrum of public health officials in the United States had made clear its opposition, on public health grounds, to such measures. Following such advice and responsive to the political pressure of gay political groups as well as their liberal political allies, some state and city governments went so far as to prohibit the use of the antibody test by employers—California, Florida, and Wisconsin were the first to do so.[21] Discrimination against those with AIDS was prohibited in a number of municipalities as the result of special legislation.[22] But most important—and despite a ruling by the Justice Department in June 1986 that the federal statute protecting individuals with handicapping conditions did not shield individuals from discrimination based on the "fear of contagion whether reasonable or not"[23]—most states had so interpreted their own handicap laws, to protect those with AIDS and those suspected of being at risk for AIDS.[24]

As it had sought to provide public health guidance to schools, employers, and hospitals, the CDC had hoped to inform the actions of federal, state, and local correctional officials responding to AIDS. What more appropriate target was there for those who believed in mandatory testing than prisons? They housed men—many of whom had histories of intravenous drug use—under conditions of confinement where homosexual activity including rape was known to occur. Ample precedent provided prison officials with the authority to enforce regulations that for other populations would be deemed gross violations of privacy. Screening would permit prison officials to identify infected inmates who could then be segregated, thus protecting uninfected prisoners from a potential threat. Guards could adopt the precautions they deemed necessary in handling those with HIV infection. Demands for such testing came not only from unions representing prison workers but from some prisoners who argued that the state had a legal obligation to protect them against the infected while they were incarcerated.[25]

But despite its efforts the CDC was forced, in March 1986, to acknowledge that sharp disagreement among correctional authorities made its goal impossible to accomplish.[26] In December 1985 draft recommendations on AIDS in prison were circulated by the CDC.[27] While acknowledging the potential benefit that could be achieved by mandatory screening, the CDC warned of "serious complications" that could be anticipated. Given the virtual impossibility of protecting the confidentiality of antibody test results in prisons and the potential for violence against inmates found to be infected, it would be necessary, for safety reasons alone, to segregate infected prisoners. But such segregation could well pose insurmountable logistical problems. Separate cells, dining halls, and indoor and outdoor recreational facilities would be needed. And even were separate facilities available, the CDC draft warned that the "magnitude of disruption consequent to widespread testing will still need to be balanced against the value of such programs in preventing transmission, which is likely to be low if intravenous drug abuse and homosexual activity infrequently occur."

The possibility that separate prison facilities would be required by mandatory testing became "the flag" that alarmed many prison officials, said the director of the American Correctional Association.[28] Indeed, in January 1986, the National Association of State Correctional Administrators voted to reject mandatory testing.[29] Opposed to the balance thus struck, the American Federation of State, County, and Municipal Employees, representing prison guards and workers, asserted that administrative inconvenience was, in the face of a deadly disease, no excuse for not taking whatever steps were necessary to halt the threat to guards and prisoners. "Prisoners should be isolated to make sure that the disease does not spread throughout the institution through homosexuality or drug abuse, to reduce the chance of violence from prisoners, and to reduce the chance of accidental exposure to body fluids."[30] No official at that point would propose publicly the distribution of condoms to prisoners as a way of limiting the spread of HIV infection. That would, of course, have required a tacit recognition that homosexuality existed in prisons and a willingness to tolerate such behavior.

The lack of consensus among the relevant constituencies compelled the CDC to abort its effort. Instead of providing guidance, it published the results of a national survey sponsored by the National Institute of Justice and the American Correctional Association that simply described how prison systems were coping with the problem of AIDS.[31] In the absence of clear direction from the Centers for Disease Control, those who supported screening were able to press their arguments unencumbered by the restraining voice of the public health community that had played so critical a role in the evolution of policy and practice in occupational settings and the schools. Legislative efforts to mandate prison testing appeared in many states. Interestingly, of the first five states that planned to initiate mandatory testing—Nevada, Colorado, Iowa, Nebraska, and South Dakota—none had diagnosed a single case of AIDS in prison at the time screening was planned.[32] New York City, New Jersey, and Florida, with more than 75 percent of the reported cases of AIDS in prisons, opposed such testing.[33] Here, as in other dimensions of the response to AIDS, there was an inverse relationship between the adoption of an "aggressive" posture and the actual burden of the epidemic in a given region. Those who opposed prison screening centered their arguments on the institutional costs that would be created by such efforts and the potential harm that might befall those identified as infected. They chose to stress the role that education could play in limiting the spread of HIV infection in prisons. Violent prisoners who could place others at risk through rape had to be isolated, not only because of AIDS, but because of the responsibility to protect inmates from such assault.[34]

If the move to impose screening on prisoners represented an attempt to force the identification of infected individuals directly under the control of the state, the effort to mandate the screening of all applicants for marriage licenses was emblematic of the desire to identify the infected among the broad social mainstream, among those least likely to be infected. Ironically, the move to impose such testing came at a time when many states had, after more than four decades, repealed their premarital venereal disease screening requirements because they had proved to be ineffective and costly public health measures.[35] That AIDS-inspired premarital screening would target populations with very low levels of HIV infection, and that the pattern of premarital sexual relations in the United States made it unlikely that uninfected partners could be protected by screening that occurred just prior to marriage mattered less to the proponents of such a policy than the symbolic significance of attempting to take any measure necessary to protect the uninfected. The vision of women at the mercy of men who either wittingly or not could infect them and the specter of infants born with AIDS as the result of such unions—both of which had informed antivenereal campaigns of the 1930s and 1940s—provided the impetus behind calls for HIV antibody screening prior to marriage.[36]

By 1987 proposals for premarital screening had been made in many states and at the federal level. Tailored to the absence of a therapeutic intervention for AIDS, such proposals typically did not stipulate that those who were infected be prohibited from marrying, only that applicants for marriage licenses be apprised of the antibody status of their partners. Opposed by civil liberties groups as an invasion of privacy—"Is it really the government's business to require mandatory testing for certain things and not for others before two people get married?" asked the Virginia Civil Liberties Union[37]—such screening was also generally rejected by public health officials, even those who strongly supported broad-scale voluntary testing.[38] For them premarital testing would entail a wasteful diversion of resources and cause unnecessary distress to the disproportionate number of people receiving false-positive results—an inevitable consequence of any screening program directed at a group with very low levels of infection.[39]

Nevertheless, proposals for mandatory premarital screening retained great popular appeal, fueled in part by the public health message that it was not just gay and bisexual men or intravenous drug users who were at risk for infection. In the balance between the rights of the infected to resist forced identification on the one hand and the social interest in taking whatever measures appeared to promise some, even remote, advantage in halting the spread of HIV infection on the other, the latter seemed much more weighty. It is a measure of the dominance of the perspective provided by public health officials in the first years of the epidemic that despite popular opinion states resisted the passage of premarital screening laws until 1987, when Louisiana became the first to enact one.[40] Illinois soon followed suit, despite the strenuous opposition of its chief health officer.[41] Within a year both states would be compelled to recognize the wisdom of those who had warned about the folly of mandatory premarital testing. The public health benefits had been astonishingly small; the cost predictably high.

Surgeon General C. Everett Koop's statement to the American people in his fall 1986 *Report on AIDS* epitomized the opposition of public health officials to wide-scale mandatory testing and the exclusionary policies that would be made possible by the coercive identification of the infected. Throughout the report Koop stressed that casual, nonsexual contact posed no risk; that the presence of those with AIDS or HIV infection in public represented no danger. Reassuringly, he asserted, "Shaking hands, hugging, social kissing, crying, coughing or sneezing will not transmit the AIDS virus. Nor has AIDS been contracted from swimming pools or bathing in hot tubs or from eating in restaurants (even if a restaurant worker has AIDS and carries the AIDS virus). AIDS is not contracted from sharing bed linens, towels, cups, straws, dishes, or any other eating utensils. You cannot get AIDS from toilets, doorknobs, telephones, office machinery or household furniture."[42] Thus, over the full range of social encounters, from the most remote to the most "intimate" of nonsexual contacts, those infected with the AIDS virus represented no hazard. Having thus dismissed as unfounded the fears that fueled proposals to exclude HIV-infected individuals from work, school, housing, and public accommodations, the surgeon general could reject discrimination based on HIV status as without medical warrant.

But despite the surgeon general's effort to preclude an irrational turn toward screening and exclusion, a sense of popular disquiet persisted. Such disquiet tapped populist distrust of the scientific elites and may even have been fostered by the apparent unanimity of the opinion-making media. Just how socially embedded the anxieties were was reflected in a referendum placed before the people of California in November 1986.

A Referendum on AIDS and Public Health: The LaRouche Proposition

In October 1985 the attorney general of California was notified by Khushro Ghandi, the West Coast coordinator of the National Democratic Policy Committee—the political arm of Lyndon LaRouche's extreme movement—and Bryan Lantz, the NDPC's Northern California coordinator, that they intended to submit a proposition on AIDS to the electorate in the November 1986 election.[43] Under their leadership, the Prevent AIDS Now Initiative Committee (PANIC) thus began its remarkable effort to obtain the 400,000 signatures needed to qualify for a place on the ballot.

LaRouche's movement, which had achieved notoriety for its conspiratorial theories linking Britain's Queen Elizabeth to the international drug trade and Henry Kissinger to the Soviet Union, seized upon the AIDS issue as providing one more opportunity to uncover the ineptitude of America's leadership to deal with fundamental crises. Critical of the refusal of public health officials to adopt harsh measures to control AIDS, LaRouche had called for mass testing and quarantine. "In order to insure that the rapid spread of AIDS is halted, nothing less than universal screening and then, under full medical care, 'isolating' or 'quarantining' all individuals who are in the active carrier state" was required.[44] In cities and states across the country adherents of LaRouche's movement had pressured local school boards to remove schoolchildren with AIDS from the classroom and demanded the screening of all food handlers and teachers, so that those who showed signs of antibody to HIV could be barred from work that would place others at risk.[45]

The proposition drafted by PANIC bore none of these strident elements in its text. Instead, California voters were to be asked to support a series of ambiguously framed amendments to the state's health and safety code. The initiative was necessary, said Bryan Lantz, because "state and federal officials are not treating AIDS as carefully as they treat other communicable diseases."[46] To protect the people of California from what the legislature had already declared a "serious and life-threatening" challenge to "men and women from all segments of society," the proposition required that AIDS be defined as an "infectious, contagious and communicable disease" and that the condition of being a carrier of the HIV virus be defined as an infectious, contagious, and communicable condition. Both were to be listed by the Department of Health Services among the reportable diseases and conditions covered by existing relevant state statutes. To preclude any recapitulation of what PANIC believed was the failure of state health officials to protect residents of California from AIDS, the proposition mandated the enforcement of all relevant statutory and administrative provisions.[47]

By the summer of 1986, the closing date for the submission of petitions, PANIC had succeeded in obtaining 683,000 signatures for what would be officially termed Proposition 64.[48] This achievement was all the more striking given the broad-scale opposition to the initiative that had gained momentum during the first six months of 1986. To those who were appalled by what they believed would be the disastrous consequences to follow if the voters of the state approved the referendum, it had to be made clear just how dangerous the superficially innocuous terms of the proposition were.

That process had begun late in 1985 when the Civil Liberties Union of Southern California undertook its first analysis of what might follow from the application to AIDS of extant statutes and regulations concerning communicable diseases.[49] Seropositive schoolchildren would be barred from school, together with all others who had communicable diseases. Antibody-positive individuals "could be" excluded from jobs that entailed food handling. Public funerals for those with AIDS or infected with HIV "might be" prohibited. Those who tested positive for antibodies to the AIDS virus not only would be reported to state health officials but would be subject to "discretionary quarantine by local health authorities." Such a reading of Proposition 64 presupposed that public health officials would apply the relevant statutes and regulations governing communicable diseases in general in an inflexible way, with little tailoring to what was known about the transmission of HIV. But given the risk that such an interpretation might be put forth by some local health officials, "it appears that all the more Draconian general provisions . . . might be applied to all ELISA positive individuals." For the Civil Liberties Union there was no question but that the "ultimate intent of the initiative appears to be to subject HTLV-III virus carriers to serious deprivations of civil liberties."

By the spring of 1986 an even more dire interpretation of what the initiative would require if approved by the electorate was made by the Orange County chapter of the ACLU: names of those who were or were even suspected of being infected with HIV would have to be reported to local health officials; those who were or were suspected of being HIV carriers would be prohibited from working as cooks, waiters, airline stewards, and possibly bartenders; school exclusion would probably be required for students, teachers, and other staff who were infected with HIV or who "conceivably even merely resided" with HIV-infected individuals; restrictions on travel might be applied to those with AIDS as well as to infected individuals; quarantine and isolation powers might be more readily used by law enforcement and public health officials against HIV carriers and those with AIDS.[50]

Opposition to the referendum came from the entire medical establishment, including the California Medical Association, the California Nurses' Association, and the California Hospital Association. In a statement to the voters, the three associations stressed the irrationality of a proposal that assumed the existence of casual transmission of HIV in the schools, the workplace, or restaurants. Only those who were expert in the scientific and clinical dimensions of AIDS were qualified to fashion public health policy, not those driven by politically motivated "partial truths and falsehoods." "Would you let a stranger with no medical training or no medical background diagnose a disease or illness that you have? Would you let a political extremist dictate medical policy?" asked the statement. *"OF COURSE NOT."*[51]

The deans of four schools of public health in the state—the University of California at Berkeley and Los Angeles, San Diego State, and Loma Linda University—signed a joint statement declaring, "Proposition 64 would foster the inaccurate belief that AIDS is a highly contagious disease, easily spread through food or by coughing, sneezing, touching or other types of casual contact." The actions that would follow from the initiative were "scientifically unwarranted [and] would do nothing to curtail the spread of AIDS."[52] James Chin, chief of Infectious Disease for the state's Department of Health Services, characterized the initiative as "absurd," "stupid," and "disastrous."[53] Finally, the state's AIDS Task Force found the proposition both dangerous and utterly without merit as a public health measure.[54]

Joining the state's medical establishment in opposition to Proposition 64 was a broad spectrum of social organizations, the state's political elite, as well as its major newspapers. The California Labor Federation (AFL-CIO) and the California Manufacturers' Association were opposed to Proposition 64, as were Democratic senator Alan Cranston and Republican senator Peter Wilson, the governor, the state's superintendent of public instruction, and the mayors of Los Angeles, San Francisco, Sacramento, and San Jose.[55]

Finally, the editors of California's newspapers repeatedly denounced Proposition 64. The Los Angeles *Times* declared that "Proposition 64 makes no sense and is based not on medical evidence but on hatred and fantasy." Unlike those who believed the state either impotent or unwilling to confront the threat of AIDS, the editors declared, "Current law grants public health officials broad authority to protect people from AIDS if they believe it contagious—including the power to quarantine AIDS victims. They have not done so because it is not necessary."[56] The San Francisco *Chronicle* saw in the possible scope of the measures that would follow from Proposition 64 "a sweeping set of dictatorial powers and prohibitions that goes miles beyond what health authorities have said is necessary (or legal) in dealing with the AIDS problem. Perhaps saddest of all, the cost of fighting the initiative in money and energy could better be spent on AIDS research and education."[57] For the San Francisco *Examiner* the AIDS initiative would, if approved, "represent a sickness of public policy almost as bad as the disease itself." It was panic that provided the basis for the more than 600,000 signatures to the proposition, and it was panic that would be fueled by the initiative's enactment.[58] Thus, said the San Diego *Union*, "Even if the initiative is ludicrous, it shouldn't surprise. AIDS is a modern horror story, tragically suited for exploitation by No-Nothings such as Mr. LaRouche. The simplistic solutions offered by the hate mongering LaRouchians appeal to society's worst instincts."[59]

To each of the attacks of the medical, political, and social elites, PANIC and its representatives had a response. To those who predicted massive screening if Proposition 64 were to be enacted and who noted that such a program followed naturally from the erroneous statements about transmission included in PANIC's own published claims (AIDS was not hard to get; potential insect and respiratory transmission had been established; transmission by casual contact was well established), it was asserted that the initiative was really quite modest. PANIC's vice president, Bryan Lantz, thus said,

"The initiative does not require mass testing unless [the director of the Department of Health Services] or other health officials think it is necessary. . . . Personally I hope that passage of the proposition encourages the state to do it, but they don't have to."[60] To those who asserted that a program of mass screening and the denial of employment in schools and food-related industries, not to speak of possible quarantines, would cost millions of dollars, PANIC's response was that such calculations represented a gross distortion of what Proposition 64 mandated. More important, "Even if the initiative did cost this much, the health and welfare of the people of California should come first."[61] Finally, to those who noted that the entire medical and public health establishment was aligned against Proposition 64, PANIC retorted that the mission of the initiative was to compel public health officials to adopt the same precautions and safeguards applied to other communicable diseases.[62] Khushro Ghandi, PANIC's president, thus said, "What we are doing in the process of this initiative is forcing the state to take those proven standard public health measures which are already law, in fact, in this state, in every other state, and in fact are generally the law in every advanced country around the world and now implement those public health laws with respect to AIDS."[63] In short, PANIC sought to portray itself as defending the tradition of public health intervention against the restraint and passivity of those who had failed to safeguard the people of California.

The strategy of characterizing the initiative in very limited terms was shared by William Dannemyer, who in July became the only major political figure in California to support Proposition 64. In a press release he noted, "All the initiative does is to treat a person who is antibody positive in the same way as a person with venereal disease is now treated, namely, the condition is reportable."[64] Though he supported the exclusion of infected children from the classroom, he argued that the proposition did not mandate such a measure but would instead grant that authority to local health officials and school boards. Dannemyer claimed that the specter of quarantine used by opponents of Proposition 64 had little to do with what the initiative called for. Distancing himself from Lyndon La-Rouche and his extreme movement, Dannemyer wrote to elected officials in California asking them to support the initiative on its merits.[65]

So ambiguous was Proposition 64 that the state's legislative analyst could not determine with any degree of certainty the ultimate fiscal impact if the initiative were to be approved by the voters.[66] Everything would depend "on what actions are taken by health officers and the courts to implement the measure." If existing laws and regulations governing the control of communicable diseases were applied and health officials continued to exercise professional discretion in determining the appropriate forms of intervention, "few, if any, AIDS patients, [or] carriers of the AIDS virus would be placed in isolation or under quarantine. Similarly, few, if any, persons would be excluded from schools or food-handling jobs." If, however, Proposition 64 were interpreted so as to place new requirements on health officers, the results would be far different, involving a massive expansion of testing, the exclusion of infected individuals from schools and food-handling positions, and the imposition of isolation.

With so ill-defined a situation before the voters, with the proposition's opponents suggesting that dire and Draconian measures would follow from voter approval, and with the proposition's proponents insisting that the implications of approval would be limited and appropriate, what could the November referendum signify? At a minimum, given the political alliance that had materialized in opposition to Proposition 64, a "yes" vote could only be read as a rejection of the claims of the medical and public health establishments that they were in fact doing everything within reason to limit the spread of AIDS. Further, a "yes" vote would be an expression of distrust and profound frustration. A "no" vote would have much broader implications. It would represent not only an expression of confidence in the state's health leadership and its policies but a rejection of the Draconian alternative—mandatory testing, workplace and school exclusions, reliance on threats of isolation and quarantine.

Given this symbolic significance of the referendum, it was no surprise that a well-organized and financed effort to defeat Proposition 64 was mounted. At stake for public health officials was their scientific authority. At stake for the state's gay leadership was the threat that a usurpation of that authority would open the doors to the mobilization of irrational public sentiment on AIDS.

On election day close to 7 million voters cast ballots on Proposition 64. Seventy-one percent opposed it; 29 percent favored it.[67] Though this was a stunning defeat for PANIC, it was a hard-won victory for those who had mobilized the effort against the proposition. Two and a quarter million dollars had been spent. The organization of the cultural, social, medical, and political elites in opposition to the proposition had required an enormous expenditure of energy. And so, despite the success, there was a darker side to this story. Just fewer than two million voters, almost one in three, had been persuaded to support an initiative linked to one of the most extreme political movements in America. The referendum had revealed how popular discontent might be exploited in the years ahead as the absolute numbers of AIDS cases mounted. It had also demonstrated the existence of a popular base that could be mobilized for a repressive turn in public policy. The specter of popular irrationality haunted public health officials as they faced the growing impact of the epidemic. This threat posed a great political challenge to such officials: to convince the broader public that the emergence of a culture of restraint and responsibility among those at increased risk for transmitting the AIDS virus required a commitment to restraint and responsibility by those with the authority to make public policy.

Reaffirming Voluntarism: The CDC and the Debate Over Compulsory Screening

Just how volatile the situation remained was demonstrated when the Centers for Disease Control announced in early February 1987 that it would host a conference of public health officials and those concerned about civil liberties to discuss the future role of HIV antibody testing in the overall strategy to control AIDS. A furor was touched off because two among the many proposals to be considered would entail mass mandatory screening: the testing of all applicants for marriage licenses (though not the prohibition of marriage by those found seropositive) and of all hospital admissions. Proposals for premarital testing were not new. But no one had ever before proposed the testing of all hospital admissions, regardless of age or diagnosis. Were these proposals a trial balloon to determine the acceptability of a major shift in the course of public policy—one that would use every encounter between public agencies and Americans as an occasion for HIV antibody testing? Was this an effort to put forth ideas being pressed within the Reagan administration and among influential conservative political groups so that the opposition to mandatory testing within the public health community could demonstrate its strength? Had a conflict within the Public Health Service itself forced the issue of more extensive, even mandatory testing onto the public agenda? Whatever the motivation, an immediate mobilization of forces took place.

In a front page *New York Times* story, "U.S. Is Considering Much Wider Tests for AIDS Infection—Broad Debate Is Sought," Lawrence Altman, the medical correspondent, predicted that the ensuing discussion and the CDC meeting "would bring clashes over attempts to protect civil liberties as opposed to protecting public health."[68] In fact, the debate over the next month would reveal that both public health officials and the defenders of civil liberties found little to recommend in the proposals for mandatory screening, that the perspective enunciated by the CDC in the fall of 1985 retained broad-scale support.

Despite the presence at the conference of public health officials with very different perspectives on such matters as the importance of reporting positive antibody test results to health departments and contact notification, a remarkable consensus emerged against the mandatory testing of those considered the primary targets of such proposals—patients attending drug abuse programs and clinics for sexually transmitted diseases, persons seeking family planning services, and pregnant women.[69] The two proposals—mandatory premarital testing and universal hospital admission screening—that had so provoked the public's attention and transformed the conference from a small meeting with an anticipated attendance of 250 into a major conference of 800, drawing the attention of the national media, received virtually no support. For those whose primary concern was the protection of privacy and civil liberties, such screening was unwarranted, given the obvious costs and the very remote prospect that either mandatory program would make a contribution to the protection of the public health. For those whose analysis was based on the importance of the efficient exercise of public health power, neither proposal, if adopted, would have resulted in a rational expenditure of resources, given the very low rates of infection among those who would be tested.

Despite the opposition to mandatory testing, there was—especially among public health officials at the conference—a perceptible shift toward the aggressive promotion of testing among high-risk groups, when appropriate pretest and post-test counseling could assure the assimiliation of the significance of serological findings and provide the necessary psychological support to those found to be positive. For those concerned about how rapidly expanded testing could perhaps inadvertently provide the basis for discrimination and social isolation, the critical question remained as it had been in mid-1985, whether an aggressive program of voluntary testing was compatible with the protection of civil liberties and the social interests of the infected.

Here too there was a remarkable consensus at the conference. The defense of confidentiality and the stress on the importance of protections against discrimination followed naturally from the rejection of mandatory testing and from the appreciation of the role of voluntary testing in the modification of sexual practices and drug-using behavior linked to the transmission of HIV infection. Only if the threats to privacy and the hazard of discrimination were forcefully addressed would it be possible to induce large numbers to be tested. It was on this common ground that the defenders of public health, civil liberties, and the rights of those most at risk for AIDS could find themselves in agreement.

Subsequent to the February conference, meetings on the future of HIV antibody testing took place between the Centers for Disease Control and representatives of the Association of State and Territorial Health Officials, the Association of State and Territorial Public Health Laboratory Directors, the Council of State and Territorial Epidemiologists, the National Association of County Health Officials, and the United States Conference of Local Health Officers. Out of the consultative process emerged the CDC's April 30, 1987 "Recommended Additional Guidelines for HIV Antibody Counseling and Testing in the Prevention of HIV Infection and AIDS," the most fully developed expression of the commitment to a policy of testing that was at once voluntary, wide-scale, and vigorous.[70]

Like the Institute of Medicine–National Academy of Sciences' report *Confronting AIDS*, and the surgeon general's *Report on AIDS*, the April 30 recommendations asserted that the testing of individuals at risk for HIV infection had to be understood as an adjunct to counseling and as part of a broad strategy of prevention based on information and education. But, unlike those who sought to confine the role of testing, the CDC believed, as it had made clear a year earlier, that testing had a vital role to play. This strategic commitment was arrived at and adhered to despite a remarkable willingness to acknowledge how little was really known about the behavioral impact of testing. In the face of uncertainty, however, the dictates of public health required action based upon reasonable assumptions. "While there is no clear evidence from scientific studies that anyone uses [test results] in determining lifestyle changes to prevent infection or transmission, it is reasonable to assume that those who have access to such information are better able to make decisions than those who do not."[71] Its own review of the few empirical studies available went even further, suggesting only "minor changes" among those who knew their antibody status *and* who identified themselves as being at high risk for HIV infection. Indeed, the premise of the CDC strategy for over a year—offering testing to those clearly identified as being at increased risk, including gay and bisexual men—was vitiated by the suggestion that "the most important public health benefit from HIV-antibody counseling and testing may come from reaching and being able to educate asymptomatic persons who would not otherwise self-identify as being at risk for HIV infection and AIDS."[72]

As a consequence, the April 30 recommendations stressed the importance of routinely offering antibody testing in many settings to individuals who might not be reached by the campaigns organized by and largely directed to the gay community. Among those included in the call for expanded routine testing were individuals seeking treatment for sexually transmitted diseases; those in drug abuse treatment and their sexual partners; women of childbearing age—including those who were pregnant—if their own behaviors or those of their sexual partners put them at risk for HIV infection, if they lived in communities where the prevalence of HIV infection was high, or if they had received a blood transfusion before routine blood testing began in 1985.[73] But such a vastly expanded routine screening program was not to be confused with mandatory testing. The counseling process that preceded testing was to include a specific informed consent. Those being urged to undergo testing were to understand that they had the "right to choose not to be tested."[74]

Not only did the CDC thus reject the early February proposals for mandatory premarital and hospital admission screening, but it raised questions about whether routine voluntary testing of those planning marriage and those entering hospitals could be justified. On the basis of "public health principles" a commitment of resources to either was unwarranted. Premarital counseling and HIV antibody testing would have "highly variable success" in uncovering infected individuals. "Most persons at high risk of infection are already sexually active and get pregnant before marriage or do not plan to be in a marriage relationship."[75] Furthermore, there was always the risk that in directing a screening program at a population with a very low prevalence of infection an unacceptably high proportion of those found positive would be false positives. The CDC thus concluded that premarital screening "generally will be of lower priority than many other programs and services designed to interrupt the transmission of HIV."[76]

Less categorical in its opposition to routine hospital admission screening, the CDC nevertheless pointed out how unnecessarily inclusive was the proposal for universal testing. There were 37 million hospital admissions a year. Approximately 10 percent were less than fifteen years of age, over 25 percent were sixty-five or older. Thus, more than one third of all admissions were extremely unlikely to be HIV infected. Only if routine testing were instituted in high-prevalence areas and offered selectively, could it be justified on public health grounds.[77]

Like the February conference, the CDC's April 30 recommendations acknowledged the importance, from the perspective of public health, of protecting the confidentiality of HIV antibody test results and the social and economic interests of those found to be infected. Not only were exclusionary policies directed at the infected unnecessary for the protection of the public health; they would subvert the efforts of public health officials to win the confidence of those at risk. "The ability of health departments, hospitals, and other health care providers to assure confidentiality of patient information and the public's confidence in that ability are crucial to efforts to increase the number of persons requesting or willing to undergo counseling and testing for HIV antibody. But of equal or even greater importance is the public perception that persons found to be positive will not experience unfair treatment as a result of being tested."[78] The care with which the issues of confidentiality and discrimination were addressed is striking. State governments were called upon to review current procedures for the protection of medical records and to determine their adequacy. The Public Health Service was urged to "seek national AIDS confidentiality legislation and/or to work with its state and local health constituencies to develop model confidentiality legislation appropriate to the AIDS situation."[79] Similarly, states were called upon to enforce relevant antidiscrimination statutes—generally those applying to the handicapped. The Public Health Service was asked to emphasize the absence of any justification for routine or mandatory screening as a condition of employment or admission to school, housing, or other public accommodations. Finally, the Department of Health and Human Services was urged to review the adequacy of antidiscrimination protections under federal law and to propose additional protections if necessary.[80]

Mandatory Screening and the Federal Government: Health Authorities in Retreat

The release of the April 30 recommendations must be viewed as an effort to make clear the CDC's position on mandatory screening at a moment when forces pressing for greater reliance on nonvoluntary testing had gained ascendency in the White House, rendering the surgeon general all but isolated within the administration of Ronald Reagan. But the turn to compulsory screening had its roots in federal policies dating from the fall of 1985. For at the very time that the CDC was attempting to demonstrate why screening and exclusion would be misguided workplace practices, the Department of Defense was preparing to initiate a program of screening for all military recruits and active duty personnel.

In June 1985 the deputy assistant secretary asked the Armed Forces Epidemiological Board—a civilian advisory panel—to consider the appropriate response of the military to HIV infection.[81] Among the issues the board was to address were whether individuals with confirmed positive antibody tests would pose public health risks in military settings, whether personnel on active duty should be screened, and whether individuals found to be positive during the screening of potential recruits should be permitted to join the military service.

Though the Epidemiological Board had not yet issued its report, the Department of Defense decided on August 30 to order the screening of all recruits.[82] William Mayer, assistant secretary of defense for health affairs, explained that this "modest . . . precaution" was being taken to protect military personnel. Those who were infected were at risk if they were administered live virus vaccines.

They posed a hazard to other soldiers if during emergencies they served as donors in soldier-to-soldier transfusions. Finally, Mayer expressed some concern about the adequacy of the studies of families that had been relied upon to demonstrate that casual transmission of the AIDS virus did not occur. Given the extremely close contact of soldiers in planes and tanks, the risk of transmission could not, Mayer asserted, be discounted.[83]

When the Epidemiological Board issued its findings in mid-September it sustained the decision to reject from service military recruits identified by screening as antibody positive.[84] They were at increased risk for disease if exposed to live virus vaccines and for developing AIDS because of the biological or physical stresses associated with military service. Unlike William Mayer, the board found no reason to believe that infected personnel posed a risk to others in tanks, submarines, and aircraft, though they were clearly unsuitable as blood donors. Thus the screening of all active duty personnel was deemed "unnecessary" as a precautionary measure. Screening of individuals was recommended prior to overseas assignment, but only as a preliminary to further medical examinations. Those who showed no sign of immunological deficiency or progressive clinical illness could be considered for world-wide duty. Guided by concerns about the costs of testing, the administrative burdens that would be created by a mass screening program, and medical considerations, the board had put forth a very circumscribed program.

At the end of October Secretary of Defense Caspar Weinberger issued a policy much more sweeping in scope than the Epidemiological Board had recommended.[85] Like the board, the secretary of defense called for the exclusion of all antibody-positive recruits. In addition to concerns about the risks posed by live virus vaccines and the inability of antibody-positive individuals to participate in soldier-to-soldier battlefield transfusions, the secretary noted the possibility that those who were infected would become sick before completing their service commitments and would as a consequence generate costs for the military's medical care system.

Rejecting the recommendations of the Epidemiological Board, the Department of Defense decided that it would test all active-duty personnel. Those found to be positive would be retained by the armed forces if no clinical signs of illness were found. Cognizant of the likelihood of charges that the military, with its explicitly anti-homosexual policies, would use test results and information obtained in medical follow-ups to weed out those with a history of homosexual activity or illicit drug use, the secretary pledged that such information would not be used against members of the armed services "in actions under the Uniform Code of Military Justice, in a Line of Duty determination, or on the issue of characterization in separation proceedings." Despite such promises, for those who were deeply suspicious of the military and who viewed with alarm the standards of confidentiality that permitted full exchanges between medical and nonmedical officials in the armed services, the new policies were a grave threat. Their concerns were only amplified as the Department of Defense extended its screening to students enrolled in the service academies and college Reserve Officer Training Corps programs, deciding to dismiss those who tested positive.[86]

Though most public health opponents of mandatory screening were deferential to the justifications put forth by the military for its policy—the Institute of Medicine and the National Academy of Sciences, so hostile to compulsory screening in *Confronting AIDS*, did not criticize military screening programs—those with a prime commitment to the protection of civil liberties were both skeptical and disturbed. And they had reason to be. Precedents were being established that would have an impact on civilian life. The secretary of defense had disregarded the counsel of the board of experts charged with the responsibility of providing advice on health matters and had even suggested that the cost of future health care was an appropriate consideration in determinations about recruitment. Certainly employers in the private sector could rely upon similar arguments for screening and exclusion. One legal critic of the military's policies thus wrote, "Civil rights advocates know that any testing produces results, results are recorded, and lists are made. They fear such lists will be used to discriminate in employment situations or, in the extreme, to create isolation or quarantine camps. If the military screening program is a precursor of civilian policy, the worst fears of civil libertarians may prove well-founded."[87]

The move toward even wider screening on the part of federal agencies proceeded despite the recommendations of the surgeon general, the Institute of Medicine, and the National Academy of Sciences. In November 1986, just one month after the publication of *Confronting AIDS* and the surgeon general's *Report on AIDS*, the Foreign Service announced that it would screen all applicants for appointment, officers, and their dependents.[88] Medical, economic, and political justifications were provided for this policy, the first undertaken by a federal civilian agency. Screening was necessary, said the Foreign Service, to identify those who would place themselves at risk by receiving live virus vaccines or by working in remote areas of the world where appropriate medical care would be out of reach in medical emergencies, and to protect uninfected individuals who might require blood transfusions from their colleagues posted abroad. Like the military, the Foreign Service asserted that infected individuals were "at considerable risk of being unable to complete their assignments due to illness" and would "pose a financial burden for the government." Finally, the Foreign Service noted that the presence of infected American representatives on foreign soil could have "disastrous" implications for the interests of the United States.[89]

To objections that the Foreign Service policy was too broad in its exclusions, based on extremely remote possibilities of medical emergencies and a hardly less credible picture of each Foreign Service officer serving as a "walking blood bank," the deputy medical director of the Foreign Service responded, "In an occupational setting is it not the employer's responsibility to protect vulnerable employees from occupational exposure? What are the medical/legal risks to an employer who ignores medical recommendations and assigns vulnerable employees to dangerous locations?"[90]

Like the military effort, a standard with general implications was being set by the federal government. In the broader society, would corporations that routinely sent personnel abroad be provided with a warrant for screening all employees and applicants for employment, denying jobs to those who tested positive? Would the Foreign Service program, like that of the military, provide a justification for those who sought to protect their economic interests by denying employment to individuals who might become sick, thus placing a burden on corporate benefit plans? For Thomas Stoddard (formerly of the New York Civil Liberties Union) of the Lambda Legal Defense and Education Fund the dangers posed by the Foreign Service policy extended far beyond the more than 15,000 people who would be screened. "It will create the impression generally that people who are positive are unable to work—an impression that is false and entirely contrary to the medical data."[91] Acknowledging the possibility of the more remote risks and striking a characteristically antipaternalistic stance, Stoddard concluded, "It is up to the employee to decide whether there are personal risks worth taking."

Most stunning in the series of moves undertaken by the federal government was the decision of the Department of Labor, announced just one month after that of the Foreign Service, to screen all Job Corps students, applicants, and staff members.[92] In justifying its decision, the department stated that it was concerned that its residential centers would become "breeding grounds" for AIDS, since many students—drawn from among the poorest youth in America—had used intravenous drugs. Those who tested positive would "if feasible" be reassigned to nonresidential locations or to a "comparable" training program. Here the threat of sexual contact among those who were infected provided the justification for compulsory screening. The implications quite obviously went beyond the 40,000 students who would be tested and suggested a broad warrant for mandatory screening in all residential settings, even where the competence and the ability of persons under the supervision of the government to protect themselves—patients in psychiatric hospitals, for example—did not arise.

But screening was proposed during this period not only for identification of infected Americans, but as a way of protecting America itself from immigrants who might carry infection to this country. Attractive to proponents of mandatory screening because it would represent an extension to AIDS of exclusionary practices already used for other diseases, such as syphilis, gonorrhea, and tuberculosis, the testing of persons applying for immigrant visas would also permit the adoption of a strong public health posture that would affect individuals not protected by constitutional provisions governing privacy. Finally, the screening of aliens could achieve its political ends without stimulating much public outcry. The federal government proposed initially in April 1986 that it be given the authority to exclude those with AIDS and to test those suspected of having AIDS.[93] "We do not propose mass screening of asymptomatic individuals. And we are not proposing routine blood testing of all visa applicants," said Lawrence Farrer, quarantine director of the CDC.[94] Opponents of the proposed exclusionary policy expressed concern that so discretionary a rule would permit the immigration authorities invidiously to target persons suspected of being homosexual. Others noted that since the United States was the advanced industrial world's primary reservoir of HIV infection the proposed policy would do little to contain the epidemic at home. It would, however, create a precedent that could have serious implications for Americans as they sought to emigrate and even to travel. But despite such objections the proposed federal rule generated little audible protest.

It was against this backdrop of federal screening initiatives that a challenge to the voluntarist perspective so carefully defined by the surgeon general and the CDC took place within the administration. Leading the surgeon general's opponents within the cabinet was Secretary of Education William J. Bennett. Already opposed to Everett Koop's advocacy of explicit and early school-based education programs to combat the spread of AIDS, Bennett believed that officials had abdicated the responsibility to protect public health by their unwillingness to impose antibody testing for purposes of enhancing the available surveillance data and facilitating the strategy of prevention. At the end of April, the secretary of education declared that "a good case could be made for requiring testing of those applying for marriage licenses, or immigration to the United States, convicted criminals before imprisonment and just prior to release, hospital admissions, and those attending clinics that served populations at high risk."[95] Gary Bauer, the president's domestic policy advisor and Bennett's former deputy in the Department of Education, made it clear that within the White House the counsels of the CDC and the surgeon general were viewed as inadequate. "I personally agree with Secretary Bennett that more testing will be needed as we attempt to combat this disease. A strong case can be made for mandatory testing in each of the areas Secretary Bennett outlined, especially for marriage licenses and immigration. After finding a cure, the prime responsibility of the government is to protect those who do not have the disease."[96] On the matter of premarital testing, Vice President Bush was already on record as supporting state action that would mandate such screening so that potential marriage partners would know about each other's antibody status.[97]

The debate within the administration over the future of antibody testing intensified during May 1987, in the weeks prior to a long-awaited Presidential speech on AIDS, to be delivered on the evening before the commencement of the Third International Conference on AIDS in Washington, D.C. It was widely known that the president favored the proposals for screening applicants for marriage licenses and immigration. Less certain was how he would decide on matters of prisoners and hospital admissions. Commenting on the resistance of public health officials to virtually all such proposals, a White House spokesman made it clear that the executive office would not be inhibited by the opposition of health professionals. "As so often happens in the area of health regulation, sometimes you have to make political judgments that can't wait for all the health data to be in."[98] By suggesting that opponents of mandatory testing were inhibited by the absence of definitive data, the White House was able to shift the terms of debate set by the public health officials, who had stressed the importance of prudence in the exercise of public health authority, and had understood the limits of compulsory screening in the struggle against a disease that required the modification of private, intimate behaviors. Furthermore, proponents of mandatory testing knew what the electorate expected from those whose task it was to protect the public health. Citing one recent poll that had found that 82 percent of those surveyed supported premarital testing, Marlin Fitzwater, the White House spokesman, noted that "all barometers of the public pulse" backed such screening."[99]

In the days before the presidential address on AIDS, the Domestic Policy Council reached a consensus that the president should advocate widespread mandatory testing. Beyond the screening of applicants for marriage licenses and immigrants, the council endorsed the testing of prisoners and hospital patients. The sole dissenting voice at the council's May 27 meeting was that of the surgeon general.[100]

When the president gave his long-awaited speech, he called explicitly for the screening of immigrants and federal prisoners and asked for a review of the feasibility of testing admissions to Veterans Administration hospitals.[101] Furthermore, he urged the states to "offer routine testing for those who would seek marriage licenses," as well as to prisoners under their jurisdictions. Justifying his commitment to expand screening, the President declared, "Just as individuals don't know that they carry the virus, no one knows to what extent the virus has infected our entire society. . . . AIDS is surreptitiously spreading throughout our population and yet we have no accurate measure of its scope. It is time we knew exactly what we were facing. And that is why I support routine testing." To those who sought solace in the president's use of the word "routine" both generally and in terms of premarital screening, Gary Bauer made it clear that the White House was committed to a firm course. "Routine testing can be mandatory or people can be given the right to opt out. . . . In all federal areas, the president is talking about mandatory testing."[102]

On the day following the president's speech, the U.S. Senate passed by a vote of 96–0 a proposal supporting the screening of all immigrants, thus backing the president but going far beyond the rule proposed by officials in the early spring.[103] Any ambiguity about whether testing would be applied to the two to three million resident aliens seeking to regularize their status under a recently announced amnesty program was resolved by Vice President Bush in his address to the opening plenary session of the Third International Conference on AIDS. They would be tested. To many in his audience who were already disturbed by the president's speech, Bush's comments were especially revealing. What standard of equity could justify denying legal status to those who—given the residency requirements of the amnesty program—almost certainly would have been infected with HIV while living in the United States? Just as the decision to screen had to be viewed primarily as a symbolic gesture designed to reassure Americans that every effort was being made to protect them, it also was perceived by critics as a symbolic affront to those who had warned about the universal extension of screening programs.

And so began the seventh year of the AIDS epidemic—with public health officials seeking to minimize the extent to which they had, in fact, been outflanked. But to those who had no need to provide a more optimistic interpretation of the new course, it was clear that the initiative that had been held by the proponents of voluntary testing under conditions of strict confidentiality had been seized by those who believed that the AIDS epidemic required the use of compulsion. Emblematic of this turn was the fact that the CDC's April 30 recommendations, with their extensively argued opposition to mandatory testing and their direct challenge to the wisdom of proposals for premarital and hospital admission screening, would never appear as a formal statement of the Public Health Service.

For those dismayed by the rout of public health officials, the future had an ominous cast. The *New York Times*, long antagonistic to coercive measures and bitterly critical of those it viewed as overstating the threat posed by AIDS, thus declared, "Testing whether called mandatory or sugared with the term 'routine' has suddenly become the politicians' cure for this incurable disease. . . . The testers fail to bring their unspoken agenda into the open. Detention camps across the country would be a shrieking departure from the American tradition; all the more reason for the subject to be openly discussed—and compared with what public health professionals believe should be done instead."[104]

Indeed there was evidence that elected officials and those seeking office across the country were beginning to reject the broad public health consensus forged by health officials, civil libertarians, and gay activists. Addressing a conservative political audience in the summer of 1987, Representative Jack F. Kemp, an early candidate for the 1988 Republican presidential nomination, called for mandatory testing of all immigrants, health care workers, hospital workers, hospital patients, and those undergoing routine medical checkups, applying for marriage licenses, or arrested for drug use or prostitution. Furthermore, he asserted, screening should be done on blood drawn from all individuals already being tested for other communicable diseases.[105] The isolation of public health officials was further underscored by what public opinion polls suggested about the views of the American people. A Gallup survey conducted in early June 1987 showed that mandatory screening was favored by 90 percent for immigrants, 88 percent for federal prisoners, 80 percent for applicants for marriage licenses. Fifty-two percent favored the testing of all Americans.[106]

But disaffection from the posture adopted by public health officials extended beyond politicians and popular opinion as measured by the polls. Some physicians and other health care workers also began to question the claims of those who had for more than two years argued against virtually all mandatory screening. With increasing self-confidence, in the latter part of 1987 medical professionals began to assert that they had a right to know whether the patients whom they were treating were infected with the AIDS virus.[107] The 1985 CDC recommendations against the screening of patients for infection control purposes had lost their persuasive force. The existence of a small number of health-care workers infected as a result of needle sticks contaminated with blood drawn from HIV-infected patients and of an even smaller number who had become infected as a result of other exposures to blood had shaken the confidence of those whose work brought them into daily contact with patients who might be carrying the AIDS virus. In the face of such anxiety no appeal to use "universal blood and body fluid precautions" to treat all patients with great caution seemed responsive.

More than the demand for the right to screen all patients, the public assertion on the part of a small number of health-care professionals—but especially surgeons and dentists—that they had a right to refuse to treat individuals who were infected with HIV represented a stunning rebuff to the carefully crafted antiexclusionary positions put forth by public health officials.[108] If physicians could demand that their patients be screened, then clearly patients could also demand the screening of health-care workers, and the exclusion of infected workers from the care of patients, no matter how remote the risks of transmitting infection with the AIDS virus.

But the behavior of those engaged in the provision of health care had far broader implications. Allowing health-care workers to screen their patients and tolerating overt or covert refusals to care for the infected would foster anxiety and irrational exclusions in other social realms. Instead of serving as a yardstick of reason against which to judge employers and school administrators, medicine would give encouragement to those whose fears, no matter how exaggerated, drove them to seek the wholesale exclusion of HIV-infected individuals from social life.

Conflicts over screening and exclusion had during the first seven years of the epidemic always involved implicit, if not explicit, efforts to balance the risks and benefits of screening, exclusion, and restrictions. They inevitably entailed judgments about how the burden of uncertainty would be borne, about how many individuals should be compelled to subject themselves to testing, and how many denied the right to participate in a full range of social activities in order to prevent the possibility of the remotest of harms. That those involved in making such judgments generally shared a common view of how, in the face of extremely remote risks, the balances should be struck did not thereby change the essentially political character of the decisions; it simply made it more difficult to discern. Only when the consensus against mandatory screening and exclusionary policies became the subject of persistent public challenge did it become more obvious that questions of fairness and equity were central to the choices that had been made and would need making.

In the next years new controversies over screening will surely arise. In each of these conflicts those who confront each other will predictably seek to appropriate the mantle of value-free decision making and will charge that those with whom they disagree have deserted the standards of science. On some occasions the risk posed by the infected will be understood to be so small and the implications of screening and exclusion so burdensome that even the most cautious will find it hard to justify compulsory testing and the imposition of restrictions; on other occasions the choices will not be so clear cut. But in each case more than "science" will be involved. Decisions about screening policy will reflect the balance of moral and political commitments to privacy, reason, and communal well-being. They will have a fundamental impact on the social context within which AIDS will be confronted and the prospects for meeting the public health challenges posed by the epidemic.

Chapter 6

Isolating the Infected

The Politics of Control

In 1987 Senator Jesse Helms, the conservative Republican senator from North Carolina, declared on a national news program, "I may be the most radical person you've talked to about AIDS, but I think that somewhere along the line that we are going to have to quarantine, if we are really going to contain this disease."[1] Three days earlier a Florida judge had ordered the confinement of a fourteen-year-old boy to a hospital psychiatric ward because he represented a danger to the public health.[2] Infected with HIV, the boy was reported to be sexually active by the state's Department of Health and Rehabilitation Services, staying away from home two to three nights a week. In both instances, the threat of AIDS had evoked an appeal to the government's most potent instrument to meet a challenge to the public health—the use of coercive power every bit as awesome as that of arrest and incarceration on criminal charges. In both instances, the response provoked by the threatened imposition of control demonstrated how efforts to call upon the historical legacy of quarantine would confront resistance founded on the prevailing understanding of the modes of HIV transmission, and beliefs about the appropriate role of the state in restricting the sexual behavior of consenting adults, the limits of power in regulating behavior that occurs in private, the boundaries of coercion in a liberal society.

To meet the challenge of understanding the implications of quarantine at a time when the use of such public health power had all but fallen into desuetude because of changing patterns of illness in advanced industrial societies and the efficacy of modern therapies that required less coercive controls to protect the public health, it was necessary to turn to the history of state responses to the epidemics of earlier periods. Bubonic plague, leprosy, cholera, yellow fever, tuberculosis—each had its chroniclers and each provided some detail of how quarantines had been used to protect the well from the threat of deadly or disfiguring illness. But the lessons to be drawn from the historical accounts were not univocal. At times quarantine had been imposed on the basis of how contemporary experts and leaders understood the nature of the threat with which they were confronted. At other moments pressure had come from "below," from a frightened populace demanding protection from the ravages of disease and disorder. There were occasions when the historical record suggested passivity on the part of those who were subject to quarantine. There were other instances when efforts to remove, isolate, or confine the infected produced resistance and social conflict. Finally, though some periods were marked by a shared understanding of how disease spread and the relative efficacy of quarantine, others were characterized by deep disagreements over both matters. During the nineteenth century, for example, a fractious controversy raged over which epidemic diseases were, in fact, contagious and over the benefits of quarantine in containing them.[3]

The nineteenth-century controversies are especially revealing because they suggest that disputes over matters of science and public health policy may be rooted in deeper ideological divisions. Liberals seeking to break the bonds of an overintrusive state whose actions were inimical to free trade often viewed quarantines as "engines of oppression, despotism and bureaucracy."[4] A British opponent of quarantine denounced it as "the most gigantic, extraordinary and mischievous superstructure that had ever been raised by man upon a purely imaginary formulation."[5] Those who viewed the state more sympathetically were less prone to such wholesale condemnation, which they perceived as deriving from a political animus.[6]

For those who feared the social toll that would be taken by any attempt to impose quarantine in the case of AIDS, the history of such efforts provided a dreary record of ineffective measures applied in ways that appeared to disregard the social and human costs entailed.

For those who believed that America lacked the will to act aggressively to contain AIDS, the history of quarantine—with all of its mishaps—demonstrated how communities had learned to protect themselves against the threat posed by contagious illnesses.

In a critical historical overview of quarantine efforts, written as a warning to America as it confronted AIDS, David Musto underscored the significance of quarantine as the creation of a boundary separating the contaminated from the uncontaminated.[7] It was fear that drove the movements for the isolation of the diseased, a fear that went beyond a simple concern about how illness spread. "The fear of disease . . . arises not just from a reflection on the physiological affects of a pathogen, but from a consideration of the kind of person and habits which are thought to predispose one to the disease. Likewise, quarantine is a response not only to the actual mode of transmission but also to a popular demand to establish a boundary between the kind of persons so diseased and the respectable people who hope to remain healthy."[8] It was a deep concern about how forces driven by such fears could influence the course of public health policy—without any regard for the lessons about the efficacy of past quarantines—that led David Sencer, New York City's health commissioner, to declare that he could not think of a single example of an infectious disease that had been effectively controlled or eradicated by quarantine.[9]

Paralleling the turn to medical and social history was an inquiry into the legal history of quarantine in an effort to determine how the courts might respond in the event of attempts to impose restrictive measures on those with AIDS or HIV infection. There was, in fact, little in the way of contemporary legal scholarship on the matter, since the problem of quarantine had virtually disappeared as a matter of litigation. Public health laws that provided the basis for the exercise of the power of quarantine had often remained unchanged for decades and were marked by the earlier era from which they had emerged. The tradition of "rather crude confinement of real or suspected cases of disease" had prevailed.[10] The lesson to be drawn from legal history was that legal history could provide almost no guide. With little case law beyond the 1920s and little legal commentary, it was possible for Wendy Parmet to entitle her analysis of how the law of quarantine might apply to AIDS "The Revival of an Archaic Doctrine."[11]

It was, nevertheless, unthinkable that the courts, which had developed such exacting standards for the protection of criminal defendants and which had rejected the unfettered discretion of the state in cases involving the control of juvenile offenders and the commitment of mental patients, would do less in the case of those who might become the targets of efforts at isolation and quarantine. Though it was suggested, at times, that the confinement of Japanese-Americans during World War II provided a chilling example of just what could occur at a moment of social anxiety provoked by a sense of national emergency, so extraordinary an example served primarily to demonstrate how extreme a situation would be necessary before so drastic a measure could be contemplated.[12] It was not plausible, in the absence of a war and national mobilization, that a court in the last decades of the twentieth century could declare, as had the Maine Supreme Judicial Court almost one hundred years earlier: "It is unquestionable that the legislature can confer police powers upon public officers for the protection of the public health. The maxim *salus populi supreme lex* is the law of all courts in all countries. The individual right sinks in the necessity to provide for the public good."[13]

In those rare circumstances when quarantine authority had been exercised in recent years—most often in cases involving individuals with tuberculosis who refused to take the medication that rendered them safe to the public—the impact of due process concerns had begun to affect the practice of public health in ways that would bear directly on how AIDS would be confronted. In West Virginia, the Supreme Court ruled in 1980 that the due-process protections required in the face of the threat of civil commitment of the mentally ill were applicable to cases involving the involuntary confinement of individuals who posed a social hazard because of infectious diseases.[14] Though it was not necessary to provide the same level of protection required in criminal cases, the court held that those whom the state sought to confine had a right to procedural safeguards, including the right to cross-examine witnesses, that would permit a robust defense in an adversarial proceeding. A year later in Los Angeles the government agreed to a far-reaching set of safeguards to protect the rights of those deemed a threat to the public health because of tuberculosis.[15] Arising out of a case in which a patient had been detained for twenty-two days in a hospital and for close to seven weeks in a prison, the new standards sought to preclude the unchecked exercise of the public health power of isolation.[16] Within twenty-four hours of detention, the patient was to be given a copy of the order of isolation providing documentation of the justification for confinement. Within seven days, if the patient contested the detention, a hearing was to be held at which representation by counsel and the assistance of an independent physician expert was to be guaranteed. In cases where the patient did not speak English, translators were to be provided. If it was determined by officials that detention for a period exceeding sixty days was necessary, a petition to the county's superior court would be required. Confinement could only continue if at least nine of twelve jurors agreed that the "patient would not reliably participate in a program of voluntary treatment such that release could constitute a probable threat to the public health."[17]

This agreement, made just one month after the first AIDS cases were reported by the Centers for Disease Control, provides an indication of the changing legal context within which the question of quarantine and AIDS would be confronted—a context characterized by the simultaneous existence of a largely unchallenged historical legacy of almost plenary public health power and some critical indications that when presented with the opportunity the courts would restrain the exercise of that power in ways more compatible with contemporary constitutional standards.

AIDS and Quarantine

Despite the existence of a broad scientific consensus about the modes of HIV transmission and the public recognition that AIDS was not a disease contracted by casual contact, there were calls, at times apparently supported by popular opinion, for the isolation of all infected individuals. This was not the first occasion in which the diction of quarantine had been used in the context of a behaviorally transmitted disease; it had been used in the 1960s when drug addiction became the source of social anxiety[18] and earlier in the century as the state sought to protect Americans from venereal disease.[19] On those prior occasions—as was true with AIDS—the targets of such preventive state control were individuals whose actions or color made them the subject of dread and contempt.

Typically, the legislative proposals for mass quarantine to control AIDS came from state legislators at the far right of the political spectrum and displayed considerable misunderstanding about the risks of HIV transmission or a remarkable willingness to consider preemptive incarceration. In Ohio legislation was introduced in 1986 that would have declared AIDS a contagious disease and required that local boards of health "immediately order the isolation of the patient in such place and under such circumstances as will prevent the conveyance of infectious agents to susceptible persons. The isolation required by this decision shall continue until such time as the attending physician certifies that the patient has recovered and is no longer liable to communicate the disease to others."[20] A bill introduced in the state of Washington declared, "When any person has been confirmed as being infected with AIDS, the local health officer . . . shall provide for the public safety as the officer deems necessary by removing any infected person found within his or her jurisdiction . . . (1) to the state hospice, if available, or (2) to a separate building . . . if it can be done without great danger to the infected person's health. . . . Alternatively [the state or local health officer] may order the infected person isolated in the person's residence."[21]

In a 1986 defense of such extreme measures appearing in the conservative journal the *American Spectator*, the logic of quarantine and preventive detention was given full expression. "There are only three ways that the spread of lethal infectious diseases stops: it may be too rapidly fatal, killing off all its victims before the disease can spread; the population affected may develop natural or medically applied immunity; it may not be able to spread because uninfected individuals are separated sufficiently well from those infected. [At this point the only way] to prevent the spread of the disease is by making it physically impossible. This implies strict quarantine, as has always been used in the past when serious—not necessarily lethal—infections have been spreading. Quarantine in turn implies accurate testing." Lamenting the failure of nerve on the part of Americans, the authors then note that "neither quarantine nor universal testing is palatable to the American public where AIDS is concerned, yet both have been used without hesitation in the past."[22]

On grounds of science, pragmatics, and constitutional values, proposals for the mass isolation of all infected individuals have found no support among those professionally concerned with the practice of public health. In a speech before the Republican Study

Committee of the House of Representatives, James Mason, then acting assistant secretary of health, asserted that since the "spread of the virus, except for very rare instances that occur through transfusions of infected blood or from mother to infant, requires voluntary, deliberate, direct intimate contact between consenting adults or the sharing of drug abuse equipment," coercive measures were not "generally" applicable to the control of AIDS.[23] Unlike those who sought to characterize the debate over mass quarantine as requiring a balancing of individual rights against the claims of the public good, Mason argued that no reasonable understanding of the demands of public health could involve recourse to quarantine. "In a case where there is clearly a danger of contagion, playing it safe by confining people for the common good would, of course, be the correct approach. . . . But AIDS is not transmitted by casual contact: therefore, restrictive measures used for other more easily communicable diseases do not seem routinely justified."

Rarely did proponents of mass quarantine consider the sheer burden of attempting to implement such a program. But it was such pragmatic matters that permitted the Council of State and Territorial Epidemiologists to voice its opposition to mass quarantine as an unthinkable strategy for the public health. Given the number of individuals presumed to be infected, the fact that the vast majority were asymptomatic, and the possibility that HIV infection might be lifelong, quarantine could not be considered a "feasible, routine, community control method."[24]

Finally, proposals for mass quarantine posed a profound threat to the most fundamental commitments of those concerned about the constitutional limits of state power. Since HIV transmission required specific behaviors on the part of the infected, mass quarantine would necessitate a willingness to confine individuals on the basis of predictions about their future dangerousness. It would be the equivalent of mass preventive detention on an unprecedented scale and would "carry in [its] sweep persons who are determined to forgo the high-risk behavior that makes transmission possible; persons who are no longer infectious because the virus had eliminated its host cells; and persons who are so debilitated or demoralized as to be unable to engage in high-risk behavior."[25] Since it was widely assumed that HIV infection was lifelong, there was no logical point at which those detained could be released—the result, "a kind of civil life commitment."[26]

Despite the broad professional opposition to mass quarantine, public opinion polls tended to suggest, at times, that popular support for such measures did exist.[27] An ambiguously worded question put to a national sample surveyed by the Los Angeles *Times* found that 51 percent of the respondents believed that AIDS should be added "to the list of diseases that must be quarantined." A more carefully framed question posed by NBC one month later, in January 1986, revealed that 31 percent supported the statement "People who are known carriers of AIDS should be separated from the rest of the population." More focused constraints on those with HIV infection were supported by those surveyed by NBC. On two occasions more than 50 percent asserted that government should restrict the sexual activity of "known carriers of AIDS." Half of those polled by the Los Angeles *Times* in December 1985 believed that government should "make it a criminal offense for a person with AIDS to have sex with another person."

The more targeted use of the quarantine power to control the behavior of individuals with AIDS who seemed unwilling to consider the public health implications of their private acts also had the cautious support of some public health officials. Unlike the overly broad proposals that "carried in their sweep" those who posed no threat to others, the prospect of controlling individuals who demonstrated their willingness to inflict harm seemed tailored to the requirements of a public health practice that was cognizant of limits both practical and constitutional. Thus did James Mason declare in the same speech to the Republican Study Group of the House of Representatives in which he had derided mass quarantine, "There are situations where restricting the freedom of individuals appears to be justifiable, as in the case of infected individuals who are irresponsibly or deliberately transmitting the disease by their actions." The appropriateness of such a limited exercise in public health authority was also recognized by the U.S. Conference of Local Health Officers, which declared, "Medical isolation of persons should be considered only as a last resort in dealing with incorrigible individuals whose activities would otherwise lead to the further spread of the disease."[28]

In the wake of the initial wave of social anxiety about the transmission of AIDS, Connecticut became the first state to pass legislation permitting the quarantine of persons with communicable diseases who were judged to be a threat to the public health. Though the bill, enacted in June 1984, did not explicitly mention AIDS, clearly it was the new threat that had motivated the legislature. The text of the legislation embodied both the commitment to control when necessary and to the strictures of a circumscribed exercise of state power. "Any town, city, or borough Director of Health may order any person into confinement whom he has reasonable grounds to believe to be infected with any communicable disease . . . and who is unable or unwilling to conduct himself in such manner as to not expose others to dangers of infections. . . . A person confined shall . . . have a right to a court hearing." Among the tasks of such a court session would be the determination of whether the confinement was necessary and was "the least restrictive alternative to protect and preserve the public health."[29]

Despite its apparent recognition of the rights of those threatened with confinement and the invocation of the language of the least restrictive alternative, the Connecticut legislation was denounced by the state's Civil Liberties Union because it would permit the state to "sweep a person off the streets on mere suspicion."[30] Alvin Novick, who was to become president of the American Association of Physicians for Human Rights, spoke of the potential for the most egregious abuse of power. "Quarantine is such a devastating blow to someone's life. If it were invoked for someone with AIDS, it would forever after deprive them of jobs [and] social life. It would be used as a statement of social oppression that is not unknown in our society, but that today is hardly tolerable. People in public health are not precluded from being ignorant or evil, and there are people in public health who are evil and ignorant."[31] Such denunciations were to become standard as the issue of quarantine was raised in other states and as gay political groups and civil liberties organizations confronted moves by public health officials to deal with the problem of the recalcitrant.

An early instance of the fury that would greet such proposals occurred in California, where in 1983—before the isolation of the AIDS virus—a careful and detailed plan for the exercise of state intervention to control the behavior of "incorrigible" individuals with AIDS had been put forth. Asked to develop a policy that would permit the state of California to intervene when an individual with AIDS demonstrated an unwillingness to modify his or her sexual behavior, James Chin, chief of infectious diseases for the Department of Health Services, proposed a protocol that involved a graduated series of warnings culminating in quarantine, that was clearly based on his experience in dealing with recalcitrant tuberculosis patients.[32] Upon documentation that an individual with AIDS had failed to follow health department recommendations and had therefore exposed his sexual contacts "who are not aware that he has AIDS," the health department would issue a verbal and written warning about the need to adhere to behavioral standards that would prevent the transmission of a "possible AIDS agent." Failure to adhere to such warnings would result in a referral to an "AIDS support group" for counseling. A continued refusal to modify behavior would elicit an order of "modified isolation" stipulating the behavioral changes that were required and outlining the quarantine procedures that would be enforced if the modified isolation were violated. Finally, if the recalcitrant individual resisted such efforts, the local health department would "quarantine the patient's residence posting a placard that indicates that a person with a communicable disease which can be transmitted by intimate contact resides in the household."[33]

Asked to comment on the legal problems that such a course might encounter, the Office of Legal Services for the state reported back to Chin that state and local health officials had the legal authority to "take such measures as may be necessary to prevent the spread of disease."[34] Therefore, such officials would be well within their mandate to take those actions necessary to prevent the spread of AIDS. Indeed, it was suggested that since the violation of "orders of modified isolation" constituted a misdemeanor and since the willful exposure of an individual to a "contagious, infectious or communicable disease" also constituted a misdemeanor, referral to the district attorney for prosecution might occur much earlier in the staged course of intervention. On the other hand, the Office of Legal Services questioned the advisability of quarantining the home and posting a warning placard. "In many instance an AIDS patient may not reside in the community or locality where he is likely to be sexually active. In many cases, public exposure of this information would serve no productive purpose and would result in an unwarranted invasion of privacy."

For those who viewed the Chin proposal as representing a dangerous step that would entail the surveillance of sexual activity and a grave risk for ever-broader efforts on the part of the state to use coercive mechanisms to control the spread of AIDS, it mattered little that the infectious diseases chief had carefully circumscribed his proposal. Coming at a time when public anxiety about AIDS was high, Chin was accused of attempting to employ "Gestapo tactics" to control the epidemic.[35] However the courts might respond to such attempts at modified isolation, critics argued that "from a public policy perspective [they would be] inadvisable."[36] At best a few individuals—probably the least articulate and the poorest—would be caught in a web of control while the vast majority of individuals who engaged in such behavior would remain undetected. The impact on the epidemic, though not on individual liberty, would be negligible. If a broad quarantine involving all HIV-infected individuals "would isolate people who were not dangerous . . . a narrow behavior-linked one would do little more than scapegoat particular individuals."[37]

All proposals for the management of recalcitrants, no matter how carefully framed, provoked inevitable questions about the due-process protections that would be brought to bear in the determinations of infectiousness, the substantiation of charges of irresponsible and dangerous sexual behavior, and the establishment of the appropriate period of confinement and control. Some believed that the risks involved in the granting of authority to state officials were simply too great and the benefits of quarantine too unpredictable to warrant the extension of public health law to the control of private sexual behavior. In Oregon, for example, though the state task force on AIDS had stipulated in 1987 that quarantine be used only as a "last resort" in "egregious" situations and only after a hearing guided by "modern due process procedures," five of the thirty task force members found it necessary to dissent.[38] "Because the HIV (AIDS) virus is not spread by casual contact," they wrote, "and because we believe established legal measures sufficiently address dangerous behavior, the use of quarantine is never appropriate as a public health measure to prevent the spread of HIV infection."[39]

Unlike those who viewed public health law and its use for purposes of social defense against disease as a humane application of the state's power without the punitive implications of the criminal law, the opponents of quarantine saw primarily the threat of an unbridled exercise of power. Thus, many defenders of civil liberties asserted that they would, as a strategic matter, prefer that the criminal law be brought to bear in response to those who knowingly and willfully put others at risk for AIDS. Commenting on the advantages of the criminal law in such circumstances, one critic wrote, "The criminal law would punish only those individuals who were found after a full trial to have committed clearly proscribed acts. A criminal statute would not rely, as might a qaurantine, on uncertain predictions of future behavior and less than full procedural protections."[40] Thomas Stoddard, an attorney closely linked to both gay rights and civil liberties organizations, underscored the limits of the criminal law. "I would prefer the state dealing with these issues through criminal proceedings because there is greater assurance of fairness and due process. There is much greater danger that the state will abuse its power under quarantine and commitment procedures."[41] Not only had extraordinary abuses occurred when the state exercised its power to confine the mentally ill—long the subject of exposé and reformist zeal—but haunting the discussion of what the American public was capable of doing in times of social anxiety was the memory of the internment of Japanese-Americans during World War II.

The assault on quarantine and the defense of the criminal sanction in the context of AIDS was part of a much broader liberal challenge to the fundamental premises of public health law with its open-ended and discretionary features. While the vision of a forward-looking, scientific, and nonpunitive law, deriving its inspiration from medicine and inspired by a rehabilitative ideal, had once stood as a critical standard against which the archaic and retributive features of the criminal law could be judged, there had been a radical shift of perspective in the 1960s and 1970s.[42] Now it was the procedurally bounded and restricted exercise of the state's power to punish that stood as a model for the reform of public health law. First had come the cleansing of criminal law of its "medical" elements, the discarding of its mistaken rehabilitative pretentions. Then the leaner criminal law began to serve as a standard against which the principles of public health law and the exercise of public health power could be judged.

Under attack by liberals concerned about civil liberties, public health law was, ironically, viewed as inadequate also by those who sought a sterner, more aggressive social response to individuals whose behavior posed a risk of HIV transmission. For conservative critics, it was the retributive feature of the criminal law that most recommended its use; it was the nonpunitive ethos of public health law that was most disconcerting. In June 1985 Jerry Falwell, president of the fundamentalist Moral Majority, called for involuntary manslaughter charges against "AIDS carriers" who knowingly infected "a non-sufferer with a deadly disease resulting in his or her death."[43] In Idaho, legislation was introduced into the state House of Representatives making it a felony punishable by up to five years in prison and a fine up to $5,000 to engage in "any activity which would cause another to become infected with [AIDS]."[44] Among the prohibited activities were "donating blood or plasma, biting or spitting, or having sexual intercourse." Drawing on the legacy of repressive antisodomy statutes, the proposed legislation included among the prohibited acts "any crime against nature." Finally, in Pennsylvania a bill making it a misdemeanor for a person with AIDS to transmit the disease through sexual conduct was introduced. Conviction of a second offense would represent a second-degree felony.[45] Wherever proposed, such legislative efforts represented an attempt to apply to AIDS the law defining public health crimes, which in some states, including New York, Texas, California, and Colorado, already made it a criminal offense for an individual with a venereal disease to have sexual intercourse.[46] Though rarely enforced, such statutes were a legacy of a period in which venereal diseases had generated considerable social consternation. Nevertheless, they stood as a symbolic statement of societal condemnation. It was from such symbolic significance that efforts to criminalize sexual intercourse by individuals with AIDS derived their attraction.

In some instances prosecutors used extant criminal laws to initiate the prosecution of those with AIDS or HIV infection. Thus, for example, in Minneapolis an HIV-infected prison inmate was indicted by a federal grand jury on charges of assault with a deadly weapon because he had bitten two guards.[47] The U.S. Army decided to court-martial a soldier on charges of aggravated assault because, though he had been told he was HIV antibody positive, he had had sexual relations with three other soldiers—two women and one man—without adequately warning them of the risks he posed.[48] These were but the first cases as law enforcement officials began to consider the question "Can AIDS Be a Deadly Weapon?"[49]

The potential role of quarantine and the criminal law in controlling the spread of AIDS became the subject of debate as the question surfaced of whether HIV-infected prostitutes represented a public health threat. For those who feared that too little was being done to control the epidemic, the HIV-infected prostitute stood as an image of uncontrolled contamination. For those who feared that the state would use the occasion of AIDS to invade the realms of privacy and sexuality, threats against prostitutes were emblematic of the much broader threats against all individuals infected with the AIDS virus.

There was indeed a historical legacy, dating from the first decades of the century, of focusing on prostitutes as the source of social contamination through venereal disease. By 1918 thirty-two states had enacted legislation requiring the compulsory examination of prostitutes for venereal diseases.[50] Prostitutes were also the target of detention and quarantine. Defending such practices, U.S. Attorney General T. W. Gregory declared, "The constitutional right of the community, in the interest of public health, to ascertain the existence of infectious and communicable diseases in its midst and to isolate and quarantine such cases or take steps necessary to prevent the spread of disease is clear."[51] At the height of anxiety about how venereal diseases could affect the well-being of the U.S. armed forces during World War I, Congress appropriated more than $1 million for the detention of venereal disease carriers. During the war, more than 30,000 prostitutes were detained under the aegis of the federal government.[52] Defending this procedure, a federal official argued that "conditions require the immediate isolation of as many venereally-infected persons acting as spreaders of disease as could be quickly apprehended and quarantined. It was not a measure instituted for the punishments of prostitutes on account of infractions of the civil or moral law, but was strictly a public health measure to prevent the spread of dangerous, communicable diseases."[53]

Seven decades later, as social anxiety about AIDS gripped American society, some prosecutors and public health officials sought to meet the challenge by restraining HIV-infected prostitutes. The Georgia Task Force on AIDS recommended that women convicted of prostitution be tested for HIV antibody and counseled about the risks of transmission. Those arrested again would face more severe penalties. When questioned about the legality of this proposal, the chairman of the task force responded, "Our sense of the matter is to let the lawyers worry about the constitutional questions . . . that are raised by people who don't want to do something."[54] In Florida a judge released a prostitute with AIDS to her home after an electrical monitoring device was attached to her so that she could not move more than 200 feet from her phone. "I wanted her off the streets, for the protection of the public, but on the other hand, I knew that jail employees were concerned."[55] Since the fall of 1986, Florida has required the screening of all convicted prostitutes for HIV infection and other sexually transmitted diseases.[56] Those testing positive who subsequently engage in prostitution may be convicted of a misdemeanor. Finally, in Mississippi, an HIV-infected but asymptomatic male prostitute with a record of sixty-six prostitution-related arrests was subjected to a quarantine order that prohibited him from having sexual relations without first notifying his partners and customers about his condition, though the state epidemiologist acknowledged that such an order would be exceedingly difficult to enforce.[57] Violation of the provisions of this order, which was not time bound, would subject the prostitute to as much as six months in jail as well as a fine.

Such efforts attracted considerable attention and raised a sense of alarm among those concerned about the imposition of coercive methods to control the spread of AIDS. But more striking was how relatively rare attempts had been to apply either public health or criminal law to prostitutes during the first years of the epidemic. Frustrated by what he believed was an enduring impasse over how to confront the problem of infected male and female prostitutes, Robert Bernstein, commissioner of health in Texas, where a celebrated case involving a male prostitute had confounded the police and health officials, exclaimed, "No one wants to talk about the problem of infected prostitutes."[58] In El Paso County, Colorado, the discovery of HIV infection among a small number of female prostitutes produced a flurry of concern on the part of local health officials. Calls to Miami, San Francisco, and Atlanta had provided little guidance about how to proceed. "As far as we can tell," said the county's health director, "no one is handling it."[59]

When public health officials in San Francisco and New York were willing to address the issue, it was with extraordinary caution. Dean Echenberg, of San Francisco's Health Department, asserted that quarantines had no role to play in the public response to infected prostitutes, male or female. "It's not like TB or typhoid. With AIDS it takes a consensual act to get infected. Public education is the most important thing."[60] In New York City, David Sencer, commissioner of health during the first five years of the epidemic, even warned about the dangers of focusing too closely on the issue of prostitution. "When we begin to mount large social studies of prostitutes, this poses civil rights problems. . . . It's not illegitimate to be a homosexual, but it is against the law to be a prostitute."[61] Here, as in so many other ways, New York City sought to "keep the city without overt panic."[62] How very different the approach to AIDS and prostitution was from the legacy of mass arrests, imprisonment, forced testing, and quarantine of the early days of the antivenereal disease drives.

In part, the difference can be explained by the changed legal situation surrounding the use of coercive powers of the state, in part by changed social attitudes toward sexuality and privacy. The mid-1980s was not 1918. Nor was it the 1940s, when, just after the discovery of penicillin, a vigorous campaign against venereal diseases was launched.[63] The difference, however, at least in relation to female prostitutes, was attributable also to the role of women in the spread of AIDS in the United States during the first five years of the epidemic. Primarily a disease of homosexual men and intravenous drug users, AIDS occurred relatively infrequently in women. By 1987, women constituted less than 7 percent of all AIDS cases. Furthermore, how infected women might transmit HIV to their sexual partners was not well understood.[64]

The first major report on the role of female prostitutes in the spread of AIDS came from Robert Redfield of the Walter Reed Army Hospital in 1985[65] and was greeted with considerable skepticism by critics who doubted the reliability of information provided to army epidemiologists.[66] Could soldiers be trusted to reveal their drug use and homosexual activity when both were grounds for dishonorable discharge? However theoretically possible female to male transmission might be—venereal diseases were always transmitted in a bidirectional manner—and whatever the distribution of AIDS in Africa indicated, where as many women as men were afflicted, the epidemiological data in the United States simply did not support the notion that women would have a significant role as a reservoir of HIV infection—so Redfield's critics asserted.[67]

Though a number of epidemiological studies had attempted to determine the level of HIV infection among female prostitutes, it was not until the spring of 1987, when the Centers for Disease Control reported on a multicity seroprevalence study, that an empirical characterization of the situation became possible.[68] A very wide range in the levels of infection with the AIDS virus was found: from 32 of 56 prostitutes—57 percent—in northern New Jersey, where heroin addiction was the single most important predictor of infection; to 1 of 92 prostitutes—1.1 percent—in Atlanta on the East Coast. In the western states the range was from 9 of 146 prostitutes in San Francisco to none of the 34 prostitutes screened in Las Vegas.

In New York City opposition to focusing on female prostitutes as a potential threat to heterosexual males merged scientific considerations—New York City's epidemiologists remained the most vocal opponents of the proposition that HIV could be readily transmitted from women to men—and political concerns about the untoward social consequences that could follow from such a course.[69] But the relative restraint that framed the response to prostitution, both male and female, stemmed also from a recognition that, given the epidemiology of AIDS, broad-scale moves against prostitutes would have relatively little impact on the rate of HIV transmission. Stephen Schultz, a deputy commissioner of the New York Health Department, warned of wasted energies. "Prostitutes pose a theoretical risk of AIDS transmission but not a practical one."[70] Attention to them would divert energy and resources from more pressing AIDS control strategies.

In the spring of 1985, when few scientific studies were available, Ann Hardy of the Centers for Disease Control told the Public Health Service Executive Task Force on AIDS that she believed there was little evidence that prostitutes were major transmitters of AIDS.[71] Even Thomas Vernon, executive director of the Colorado Health Department, and an advocate of using sanctions against HIV-infected individuals where necessary, declared, "Frankly, the effective control program is not going to be isoloation and quarantine. . . . It's going to be a message that says, 'Every time you sleep with a prostitute, you are sleeping with her last half-dozen sex partners and all the diseases that those partners might have brought.' "[72] Commenting on the fate of an incarcerated male prostitute who would ultimately become the subject of a quarantine order, the executive director of the Mississippi Gay Alliance noted that attempts to focus on prostitutes would miss the far more troubling pattern of sexual behavior in noncommercial settings. "I don't think that what this guy in jail is doing is any worse than what a lot of other people are doing. . . . The only difference is that he is getting paid for it."[73]

That wholesale attempts to test prostitutes coercively for HIV infection and to use the force of law to prohibit the infected from engaging in the sale of sex had not occurred in the first years of the AIDS epidemic mattered less to those committed to the protection of civil liberties than the fact that such efforts had occasionally been made. Indeed, civil libertarians believed that it was only a matter of time before broader efforts would be undertaken. When the CDC first addressed the issue of AIDS and prostitution in March 1987, it had simply suggested that efforts to halt the spread of HIV infection from prostitutes might include "additional control measures by local health departments and law enforcement agencies."[74] Five months later, in August 1987, when the Public Health Service issued a broad report on HIV screening, it stated more forcefully, "Male and female prostitutes should be counseled and tested. Particularly prostitutes who are HIV-positive should be instructed to discontinue the practice of prostitution. Local or state jurisdictions should adopt procedures to assure that these instructions are followed."[75] This trend underscored the importance of articulating the appropriate principles of privacy in matters of sexuality before the wholesale abrogation of rights began to occur. It was this concern that influenced the American Civil Liberties Union as it confronted the issue of state interference with consensual sexual activity, using the case of the "willful prostitute" as the paradigmatic problem with which it had to deal.

The Civil Liberties Union and Quarantine

Though the American Civil Liberties Union had never developed a fully formulated position on the use of the quarantine power in the face of infectious and communicable diseases, the evolving perspective of those committed to civil liberties on matters such as the confinement of the mentally ill, due-process protections for those charged with criminal offenses, the limits of the state's power in dealing with victimless crimes, and matters of sexual expression presaged the stance that would be adopted when AIDS posed its challenge. When the Northern California branch of the American Civil Liberties Union adopted its wide-ranging policy "AIDS and Civil Liberties" in March 1986, it denounced the "routine generalized" quarantine of individuals with frank disease or of those who were asymptomatic but seropositive as "inappropriate," as a "grave" threat to civil liberties, and utterly unjustified by the medical understanding of the transmission of HIV.[76] This rather unexceptional statement was, however, remarkably silent on the issue that was far more critical than that of wholesale quarantine—the use of state power to control individuals who demonstrated by their behavior an unwillingness to consider the hazard they posed for transmitting a lethal infection. But this was no oversight. The committee that had drafted the position on AIDS for the consideration of the board of the Northern California branch of the ACLU had intentionally omitted any discussion of circumstances "in which quarantine might be an appropriate government response to control the spread of AIDS."[77] Committed to the protection of civil liberties, it was not the "ACLU's business to propose when it might be permissible for the government" to violate the rights of those with AIDS or the carriers of HIV infection. Neither the statement on mass quarantine nor the decision to avoid a consideration of more focused efforts at control provoked substantial discussion as the board unanimously approved its committee's work.

Paralleling the efforts of the Northern California branch of the Civil Liberties Union to fashion a broad statement on AIDS was that of the national ACLU. The Privacy Committee, under whose aegis the policy was being developed, did receive a draft proposal acknowledging that quarantine or detention could be relied upon "when there is reasonable cause to believe [a] person poses a substantial and immediate threat to the health of others and willfully refuses to tailor his or her conduct accordingly," but it, like the California committee, chose to reject such a posture.[78] In its deliberations, the Privacy Committee considered the issue of the "willful prostitute" as the paradigmatic case of an individual who willingly and knowingly infects others with the AIDS virus.[79] While it did not "condone" such acts, described as the "rare scenario," the committee rejected the use of the criminal law as a response to such behavior, since it viewed any criminal sanction on sexual activity as violating individual privacy. On the other hand, the committee was willing to acknowledge that an individual infected by a willful prostitute could bring suit for damages in a civil action. What distinguished AIDS from other communicable diseases—where the Privacy Committee had just acknowledged that coercion including the use of isolation, quarantine, and the criminal sanction might be applied under appropriate circumstances and under carefully defined procedural protections—was that sexual behavior was involved. In that realm a prohibition on governmental intrusions had become a virtual orthodoxy for the Civil Liberties Union.

And so when the ACLU's Board of Directors met in mid-April 1986, it had before it a proposed AIDS policy that not only denounced routine quarantine as a "severe deprivation of liberty [that was] never an appropriate public health measure to deal with AIDS in light of the modes of transmission of the disease," but rejected state intervention of a more focused kind directed at behaviors clearly implicated in the transmission of the disease. "The government may not restrict consensual activity among adults, even where one or both parties has AIDS or has been exposed to the virus. This includes, but is not limited to, criminalization of sexual activity. . . . Such government actions intrude deeply into the right of privacy."[80]

Some members of the board, which included a broader array of perspectives on civil liberties than that found on the Privacy Committee, were deeply troubled by the question of whether the state could use its power to discourage those with AIDS or HIV infection from having sexual relations without first informing their partners of the risks involved. Those who favored, or at least were not opposed to the use of governmental sanctions, argued that when individuals consented to sexual relations they did not also consent to placing themselves at risk for AIDS. Hence the government could legitimately punish those who "knowingly or recklessly" infected others. The invocation of privacy did not provide a warrant for inflicting harm.

Those opposed to the recognition of such state authority saw in it a profound challenge to the most fundamental precepts of civil liberties. State sanctions would open the way to the intrusion of the full apparatus of the criminal justice system into intimate sexual relations, including those occurring in the privacy of the home. Search warrants would be issued. Police investigations would be conducted. Grand juries would hear charges on matters involving consensual sexual activity. No civil libertarian, committed to the protection of privacy, could countenance "governmental intrusion[s] into the most intimate and private aspects of people's lives." Furthermore, the untoward consequences would be compounded by the epidemiological reality of AIDS. Permitting the state to impose sanctions would inevitably "increase the harassment and oppression of high-risk groups," especially gay men and intravenous drug users. Finally, such efforts would not serve the public health ends they putatively were designed to advance. The gay community would be "forced" underground, thus inhibiting the fight against AIDS.

The ACLU's board voted explicitly to reject the use of the criminal sanction to protect those who might unknowingly be infected by individuals who knew themselves to be carriers of HIV. But at the same time it went on to subvert its position. Demonstrating its own confusion about how to proceed, it endorsed a proposal on consensual sexual activity that appeared to limit opposition to the use of the state's sanctions—including the criminal law—to situations in which individuals had given their "informed consent" to possible exposure to HIV infection. "Without such informed consent," said a board member, "the privacy interest is not present." To forestall the adoption of a policy they viewed as anathema, the opponents of the informed-consent proviso—"conditional privacy is a contradiction in terms"—successfully employed a parliamentary maneuver to refer the issue back to the Privacy Committee, ostensibly to provide greater clarity for the board in its deliberations.[81]

In the fall of 1986 the Privacy Committee, mindful of the confused parameters set by the board's actions, met twice to consider the issue of AIDS and consensual sexual activity.[82] The language of informed consent was found by the committee to be incompatible with the protection of the privacy of sexual relations. Opposition to the criminalization of sexual activity, "something the ACLU has never countenanced," led the committee to reject not only any endorsement of sanctions in the case of those who knowingly infected others but any reference to how extant assault and battery laws could be used in such situations. Though it viewed the invocation of civil liability as less threatening, "since it involves no threat of *a priori* government regulation of sexual activity," and though it recognized that noting the availability of tort actions would satisfy the board's concern about the protection of the potential victims of HIV infection, the committee ultimately chose to remain silent on even this matter. Those who were the victims of HIV-infected individuals needed no guidance. They would "inevitably invoke civil liability on their own." Even an explicit reference to tort action was thus deemed a dangerous invitation to further state intrusions. Only public education "aimed at those with AIDS and those who might be their sexual partners" was deemed completely consistent with the ACLU's concern for privacy. The committee thus proposed to the board the following resolution: "While there is a need for public education encouraging individuals who have been exposed to the HTLV virus to act so as not to transmit the virus, and for education as to the risk of sexual activity with those who have AIDS, nevertheless, the right of individual privacy which extends to the sexual acts of consenting adults prohibits government regulation including criminalization of sexual activity and restrictions on non-public places where sexual activity takes place."[83]

When the ACLU's board once again took up the issue in January 1987, little new emerged during the debate.[84] With limited support for the use of the criminal sanction and with concern about how the incorporation of the language of informed consent could provide a warrant for such sanctions, the board finally elected to endorse the decision of the Privacy Committee. To demonstrate its concern for the potential victims of unconsented exposure to HIV, the board did, however, append an explicit, though weakly phrased acknowledgment that civil damages could be brought under such circumstances. "[The right of privacy] does not necessarily bar civil remedies in tort."

Unlike those who questioned the utility of meeting the challenge of AIDS by isolating and controlling individuals whose behavior exposed others to the threat of disease, or those who warned that recourse to coercion would subvert the attainment of the broad public health goal of mass behavioral change, the ACLU staked out a position on the basis of principle. Where matters of sexuality were involved the principled commitment to privacy was so stringently defined that even the willful or malicious infliction of injury could not provide a warrant for state intervention. Such a conception of privacy entailed a disregard for not only the rights of the injured but the health of the public as well. It was a conception of privacy that reflected the triumph of an ideology of asocial individualism.

The Politics of Quarantine: Texas, Colorado, California

The first full public airing of the issue of how to control the behavior of HIV-infected individuals who demonstrated little regard for the well-being of their sexual partners came in Texas in the fall of 1985, when the commissioner of health, Robert Bernstein, announced that he would ask the state's board of health to add AIDS to the list of quarantinable diseases that already included cholera, tuberculosis, gonorrhea, syphilis, and other communicable conditions.[85]

Bernstein's move to obtain the authority to impose restrictions on individuals with AIDS who "for some reason [were] spreading the disease knowingly" was made with a full appreciation of the very limited role it would play in the overall strategy to control AIDS in Texas.[86] "It probably won't be used much, but it does give us another tool under certain circumstances to be able to control an infection."[87] The decision to seek quarantine power in the face of AIDS came after a number of well-publicized events in Texas. In Houston, Fabian Bridges, a black man with AIDS who would become the subject of a nationally broadcast documentary in the spring of 1986, had become the object of public alarm when he declared that he would continue to engage in sexual activity, including prostitution. The realization on the part of the city's health commissioner, James Houghton, that he did not have the power to impose an order of quarantine and the failure of police efforts to limit Bridges' actions had forced public officials to confront the limits of their practical and administrative authority in dealing with such cases.[88]

Spurred by the situation, the chief health officer of the San Antonio Metropolitan Health District, backed by the county's district attorney, sent a warning letter to each individual with AIDS in his district. "While local patients with AIDS have, until now, been acting responsibily in avoiding those practices which can lead to transmission of the AIDS virus to others, I now have reports of at least three (3) diagnosed AIDS patients [who] have indicated their intent to act recklessly in their contacts with others, without regard for the health implications which such conduct has for those who unsuspectingly become involved. . . . You are hereby ordered to refrain from any activity which could lead to the spread of the AIDS virus."[89] Included among the prohibited acts was sexual intercourse with anyone not diagnosed as having AIDS, the sharing of drug-use paraphernalia, and donations of blood and body tissue. Furthermore, all individuals with AIDS were ordered to inform their physicians and dentists about their condition. Failure to abide by these requirements would be met by the initiation of criminal proceedings, which under Texas law would involve a third-degree felony, punishable by a maximum of ten years' imprisonment.

An outcry from gay and civil liberties groups greeted the San Antonio letter. Texas Civil Liberties Union Executive Director Gara La Marche warned the district attorney, whose enforcement authority was to be called upon by the health department, of the dangers that would follow from politicized moves like those he was considering. Utterly unacceptable invasions of privacy would be required in any attempt to act upon the threats being directed at individuals with AIDS. "[How do you] plan to enforce this new policy? Will AIDS victims be in jeopardy of quarantine or criminal prosecution if they engage in any sort of intimate contact or just in non-safe practices—i.e., anal intercourse? How do you plan to determine whether AIDS victims have violated these restrictions?" Acknowledging the impact of the Fabian Bridges case, La Marche cautioned about developing policy on the basis of an extraordinary and isolated event. To do so "always runs a great risk of violating individual rights."[90] To those who were appalled by the tone of the letter, its threat, and the scope of its provisions, Courand Rothe, San Antonio's director of health, stated, "I'm not interested in putting people in jail. I just want to control this disease."[91]

This then was the context within which Bernstein's proposal was made to the Texas Board of Health. Rising social anxiety sparked by the Bridges case had produced pressure for action on the part of public health officials. "You've got to look at the public's reaction," said the state's chief epidemiologist. "People want to have some reassurance that public health agencies are in control of the situation."[92] On the other hand, the first moves, like those undertaken in San Antonio, suggested that when public health officials did act, they might do so in ways that threatened profound invasions of privacy. Of paramount importance to those concerned about the rights of gay men and more generally the right of sexual privacy was the possibility that policies designed to manage "very rare cases" would ineluctably lead to more extensive controls over individuals with AIDS, as well as those infected with HIV or at risk for infection.

But the significance of Bernstein's move went beyond the limited situation in Texas. For those concerned about the adequacy of the public health response to AIDS, Bernstein's effort represented an important step. Kristine Gebbie, administrator of the Oregon

Health Department and chair of the AIDS Task Force of the Association of State and Territorial Health Officials, lauded the announcement of the Texas health commissioner. Bernstein, a former president of ASTHO, had taken the first public action on a matter "privately under discussion by many health officials."[93] For those concerned about how moves in Texas could provoke a rash of quarantine proposals, the significance of the debate in that state was far-reaching. Thus Nancy Langer, speaking for the Lambda Legal Defense and Education Fund, said, "We don't want that kind of misconceived policy to come to the attention of other health commissioners around the country. This is going to attract a certain amount of notice and other people could decide that they want to get on the bandwagon."[94]

Those who opposed the call for quarantine power did not deny that there were indeed some individuals who, though afflicted with AIDS, continued to behave in ways that put others at risk. But they emphasized how rare such cases were. "No one knows better than [those with AIDS] how terrible the disease is, and they wouldn't want to spread it," said Jeff Levi of the National Gay Task Force.[95] Indeed, despite the fact that no one knew how many persons diagnosed with AIDS did engage in unsafe sexual behavior, both proponents and opponents of the quarantine power seemed implicitly committed to underscoring the exceptional nature of the problem, the former in order to contain anxiety about how broad-scale the control efforts would have to be, the latter to prove that new policies of control were unnecessary, a response to an exceedingly marginal issue. Neither side in Texas sought a full airing of the issue of infected asymptomatic individuals and their behavior.

Bernstein's antagonists acknowledged that it would be necessary to intervene in cases of irresponsible behavior on the part of individuals with AIDS. What they either rejected on principle or were extremely reluctant to admit was that the state's coercive power might, on occasion, be called for. "Social services" were needed, not "police force."[96] Indeed, an adequate program of education was central to both communal prevention and individual behavioral modification. Speaking for the Austin Lesbian-Gay Political Caucus, Bill Foster underscored the themes that were to be repeated over the next month. "The inclusion of AIDS as a communicable disease under the state quarantine law may allay fears of the general public, but would, in fact, be nothing more than a smokescreen and a misdirection of public resources. Everybody wants these people off the street. We think by having a place in the community where these people are counseled and made to feel that they have a home would give as good a chance . . . as waiting around for them to have sex and arresting them."[97]

In the face of a rising tide of opposition from gay political leaders, civil liberties groups, and their political allies, Bernstein called a special meeting for the end of November 1985, at which he hoped to mollify his critics. Sensitive to the concern of those who feared that all individuals with AIDS would be subject to surveillance and control, Bernstein stressed his limited purpose. "We have no intentions whatsoever of isolating the average AIDS patient. . . . It's only a means of dealing with an AIDS-infected person who might not behave properly."[98] Aware of the fears generated by the very word "quarantine," the health commissioner sought to allay anxiety by acknowledging that the term was inapt. Since quarantines had been used historically to control the spread of illnesses that were easily transmitted and had served to warn "Don't come near this house," gay leaders were understandably worried that the public would disregard the lessons about how the AIDS virus passed from one person to another. Hence Bernstein declared, "We'll use a word like 'isolate,' which is a medical term." Finally, to provide reassurance to those who feared that empowered by quarantine authority, county health officials would launch campaigns against AIDS patients bearing little relationship to the very circumscribed program being proposed, Bernstein stipulated that he would maintain ultimate authority over decisions to seek isolation of recalcitrant individuals. "With 254 counties, all with health officials, something might happen that would violate, at least the spirit, of what we are trying to do."[99]

Coming from that session, Bernstein announced to the press that he had been able to win over those who had been so critical of his effort. Local newspapers did, in fact, convey the impression that some leaders of the gay community were pleased by the commissioner's stated intention to put forth a carefully limited proposal to the Texas Board of Health in mid-December. But whatever the understanding and perspective of some gay leaders at the time of the meeting with Bernstein, the politically organized elements of the gay community quickly moved to dispel the impression of cooperation. Representatives of the gay community had agreed prior to the meeting that quarantine was "unacceptable and non-negotiable."

But the commissioner had "failed to hear or to understand what our representatives were saying. In the final analysis, Dr. Bernstein manipulated this meeting and the media. At his news conference, [he] told the media that there was 'no opposition from the gay community on the issue of isolation' (his new euphemism for 'quarantine'). This comment came after a two-hour meeting where the chilling effects of quarantine were spelled out to him."[100]

To mobilize opposition to Bernstein from the gay community across Texas, the Lesbian and Gay Rights Advocates called upon its organizational affiliates to launch a letter-writing campaign to the State Board of Health that would stress the counterproductive consequences of pursuing quarantine (which would "undermine most devastatingly the public health and epidemiological network that is critical to control AIDS") and underscore that such a course would only create an "erroneous impression that something is being done about AIDS."[101] In fact, resources would be diverted from "proven, workable" approaches to dealing with AIDS. Education and counseling were the first lines of defense.

Though considerable attention was devoted in the pronouncements of gay groups to the deleterious consequences for the public health that could follow from any attempt to invoke the powers of quarantine, it was an ideological opposition to the intrusion of the state into matters affecting sexual behavior that animated the opposition. A history of repression and the existence of sodomy laws across the United States made the prospect of government intervention anathema. The bathhouse controversy had underscored the rejection by gay leaders of the judgments of public health officials, who sought to regulate consensual sexual activity in commercial settings. Opposition to the recourse to quarantine went further. It represented a rejection of the imposition of state sanctions even when a failure to warn one's sexual partners about the threat of HIV infection undermined the very conditions of consent. So thoroughgoing was the ideological commitment to individualism that gay leaders were compelled to embrace a perspective within which sexual partners were to view each other as potential agents of harm. Not trust, but self-defense, was to provide the basis for protection from the threat of HIV transmission in the most private of settings. This was an individualism that would, ironically, subvert the very meaning of intimacy.

Providing a skillfully worded summary of the arguments that

would in one form or another appear in each denunciation of Bernstein's proposed course was an article in the Austin *American Statesman* by Jeff Levi of the National Gay Task Force. Quarantining AIDS patients, even the few irresponsible patients, would have no impact on halting the spread of AIDS, since such an effort would have no impact on asymptomatic carriers, who could only be identified through the mass mandatory screening of the entire population. Only education of the sexually active, both heterosexual and homosexual, would "eliminate" the spread of HIV infection by teaching individuals about how they might protect themselves. An understanding of how HIV was transmitted was the ultimate source of defense both for individuals and for society. Thus, in the face of a grave social threat, Levi asserted that "taking personal responsibility for health is a far more sensible approach than seeking to scapegoat those already ill, through quarantine."[102] Not only was Bernstein's proposal a mistaken course in terms of prevention, but his efforts might undermine the state's epidemiological work by creating a profound disincentive to the reporting of AIDS cases to state health officials. Patients with early signs of AIDS might be so frightened that they would delay both needed treatment and the counseling that was so critical for the interruption of the spread of AIDS. Finally, for the "exceptional case" of the irresponsible AIDS patient, Levi proposed counseling and compassion rather than the imposition of control through quarantine procedures. Indeed, the case of Fabian Bridges demonstrated how effective such a community approach could be. State officials who sought quarantine powers were responding to public hysteria and the pressure to demonstrate that they had the threat of AIDS under control. But the panic would only return more dramatically when it became clear that quarantine had brought only false hope.

Responding to the appeal of the Lesbian/Gay Rights Advocates, letters of protest came not only from gay political and AIDS-related organizations in Texas but from the National Gay Task Force[103] and the Washington-based AIDS Action Council.[104] At the behest of the NGTF, the president of the United States Conference of Local Health Officers wrote of its own deliberations on the issue of quarantine. "It was the consensus . . . that quarantine of AIDS patients should be contemplated with the utmost caution." A resolution of the conference thus stated, "Basic civil and human rights should not be compromised by misguided public health practices." Without condemning Bernstein's initiative, the Conference president warned, "We urge you to weigh carefully the long-term implications in including AIDS among quarantinable diseases."[105]

On December 15, the Board of Health in a 12-5 vote gave tentative approval to Bernstein's proposal, thus commencing a thirty-day period for public comment before final action could be taken.[106] Among those casting votes in opposition was the board's president, who though appreciative of Bernstein's concerns, expressed discomfort about the reliance on a quarantine statute that he viewed as "archaic."[107] For the Lesbian/Gay Rights Advocates who had orchestrated the opposition to quarantine, the board's action came as a bitter rebuff. "We had hoped that the board would have made a different decision today so that we could get on with the projects under way in our communities dealing with the illness. Instead, our time and energies will have to be directed towards the Board of Health to educate them of our concerns."[108]

When at last public hearings were held on the proposed rule, twenty-one individuals came forward to testify, only one of whom supported the proposal for quarantine. James Houghton, director of Houston's Health Department, whose plea to Commissioner Bernstein had been so critical to the decision to fashion a new rule for AIDS, stated that the new measure was no threat to the gay community.[109] Focusing on the fears expressed during the prior three months, he urged gay leaders to calm the unwarranted distress provoked by Bernstein's effort. "I would beseech you not to stimulate fear where there is no need for fear, [not to] stimulate hysteria where there is no need for hysteria." Opposing the proposed rule were representatives of gay groups from across the state and the Texas Civil Liberties Union.[110] Mathilde Krim, a nationally prominent leader in the effort to mobilize resources for research into the treatment of AIDS, flew to Texas to voice her concern.[111] The arguments advanced by Commissioner Bernstein's opponents were by this time all well known. What was striking was the bitter antagonism that had been engendered by the proposal. For Bernstein, it was his opponents who were "fanning the flames of fear" by focusing on matters that were "not germane to the relatively minor thing we are trying to do."[112]

But despite this denunciation, Bernstein made a stunning about-face just three days after the public hearings. At a January 16 press conference he announced that he would ask the Board of Health to withdraw from consideration his proposal for medical isolation.[113] Virtually repeating the arguments made by those with whom he had been locked in conflict, Bernstein explained that the potential benefits that would be obtained by the infrequent use of the quarantine authority were outweighed by the effect that enactment of the proposed rule would have on the relationship between the health department and the gay community. Confronted with an epidemic that could be brought under control only by the modification of the behavior of those at risk of infection, Bernstein had been compelled to acknowledge the importance of preserving an open and cooperative relationship with the gay community. "We consider the relationship of this department and the gay community as important—vitally important—to influence the incidence of AIDS. . . . That relationship would suffer out of all proportion to the value gained. . . . We have no vaccine for the disease. We have no treatment. The only thing we have is education in the high risk groups. The gay community has to be part of that education process."[114] Whether the threat to the overall program of AIDS prevention was brought home to Bernstein in the course of the hearings by the president of the Board of Health, who warned that the commissioner no longer had a majority,[115] or whether the politically divisive atmosphere had moved the governor to press Bernstein to withdraw his proposal, gay opponents had, in effect, exercised a veto.[116]

In withdrawing his proposal, Bernstein also acceded to the demand of his opponents to reactivate the state's AIDS task force and to expand its membership to incorporate the full participation of the gay community. Among the group's missions was to be the fashioning of an alternative to the proposal that had proved so politically disastrous. "We haven't abandoned the idea of finding a way to restrain irresponsible people with AIDS from knowingly spreading this deadly disease, but I am convinced that we can and will find a more acceptable method for handling this rare problem."[117]

To those who had fought Bernstein since late October, his decision came as a welcome surprise, not only because it represented a victory in Texas, but because of the message it sent to the nation. Gara La Marche of the Texas Civil Liberties Union hoped that the Texas decision "would be a turning point in the wave of public fear and hysteria that has accompanied the AIDS issue."[118] Jeff Levi of the National Gay Task Force believed that the outcome in Texas would serve as a warning to health officials across the country. "It will cause anyone else considering this route to think twice."[119] For Ben Schatz of the National Gay Rights Advocates, the victory in Texas was important because it would "help to mobilize people in other states to fight similar legislation."[120] But for those who were appalled by what they viewed as an unwarranted capitulation to gay political pressure, Bernstein had simply reached an "accommodation with the sodomites."[121]

Spurred by the challenge that surfaced during the controversy over AIDS, the health department undertook in the following year a major statutory revision of the state's Communicable Disease and Control Act. Most critical was the incorporation of a new article with provisions that carefully detailed a range of safeguards absent from the older statute—the right to representation by counsel, the right to a timely hearing, and the right to jury trial.[122] Unlike the pre-revision act, which like public health laws enacted in prior decades provided only the option of quarantine in the face of "incorrigible" individuals afflicted with communicable diseases, the proposed law acknowledged the importance of employing the "least restrictive alternative" to protect the public health, of using outpatient care as an alternative to isolation.

In all, the revised statute reflected the influence of due-process considerations in the fashioning of contemporary public health law, which for so long had remained insulated from the transformations in American jurisprudence. The conditions under which the revised communicable disease statute emerged also reflected the profound impact of political conflict in the making of public health policy. One year after it had successfully blocked Commissioner Bernstein's effort to extend the quarantine power to some individuals with AIDS, the coalition of gay groups offered its support to the health department's proposed statute."We feel it is a necessary tool for public health officials to have—and politically it is the least restrictive law that we could possibly have. Without this proposal being adopted, we expect that something much more onerous would be proposed by the right wing of the legislature."[123]

If in Texas the issue of quarantine provoked bitter controversy and then accommodation with opponents of state control over individuals who behaved in ways that threatened to spread AIDS, in Colorado a year-long political struggle ultimately led to the passage in 1987 of an AIDS bill that included provisions for quarantine, despite the opposition of gay groups. The saga of Colorado's effort began in February 1986, when conservative state representative Dale E. Erickson proposed legislation that many considered utterly devoid of appropriate confidentiality protections and lacking any appreciation of the importance of due process when deprivations of liberty were threatened.[124] In a letter to his colleagues in both houses of the Colorado legislature, Erickson had written, "Until now, neither Congress nor any state has proposed legislative action to provide for the isolation or control of this dreaded disease. Present consensus seems to favor legislative attention to isolate and control, where possible, this virus. Historically, legislation for the control of scarlet fever, smallpox, venereal disease, tuberculosis and other communicable diseases, have proven effective until remedies were perfected. . . . If quarantine of some individuals is necessary, then let's use the proven measures of previous legislation. There is nothing heinous in this approach, only long-proven, accepted common sense."[125]

Passed by the lower house, Erickson's bill underwent substantial revision in the state senate. Provisions derived from model legislation designed to protect the confidentiality of venereal disease reports to state health departments were added, so that reports of AIDS cases and HIV test results would not be subject to subpoena, search warrant, or other discovery proceedings. Furthermore, legislative reformers, backed by Thomas Vernon, the executive director of the State Health Department, saw in the legislation an opportunity to revise the very broad standard statutory language that provided the basis of quarantine in Colorado[126]—"[The Department shall] exercise such physical control over property and the person of the people of this state as the Department may find necessary for the protection of the public health."[127] In fact, Vernon believed that in confronting AIDS it would be possible to make modifications in "laws written early in this century [that were] no longer consistent with the evolution of due process rights and practices."[128]

The senate-imposed amendments would have required that verbal and written warnings be given prior to the issuance of an isolation order; that the state bear the burden of proof in demonstrating the necessity of control for the protection of the public health; that the level of control imposed be consonant with the least restrictive alternative standard; and that court review be available at each stage of the process.[129] Nevertheless, gay groups saw in the bill "a direct, clear challenge to the civil liberties of thousands of Coloradans."[130]

Despite such opposition, the senate passed the revised bill. Ironically, it was ultimately defeated when Representative Erickson, appalled by the liberal procedural amendments to his initial legislation, asked his colleagues in the house to reject the bill because it no longer reflected his purposes.[131]

It was one year later that the Colorado legislature finally enacted a statute—supported by the governor as well as Thomas Vernon—that included a statutory basis for the reporting of HIV antibody test results, penalties for those who failed to notify the health department of such findings, and the use of "restrictive enforcement measures . . . only when necessary to protect the public health."[132] This legislation was, if anything, more explicit in its enumeration of the conditions under which quarantine authority was to be imposed—"restrictive measures . . . shall be used as the last resort when other measures to protect the public health have failed, including all reasonable efforts which shall be documented to obtain the voluntary cooperation of the individual who may be subject to such an order"—and more exacting in its specification of the procedures to be followed when such controls were to be enforced. A number of gay leaders had cooperated in the drafting process that had produced this legislation. For some of them the incorporation of the full range of due-process protections was important not primarily because such provisions would make the bill more compatible with respect for civil liberties, but because they would so overburden the statute as to make it unworkable.[133] Most, however, opposed the legislation. In part this was because of the HIV reporting provisions, which remained anathema. But equally important was the explicit extension of the quarantine power to AIDS and HIV infection.

In California, the political conflict surrounding the issue of the restricted application of quarantine to "recalcitrants" resulted in a June 1987 decision by the California Conference of Local Health Officers—CCLHO—to reject a proposal that would have endorsed the exercise of such authority. Though the proposal was characterized as an action of last resort in the exercise of public health powers, the state health body had yielded to strong opposition and had ceded responsibility to the criminal justice system for those with AIDS who could not be convinced to change their behavior.

Two years earlier the local health officers had confronted the issue when Robert Benjamin, the chief communicable diseases official from Alameda County (across the bay from San Francisco) reported to his colleagues that he was aware of an individual with AIDS who had been treated repeatedly for rectal gonorrhea at venereal disease clinics. "He admits," said Benjamin, "to having three to five sex partners a week. We've said to him that the likelihood is good you're giving *it* away."[134] Cautioned and counseled for more than a year, the individual would not change his sexual behavior. When his case was presented to the CCLHO, other health officers reported similar cases. All were perplexed about how to proceed.

A week following the conference session, Benjamin met with gay leaders to solicit their advice. "I'm here because we need your help and we don't know what to do."[135] For him, none of the options involving the use of quarantine—technically termed isolation in California—seemed appropriate to the case of AIDS. The strategy of staged warnings laid out by James Chin, the state's director of infectious diseases, early in the course of the AIDS epidemic was deemed inappropriate. Months later, Benjamin outlined his opposition to the use of coercion on grounds of pragmatics and philosophical outlook.[136] In the case of tuberculosis the control of recalcitrants was a public health practice, however infrequent. Why was AIDS different? "You don't have to consent to anything to get TB. . . . You just have to breathe the air. . . . To quarantine this one individual would not be effective in stopping the spread of this disease. There is more than one of him out there." Underscoring the significance of self-exposure to hazards in the context of AIDS, Benjamin noted that the only solution was for each individual to assume responsibility for his own health, "to be damn certain [that] if they choose to go to bed with somebody, they are protected."

But if Benjamin was not willing to pursue the option of isolation, others in California's public health apparatus were. In January 1987, the Epidemiology and Disease Control Committee of the CCLHO presented a proposal for the "Management of Willful Agents of Infection with Human Immunodeficiency Virus."[137] As public health officials had often noted when opposing extreme legislative measures for the protection of the public from AIDS, no new statutory authority was necessary. California law already provided the necessary authority to control "recalcitrants." What was needed was guidance on how to proceed in a socially volatile climate. The January proposal sought to provide that guidance, in a way that brought to bear public health powers while "offering protection [for] the rights of the involved individuals."

The proposal was sensitive to the political and constitutional requirement that state intervention be carefully tailored to guarantee that the level of threatened control not exceed the limits imposed by the least restrictive alternative standard. It stressed that legal action to restrict individuals be taken only after all efforts to gain voluntary compliance had failed. Modified isolation—imposing restrictions on the *behavior* of individuals—was to precede isolation itself, which would restrict the movement of those who violated the mandated behavioral restraints. "In those instances, [when] persons willfully and knowingly engage in behaviors which place others at risk . . . without the knowledge and consent of others, the local health jurisdiction has the responsibility to intervene. [If] it becomes necessary to consider the use of isolation power, it is essential [that] the procedure allows due process for the individual under consideration."

A hearing before a health officer was to be held, before which the individual threatened with isolation was to be guaranteed the right to representation by counsel, cross-examination of witnesses, and assistance of an interpreter and an independent medical expert. If the hearing officer found that there was "reasonable cause" to believe that the individual was infected with HIV, could not be expected to reliably participate in a program of voluntary restraint, and therefore represented a "probable threat" to the public health, an order of isolation could be issued.

Despite the attempt to couch the proposal cautiously in terms of a phased process of warnings and controls and the effort to incorporate the procedural safeguards developed in the course of dealing with recalcitrant tuberculosis patients, the plan provoked an immediate and sharp protest from the gay community. The *Bay Area Reporter* headlined: "State Quarantine Plan Proposed—Includes Antibody Positive People: Calls for Isolation Facility."[138] Bruce Decker, a prominent Republican gay political leader and chair of the state's AIDS Advisory Committee, warned, "Public health clinics may become clinics for self-incrimination. . . . We may be creating kangaroo courts above the law [which can be used] to incarcerate patients for the rest of their lives."[139] Like those who had opposed other quarantine proposals, local gay leaders warned that California's effort to isolate individual recalcitrants would be a political gesture with little public health benefit. Ben Schatz of the National Gay Rights Advocates declared, "The quarantine issue is a smokescreen. It is a superficial way—and an appealing way—to make it appear as though health officials are taking firm action against AIDS when they are not. . . . It's an emotional and political response. It's not a medical response."[140]

But gay representatives were not alone. Like Robert Benjamin of Alameda County, other public health officials raised concerns about the proposal. Most significantly, such protests came from the two centers of the AIDS epidemic in California—San Francisco and Los Angeles, where public health officials had developed strong ties to the gay community. San Francisco's associate health director Tom Peters warned that the proposed plan would be subject to great abuse and that efforts to impose isolation would drive patients underground. "We look askance at any proposal that gives out the message that when you need help, you'll get handcuffs instead of a stethoscope."[141] Education of the "many," not expenditure of energy and resources on controlling the "few," was necessary. Shirley Fannin of Los Angeles, who had publicly opposed closing the bathhouses in San Francisco and New York City, also warned about the diversion of energy from more effective efforts at education.[142]

Thus, opposed by gay leaders whose cooperation was critical to a broad-based program of community education and by health officials who had worked so hard to foster such cooperation, the CCLHO Committee on Epidemiology and Disease Control was compelled to reconsider its January proposal. Five months later, a radically revised document was prepared for consideration, one that echoed the concerns of those who had denounced the earlier effort.[143] Focused more narrowly on those with AIDS or ARC rather than all HIV-infected individuals and limited to the "rare individuals" who knowingly exposed those with no knowledge of the risks presented by their sexual partners, the new proposal nevertheless acknowledged that any effort to impose orders of isolation would be counterproductive from a public health perspective.

Confronted with recalcitrant individuals, local health officers would have to determine the appropriate course of action by asking, "Is it worth it?" The calculation had to be made on the basis of the estimated impact on the broad program of AIDS control. "To move to invoke current law to reduce the public health threat caused by the actions of one or a very few individuals will do no overall good if other aspects of the local jurisdiction's AIDS programs suffer disproportionately. The effect of such an action may do more harm than good." The pragmatics of public health thus dictated a response quite different from that which the logic of public health might suggest. As a consequence, the revised plan rejected the use of orders of isolation in the case of AIDS. Failures to abide by orders of modified isolation—restricting dangerous behaviors—were to be referred to the criminal justice system. There, existing statutes already made it a misdemeanor knowingly to expose an individual to an infectious disease. Violation of a public health order to desist from behaviors or actions that posed a risk to others was also the subject of extant criminal sanctions. It was thus the criminal law of California, rather than the health law, that was to be the guarantor of the public health and of individual rights.

That on each occasion the prospect of formally extending the authority to quarantine to the case of AIDS provoked a sharp response from the advocates of civil liberties and gay organzations is less remarkable than the relative success with which such protests met. Officials who advocated the imposition of restraint on HIV-infected individuals whose behavior posed a risk to the health of others were compelled to retreat or modify their proposals radically in ways that carefully incorporated the exacting demands of due process. This outcome was the result not so much of the power of gay groups and civil liberties organizations, but of the recognition that a refusal to accommodate the concerns of the organized gay community could profoundly affect the relationship of trust and cooperation so critical to the control of a disease transmitted by the consensual sexual behavior of hundreds of thousands of men and women.

Like the bathhouse controversy, the struggle over quarantine had taken on an important symbolic dimension. For the advocates of even limited quarantine, it was important to articulate the presence of public health values, though they knew that as a practical matter efforts to control the infected who were easily identifiable would have only marginal significance for the epidemic. For the defenders of civil liberties, it was critical to protect the realm of privacy and sexual behavior from state authority, even when such authority was exercised under egregious circumstances.

Accommodation—when it was reached—in the public discussion

of quarantine was virtually always accompanied by the repetition in almost talismanic form of the proposition that individuals who knew themselves to be HIV-infected but persisted in behaviors that posed a risk to others were exceptional, that the problem of the incorrigible or recalcitrant was "extremely rare." When the story of Fabian Bridges was aired on television, it provoked a storm of protest from gay groups. They feared that the graphic portrayal of one man with AIDS who, out of his own needs, or desperation, perhaps as a result of HIV-related dementia, continued to engage in sexual activity, sometimes as a prostitute, would convey to the large audience an impression that this behavior was typical. Some gay leaders refused an invitation to appear on the television panel to discuss the issues raised by Bridges. Others did so only on condition that the basic premise of the show be open to challenge. They argued that the portrayal of Bridges did more harm than good. In a carefully worded introduction, the program's host told her audience, "This is a story of one man—not the typical story of a person with AIDS in our view. His choices are rare. He tried the limits of our system."[144]

There is no way of knowing whether such cases are, in fact, extremely rare. What is true is that neither the capacity for surveillance nor the most elemental notions of the constitutionally limited state permit us to do much to monitor and prevent such actions when they occur in private settings. By formulating the issue in terms of the "exceptionally rare case," the limits imposed by sheer pragmatics and a commitment to the protection of privacy could be made more socially bearable.

This is the context within which so much stress has been placed on the role of education as an instrument for imbuing a sense of moral responsibility in those who are infected with HIV or those who do not know their serological status but are at increased risk of infection. It is also the context within which so much emphasis has been placed on the role of education in warning individuals about the need to protect themselves. In the face of the serious social threat posed by AIDS, the preeminent strategy of defense has of necessity entailed reliance on individual choices made in private. Only in helping to foster a culture of responsible behavior could public health officials hope to shape those choices in a fundamental way. Not understood by those who opposed—under any circumstances—reliance on coercive mechanisms to control individuals who willfully placed others at risk was the role that carefully defined sanctions could play in the development of such a culture.

Chapter 7

Prevention Through Education

The Politics of Persuasion

At every encounter with the threat of coercive public health measures—calls for mandatory screening and proposals extreme or limited, for the isolation of those capable of transmitting HIV infection—gay leaders, civil libertarians, and a broad alliance of physicians and public health officials who were committed to a voluntarist health strategy for combating AIDS demanded that education provide the central, if not the sole, element in the preventive response. More money, more inventiveness, more boldness were necessary if individuals were to be taught how to protect themselves from HIV infection, if they were to learn how to protect their sexual partners or those with whom they shared intravenous drug equipment, if they were to prevent the birth of babies with AIDS.

Here was a public health strategy that was utterly compatible with the protection of the private realm, a strategy for the modification of private acts with dire social consequences that did not employ the coercive power of the state. It was a strategy dictated by political and moral commitments as well as by the unique epidemiological features of an epidemic that spread in the context of intimate relationships. In the face of a dire public health challenge, it appeared that public health officials had little alternative but to turn to the weakest and least-well-understood instrument of social intervention. Commenting on the challenge of combating a modern epidemic for which neither vaccine nor effective therapies were available, two officials at the Centers for Disease Control wrote in 1986, "HTLVIII/LAV infection is the first modern transmissible disease causing significant morbidity and mortality for which health education and risk reduction are the main instruments available to carry out a public health control effort. This reality colors every consideration in the development and implementation of strategies for control."[1]

No one denied that education in its various forms, from mass public health campaigns to private counseling, had a critical role to play in combating AIDS. What was cause for bitter conflict was the extent to which education ought to represent the sole element in the strategy of prevention; the explicitness with which governmentally funded programs would address matters of sexual behavior and intravenous drug use; the extent to which it would be possible to use language that many would find offensive, pictures that many would consider pornographic. If the political controversies that surrounded screening and quarantine centered on the limits that should govern public intrusions into the realm of privacy, those that surrounded education involved conflicts over how the public realm would be affected by the open discussion of the most private acts of gay and bisexual men, intravenous drug users, and their sexual partners.

Despite the very early and broad appreciation of the role that risk reduction education might play in the control of AIDS, the federal government did virtually nothing to fund such efforts in the first years of the epidemic. Part of the more general inadequacy of the government's response—funds for research were also critically below what was needed—the failure to support educational efforts was nevertheless striking. Thus, in its *Review of the Public Health Service's Response to AIDS*, the Office of Technology Assessment of the U.S. Congress wrote in February 1985, "So far, efforts to prevent AIDS through education have received minimal funding, especially efforts targeted at groups at highest risk."[2] How little had been done to underwrite the efforts of the gay community groups that had borne the burden of educating homosexual men about the risks of AIDS was tellingly underscored by the fact that in fiscal year

1984 the Public Health Service made an award of $150,000 to the U.S. Conference of Mayors so that it might fund community groups engaged in prevention activities.[3] Virtually nothing was done in those years to support the education of intravenous drug users and their sexual partners.

Gay leaders, the liberal media, and political leaders with close ties to gay constituencies repeatedly attacked the failure of government to act upon its own designation of AIDS as the nation's number-one health problem. Gary McDonald of the AIDS Action Council, a coalition of gay political and AIDS service organizations, said in early 1985, "There is so much knowledge about the disease and about safe sex practices to prevent the disease that we need to get out to the groups at risk, but the government has given only paltry sums to do the job."[4] As late as June 1986, the Los Angeles *Times*, a persistent critic of the federal AIDS effort and a strong opponent of coercive measures, could write, "Stopping AIDS requires changing private behavior that is driven by deep biological urges—behavior that has enormous personal and social consequences. The government needs to spend whatever it takes to drive the message home to everyone in a high risk group for AIDS: behavior must be changed. This is a matter of life and death."[5]

The failure of the federal government to provide aggressive leadership in the funding of education was mirrored at the state and local levels. The collaborative efforts of the San Francisco Department of Health and the local gay community, though limited, provided a model for innovative campaigns that few cities were to emulate. In New York City, where the commissioner of health, David Sencer, was skeptical of what education could achieve[6] and concerned about how an anti-AIDS campaign could itself provoke a sense of social alarm, very little was done, despite pressure from within the Health Department to undertake a vigorous program. Gay leaders denounced the city's effort as lethargic at best.[7]

When the National Academy of Sciences and the Institute of Medicine issued the report *Confronting AIDS* in the fall of 1986, they stressed the importance of education and were sharply critical of the efforts made during the first five years of the epidemic. "Because no vaccine is likely to become available in the near future and because of the seriousness of the disease, the only prudent course of action is an immediate major effort to stop the further spread of infection through public health measures, particularly education.

Any delay will bequeath to future policymakers a problem of potentially catastrophic proportions and will condemn many thousands of individuals to infection and death."[8] Faced with the enormity of the epidemic's potential toll, past and current efforts could only be described as "woefully inadequate."[9] How vast an expansion in the public effort was required was underscored by the report's estimate of what would be needed within five years. By 1990 upwards of $1 billion a year, most of it in the form of federal expenditures, would be necessary for education and other preventive public health measures.[10] Such a program of public education would have to go beyond the mere transfer of information about how HIV was transmitted. More critical would be the process of "inducing, persuading, and otherwise motivating people" to modify their behaviors in order to protect themselves from infection.[11] Though *Confronting AIDS* reflected an appreciation of how difficult such a process might be, and recognized the very mixed results of other efforts designed to motivate changes in behaviors linked to disease and death ("The literature on behavioral risk modification generally concedes the extraordinary difficulty of modifying behavior, even when there is a clear demonstration of risk"),[12] it asserted that in the case of AIDS educational efforts could be "entered into with a strong degree of conviction and hope."[13]

Safer Sex and Sexual Moralism

The inadequacy of federal funding for educational efforts designed to limit the spread of AIDS had roots, however, that went deeper than the fiscal constraints that hobbled national efforts to control the epidemic. The very prospect of a major government effort to underwrite risk reduction education was mired in controversy from the outset. How could it have been otherwise? How could government agencies teach gay men about "safer" sexual practices when homosexual acts were criminal offenses in twenty-four states and the District of Columbia? How could such agencies teach addicts about the sterilization of drug paraphernalia when the use of heroin and cocaine constituted criminal offenses in every state? Commenting on the failure of government to act more directly, imaginatively, and vigorously, the *New York Times* wrote, "Why not teach prostitutes and their customers that practices like the use of condoms would help block the virus's transmission? Because that would condone prostitution. . . . Why not educate intravenous drug abusers about the risk [of sharing needles], provide more drug treatment centers and supply clean needles in an effort to retard the virus's transmission on dirty syringes? Because that would sanction drug use. . . . These are substantial objections, but shouldn't all of them yield to the need to curb AIDS?"[14]

Inevitably, even when public health departments sought to fund AIDS education through intermediaries they were forced to confront the question of how explicit their contractors could be in their instructions and were compelled to consider the acceptability of the language used in educational material designed to foster the modification of sexual behavior. In 1985 AIDS Project Los Angeles, under contract with the state of California, began to distribute a brochure entitled "Mother's Handy Sex Guide," the cover of which had a photograph of a seductively seated man wearing nothing but an athletic supporter. The warnings contained in the pamphlet were direct: "When you share urine, shit, cum, blood and possibly saliva, you are at greatest risk for getting AIDS." Under the heading "Playing Unsafely," the pamphlet listed "Fucking without a condom. Your partner coming in your mouth. Water sports. (Pissing) in the mouth or on the skin with cuts or sores." The bulk of the material included in "Mother's Handy Sex Guide" was devoted to three erotic gay fantasies that depicted sexual encounters that involved mutual masturbation and anal intercourse with the use of condoms—safe or "relatively safe" sexual acts. When a conservative member of the Los Angeles County Board of Supervisors became aware of this material, he was outraged. "It goes beyond all boundaries of good taste and decency. . . . The material is not educational, it's hard core pornograph[y]."[15] As a result of this controversy, the state created a Materials Review Committee that ultimately issued guidelines designed to limit the extent to which sexually explicit material would be distributed by publicly funded projects. "It is preferable," said the committee, "to use clinical or descriptive terms describing sexual contact or behavior . . . rather than their slang or 'street language' equivalents." Photographs and other "visual messages" were not to be explicitly suggestive.[16]

With farther-reaching implications was the decision of the CDC to impose similar contraints on the educational material developed under grants it would make for risk-reduction efforts. As a result of what was widely reported to be intervention from the White House, the CDC moved to prohibit the funding of material that might be deemed offensive by broad community standards. Michael Lane, director of the Center for Prevention Services, under whose auspices the education projects would be funded, underscored the delicate political situation with which he was confronted. "We are carefully considering," he said, "how explicit the message must be in order to educate risk groups. Clearly AIDS is a problem which requires bold and unprecedented approaches. However, every aspect of AIDS activity receives intensive public scrutiny. Accountability for the appropriate use of public funds . . . must be kept in mind."[17] More bluntly, James Mason told Alvin Novick—who as president of the American Association of Physicians for Human Rights had protested the anticipated imposition of constraints—"You would be naive to think that we can spend tax dollars to eroticize homosexuality."[18]

When the Centers for Disease Control issued its guidelines in 1986, it sought to portray its restrictions as a politically prudent compromise between the importance of candor, "which may provoke criticism by some in society," and the need to be answerable for the use of federal funds. To assure that educational materials and programs funded by the CDC did not generate sharp protest, local review panels were to be established to consider all proposed projects. Those panels were to determine the balance between the need to communicate and the need to avoid offense. To assure that the panels, in fact, did reflect the broadest community representation—that they were not dominated by gay groups or their allies—approval of their membership from state and local health officials was required. Guiding these panels, the CDC asserted, was to be a set of basic principles: the terms used in all educational material were to be understandable by those to whom it was directed but not offensive when judged by a "reasonable person." Pictorial material was to avoid the display of the "anogenital area of the body or overt depiction of the performance of 'safer sex' or 'unsafe' sex practices."[19]

With so broad a mandate, the locally constituted groups could impose rather severe restrictions on the material used for education. On the other hand, in states and cities where health officials had close working relationships with gay community-based AIDS groups and political organizations, local review might be quite liberal. Nevertheless, the restrictive intent of the guidelines was clear. It was that intent, fear about how the regulations might be implemented, and great anxiety over the censorship of the content of public health messages directed at those who engaged in homosexual relations that provoked the denunciation of gay leaders. Counterproductive and an exercise in moralism, the restrictions, it was asserted, would hinder the most critical and difficult undertaking in the effort to control the epidemic. "Sex education," stated Jeff Levi of the National Gay Task Force, "must be explicit if it's going to be effective. I'm not sure this new approach reflects an understanding of what has to be done."[20] Neil Schram, former president of the American Association of Physicians for Human Rights and chair of the Los Angeles AIDS Task Force, underscored the extent to which the CDC guidelines would subvert the prospects of success in getting people to modify their sexual behavior, "one of the most difficult public health procedures we have faced in our lifetime."[21]

Though the CDC guidelines initially had a chilling effect on the content, style, and language of programs seeking federal support, it became clear soon after their promulgation that it would, in fact, be possible in some states to create panels that were quite sympathetic to the concerns voiced by gay leaders like Levi and Schram, panels that would concur with the perspective of those who believed that the modification of behavior required more than the presentation of clinical information, that the task of "inducing, persuading and otherwise motivating people" might require the use of erotically charged material.[22] Indeed, Richard Dunne, executive director of the Gay Men's Health Crisis, the largest AIDS service organization in New York City and a recipient of federal funds, declared that the guidelines were "something we can live with."[23] Ironically, the prospects for the creation of relatively liberal panels was greatest in those states with large, well-organized gay communities—states where the level of HIV infection was already high. In those states with smaller gay communities, where the epidemic of HIV infection was still relatively contained and where imaginative and vigorous campaigns would be necessary to prevent the replication of the seroprevalence rates of New York and San Francisco, the prospects for the appointment of liberal panels was far from certain.

But the assault on the public funding of safer-sex educational material went beyond revulsion provoked by the use of "street language" and sexually explicit drawings and photographs. To those who believed that AIDS was the consequence of the erosion of traditional values, of a sexuality unrestrained by heterosexual monogamy, the very premises of the AIDS educational efforts being encouraged by public health officials under pressure from gay leaders were profoundly flawed. It was in the reactions to the Surgeon General's *Report on Acquired Immune Deficiency Syndrome* published in October 1986 that the intensity of such ideological opposition was to be revealed, that the political power of the opposition was to be demonstrated.

To those who had feared that the surgeon general would use the opportunity of his statement on AIDS to the American people to advance the conservative social agenda of the political constituency to which he had been popularly linked, the report came as a welcome surprise. To those who had anticipated that their ally in the social movement against abortion would seize the opportunity to stress the importance of traditional sexual morality, it represented a betrayal.

"Some Americans," wrote the surgeon general, "have difficulties with the subjects of sex, sexual practices, and alternative lifestyles. Many Americans are opposed to homosexuality, promiscuity of any kind, and prostitution."[24] Acknowledging such distaste and antipathy, Koop noted that his report would have to deal with such matters. He did so with the intent of educating Americans about the necessity of changing individual behavior "since this is the primary way to stop the epidemic." In carefully chosen words, Koop went on to note that his report would discuss the positive and negative consequences of certain behaviors from a "health and medical point of view." By adopting a clinical posture, Koop could thus say what might otherwise have been utterly unacceptable. He could bracket traditional and conventional moral claims in the name of health and life.

There was, in fact, a rather straightforward response to the threat posed for the individual and the nation. "The most certain way to avoid getting the AIDS virus and to control the AIDS epidemic in the United States is for individuals to avoid promiscuous sexual practices and to maintain mutually faithful monogomous sexual relationships and to avoid injecting illicit drugs."[25] But the control of AIDS was not so simple. In some populations where the level of infection with HIV was high, the avoidance of promiscuity was no longer protective. And Koop knew that there were individuals who would give up neither a life of multiple sexual partners nor intravenous drug use. They needed to be reached if AIDS was to be brought under control.

In direct, unadorned language Koop warned Americans both homosexual and heterosexual about the risks of AIDS. Sexual contact including "penis-vagina, penis-rectum, mouth-rectum, mouth-vagina, [and] mouth-penis," all could serve as routes of transmission.[26] Partners who were uncertain of each other's past sexual and drug-using histories could no longer assume that they could engage in sexual activity without the risk of infection with the AIDS virus. In the face of uncertainty, only an antibody test could provide a definitive answer. For those who tested positive, or who though untested had engaged in "high risk activity," the surgeon general counseled honesty with their sexual partners. "If you jointly decide to have sex, you must protect your partner by always using a rubber (condom) during (start to finish) sexual intercourse (vagina or rectum)."[27] Emphasizing the break with conventional reticence and the importance of candor, a picture of a rolled condom next to the packet from which it had been removed appeared on the page with these "safer sex" recommendations.[28] A similar boldness characterized Koop's discussion of intravenous drug abuse and AIDS. "No one should shoot up drugs because addiction, poor health, family disruption, emotional disturbance and death could follow."[29] But the surgeon general knew that such a warning would have little meaning for those already addicted. For them, the most important message was that they use clean, previously unused needles and syringes.[30]

Not only adults but adolescents and children had to be warned about AIDS. Ineed, Koop urged that education about AIDS and HIV infection start "at the lowest grade possible."[31] Every health and hygiene program had to include sex education and all such education had to "include information about heterosexual and homosexual relationships." With a bow to those of conservative social temperament and reflecting his own deeply held beliefs, Koop asserted that it would be important to teach boys and girls to "say no to sex and drugs." But there could be no doubt that if the education ended with that message, it would be inadequate in the face of a deadly epidemic.

The surgeon general's report provoked a bitter reaction from conservative and antihomosexual California congressman William E.

Dannemyer. In a letter to Koop that joined religious concerns with a challenge to the scientific foundations of the surgeon general's report, Dannemyer underscored in an extreme way the profound gulf that existed between the public health establishment and those who believed that officials involved in the forging of public health policy on AIDS were guilty of a betrayal of the nation's moral traditions and its future well-being.[32]

Most disturbing to Dannemyer was the adoption in Koop's report of a "health and medical point of view." The surgeon general had provided clear moral leadership on the "right to life" issue for both the unborn and the handicapped child. Why had he abandoned this perspective when dealing with AIDS? "This is not an issue which can be addressed from a neutral point of view, either morally or ethically. To attempt to do so is to tacitly endorse the moral position of those who consider homosexuality an acceptable alternative lifestyle." AIDS was not the occasion to abandon the Judeo-Christian assertion of the primacy of heterosexuality. Rather, it provided the opportunity to reaffirm Biblical proscriptions on homosexuality. Public health authorities could not "merely" relate the health and medical consequences of sexual behavior. They had a duty to acknowledge the inseparability of "human sex, conscience, morality and ethics." Classroom education could not simply inform children about the medical hazards associated with some homosexual acts, but had to stress the "moral and ethical reasons which exist for avoiding homosexuality. . . . By inference you are . . . disavowing, by failure to assert or by denying by omission, the heterosexual ethic which is the foundation of our civilization."

Framed in the diction of the antisecular right wing of American politics, Dannemyer's concerns found an echo within the administration of President Ronald Reagan. Leading the surgeon general's opponents within the cabinet was Secretary of Education William J. Bennett, who like Everett Koop was well known for his conservative social commitments. Disagreements between the two occupied the attention of the Domestic Policy Council on at least two occasions in January 1987.[33] Koop's views were clear. Education had to begin with young schoolchildren. Though he stressed sexual abstinence for the unmarried, he believed that it was important to provide protective information to those who would not adhere to such standards. Bennett and his allies saw in Koop's recommendations a failure to assert the primacy of abstinence and the extension of the liberal trend to provide "value-neutral" sex education to the young. "With AIDS," said Bennett, "harsh nature becomes the unwitting ally of responsible morality."[34] At best, Koop's message was laced with moral ambiguity.

In an effort to heal the public rift, Bennett and Koop issued a joint statement at the end of January that, it was hoped, would provide at least the appearance of a common ground within the administration. "With the appropriate involvement and approval of parents and the local community, schools should help teach young children about the dangers of AIDS . . . but an AIDS education that accepts children's sexual activity as inevitable and focuses only on 'safe sex' will be at best ineffectual, at worst itself a cause of serious harm. . . . Young people should be taught that the best precaution is abstinence until it is possible to establish a mutually faithful monogamous relationship."[35] But the statement was silent on the core of the dispute: how to convey instruction about protecting oneself and one's sexual partner if abstinence was unacceptable. What most pleased conservative opponents of Koop was that he appeared to have retreated in the face of what was clearly emerging as the dominant stance of the administration.

In mid-February, Attorney General Edwin Meese informed the Domestic Policy Council of the president's decision on the principles that should guide federal AIDS educational efforts.[36] Federal authorities should not dictate the content of school programs but should provide "accurate health information" to local officials, permitting them to determine, in a manner consistent with parental values, the substance of AIDS education. Thus, the surgeon general's effort to provide a leadership role in the fashioning of local school board decisions was thwarted. More important was the outright rejection of Koop's effort to bracket the moral issues surrounding sexuality so that he could speak as a physician from "a health and medical" point of view about sexual behavior, both homosexual and heterosexual. "Any health information developed by the federal government that will be used for education should encourage responsible sexual behavior . . . based on fidelity, commitment, maturity, placing sexuality within the context of marriage. . . . Any health information provided by the federal government that might be used in schools should teach that children should not engage in sex and should be used with the consent and involvement of parents." Bennett and his supporters had succeeded in outflanking Koop by placing their stamp on future AIDS education initiatives by the Centers for Disease Control.

Finally, the influence and constraining impact of moralism was further revealed in the spring of 1988, when the U.S. Senate overwhelmingly voted to support an antihomosexual amendment put forth by Senator Jesse Helms. Enraged by a sexually explicit "safer sex" comic book produced by the Gay Men's Health Crisis—a recipient of federal funds—Helms had denounced the "promotion of sodomy" by the government. The threat of AIDS would never be met effectively "as long as [the U.S. Senate encourages] groups that advocate homosexuality, which was the original source of the AIDS virus."[37] And so the conservative Republican senator proposed a restrictive measure that would preclude the use of federal funds "to provide AIDS education, information, or prevention materials and activities that promote or encourage, directly or indirectly, homosexual activities."[38] Less surprising than Helms's move was the ease with which he was able to elicit support from his colleagues. Whatever the ultimate impact of the amendment, its passage underscored the persistence of an antagonism to homosexuality that would, on practical as well as symbolic levels, hinder the American struggle against AIDS.

Safer Drug Use and the Problem of Drug Abuse

Like the efforts to foster the modification of sexual behavior among gay men, attempts to address intravenous drug users about the risks they posed to themselves and their sexual partners as a result of their behaviors were embroiled in controversy from the outset. If "safer" sex literature provoked conflict because of explicit language and the tacit toleration of homosexuality, messages to addicts about the importance of avoiding contaminated drug paraphernalia suggested a temporary truce in the seven-decade medicolegal effort to suppress the illicit use of drugs. The first major encounter over how to address drug users at risk for HIV infection and transmission occurred in Los Angeles and was provoked by the distribution by public health officials of a pamphlet entitled "Shooting Up and Your Health." Warning about the hazards associated with intravenous drug use, the pamphlet nevertheless rejected the condemnatory stance of those who sought to extirpate such behavior. "There are always risks associated with any use of drugs by injection. The only way to avoid these risks is not to use needles. If you continue to inject drugs, the following measures will reduce your risk. DON'T SHARE NEEDLES! Sharing drugs can share diseases too. Obtain your own 'works' and don't let anyone else use them. CLEAN YOUR OWN WORKS. Wash them with alcohol after each use, then leave them to soak in alcohol until the next use. CLEAN YOUR SKIN with alcohol before injecting."

Brought to the attention of the county's Board of Supervisors at the same time that the pamphlet "Mother's Handy Sex Guide" was stirring outrage, "Shooting Up" was denounced as "impl[ying] the official approval of the government of the county and city of Los Angeles toward drug use."[39] One conservative supervisor saw in it another example of "radical liberals using taxpayers' dollars to subsidize deviant behavior and another example of bureaucrats gone crazy." Bowing to the fury, officials withdrew the pamphlet, acknowledging that it had been "inappropriate" to inform addicts about how best to use drugs.

Controversy, though less public in form, also surrounded a program in New Jersey—the first state where more than half the reported cases of AIDS were among intravenous drug users—to use ex-addict street workers to inform drug users not only about the risks of AIDS and the importance of seeking treatment, but about the need to avoid unsterile needles if they continued to use drugs.[40] Ultimately, however, the state health department did produce a flyer directed at addicts that was, if anything, more explicit than "Shooting Up and Your Health" in providing information about the sterilization of intravenous drug paraphernalia. "Buy a new needle in a sealed package, clean it . . . before use and don't let anyone else use it. If you must use someone else's works, first rinse the works several times by pulling water up into the syringe and squirting it out through the needle." The flyer then went on to describe in some detail how to sterilize equipment by three methods: boiling water, rubbing alcohol, and the use of bleach and water.

For those who saw the prevention of drug abuse as their professional mission, the publicly funded distribution of such literature was often very troubling. In 1985 representatives of the National Institute on Drug Abuse repeatedly voiced such concerns at meetings of the Public Health Service's Executive Task Force on AIDS. "NIDA does not feel comfortable sending information which tells drug abusers not to use dirty needles or share needles. NIDA's position is based on [the clear] message, "Do Not Use Drugs."[41] Ultimately, however, public agencies could not avoid the imperatives of an anti-AIDS campaign among drug abusers. Unlike the situation that prevailed among gay men, where voluntary and community-based organizations could assume responsibility when public agencies abdicated it, for addicts, if publicly funded agencies did not act there would simply be no action.

Despite the critical dimensions of the AIDS problem among drug users in New York and other East Coast cities and the recognition that the problem could spread—if more slowly than AIDS among gay men—to other regions, the response of state and federal authorities during the first six years of the epidemic can only be characterized as extraordinarily feeble. Long waiting lists for entry into drug abuse treatment continued to exist in the seventh year of the epidemic. Educational campaigns were far from adequate. Poor, socially disadvantaged addicts could not themselves, if they had so desired, press for the resources that were necessary. Professionals responsible for the treatment of addiction had been only marginally effective.

Though the public health effort was inadequate, evidence did begin to surface indicating that knowledge about the risks associated with the use of unsterile needles had begun to penetrate the subcultures of drug abusers as early as 1984. In the summer and fall of that year in New York City, researchers found that used needles were being repackaged and sold as new. They concluded that "the demand for new needles has reached a point where it can now support a supply of counterfeit new needles."[42] In the spring of 1985, researchers working for New York State observed a street seller chanting, "Get the good needles, don't get the bad AIDS."[43] A report on intravenous drug use in the Haight-Ashbury district of San Francicso, where the level of HIV infection was much lower than in New York and New Jersey, also found growing interest in clean needles among drug users.[44]

Thus it appeared that the portrayal of addicts as uniformly and relentlessly impulse ridden and refractory when warned about the dangers to their own health was inaccurate. The importance of reaching into the subcultures of addiction became all the more important. But in addition, the evidence began to suggest to some that the legal prohibitions and restrictions governing the sale and possession of hypodermic needles and syringes were contributing to the transmission of HIV infection. Clean needles might do for addicts what condoms could do for the interruption of the spread of AIDS through sexual contact. In July 1985 a study conducted by the New Jersey Department of Health concluded, "Making sterile hypodermic equipment available to IV drug users will reduce needle sharing and hence viral transmission by this mode."[45] But any such innovation, warned the report, would have to be part of a much broader outreach effort directed at drug abusers.

To raise the issue of providing access to sterile needles to drug users was, however, to court political disaster. Like the provision of condoms to prisoners—an option that was rarely even mentioned—so that homosexual intercourse would not carry with it the risk of AIDS, the provision of sterile needles would involve the facilitation of illegal behavior. Proposals for the reform of drug paraphernalia laws were thus bound to arouse the opposition of the law enforcement establishment and the public, so easily moved by fear of moral decay. How could a society committed to the elimination of the "scourge of drug abuse" at the same time facilitate the injection of illicitly obtained substances? Would the elimination of the barriers to the acquisition of such equipment encourage drug use and hence the spread of addiction? Was the challenge posed by AIDS of sufficient magnitude to warrant such a dramatic about-face in public policy?

In New York City discussions of this issue between Mayor Edward Koch and the commissioner of health, David Sencer, led to a decision to have the chief health official himself propose a radical change in the laws governing hypodermic needles, thus freeing the mayor from the political liability that might well be created by such a suggestion.[46] In the summer of 1985 the commissioner sent a memorandum to the mayor—"leaked" intentionally—urging the course of bold reform. "Addicts," said Sencer, "understand the risks associated with the sharing of needles and syringes. They have a desire to obtain sterile equipment." They were, however, frustrated by extant legal prohibitions. "I believe it is time to reevaluate this aspect of society's approach to drug abuse, because by forcing addicts to use others' needles and syringes, we are condemning large numbers of addicts to death from AIDS. A live addict may be amenable to treatment of his drug abuse. An addict infected with [the AIDS virus] continues the spread of AIDS, not only to other addicts but to their sex partners and, tragically, to children born of such parents."[47] Sencer estimated that there were in New York City 200,000 addicts, only 30,000 of whom were in treatment. Half, he estimated, were already HIV infected. The other half could benefit by a bold act of prevention. "Shouldn't we attempt to practice preventive medicine and do something to interrupt the transmission of the virus? I think we should." Rather than suggesting that the city itself act to dispense drug injection equipment, the commissioner proposed that drug abuse treatment programs be permitted to exchange sterile needles for those already used, "without the threat of surveillance"; that the state repeal the statutory restrictions on the sale of needles and syringes; that law-enforcement agencies adopt a policy of nonenforcement for violations of the laws prohibiting possession of drug-injection paraphernalia. The mayor was urged to begin discussion with city and state agencies about their reactions to this set of proposals immediately, "because of the urgency of the AIDS problem."

The *New York Times* cautiously supported the Sencer proposals. Aware that some believed that lowering the barriers to needle possession would encourage drug abuse, the editors wrote, "The medical case is entitled at least to presumptive initial support. . . . Lowering [the restrictions on needle possession] before an overriding health concern does not weaken the moral stand against drug abuse. AIDS is a wildfire plague and no reasonable means of halting it can be lightly ignored."[48] As anticipated, Sencer's proposal did, however, meet with very forceful opposition. Carol Bellamy, who had adopted the posture of a political reformer in her electoral challenge to the mayor, termed it "one of the most hare-brained ideas I've heard from city government."[49] More important, the city's police and district attorneys denounced the idea as a threat to drug control programs.[50] Concern was also expressed at the federal level by officials at the National Institute on Drug Abuse.[51] In the end, the mayor bowed to the judgment of those who had asserted that Sencer's initiative would have a disastrous impact on the city. "How can I support something that the police and law enforcement leaders are totally against?"[52]

A year after Sencer had made his first proposal on needles, the New York State Health Department expressed its willingness to consider a demonstration project that would, without the need for legislative action, provide for a controlled experiment on the distribution of sterile equipment for drug users.[53] In the interim, support for such a trial had come from the Institute of Medicine and the National Academy of Sciences. *Confronting AIDS* had bluntly argued that even if treatment facilities were adequate to meet the demand by those in need of assistance, the problem of HIV transmission among drug users would not be solved. "Clearly it will not be possible to persuade all IV drug users to abandon drugs or to switch to safer noninjectable drugs. Many may wish to reduce the chances of exposure to HIV infection but will neither enter treatment nor refrain from all drug injection." For them, held the report, experiments with public policies that would encourage the use of sterile needles and syringes "by removing legal and administrative barriers to their possession and use" were vital.[54]

In the wake of this report there was apparently some interest in conveying an image of flexibility and open-mindedness. Even Mayor Koch, who had yielded to the voice of alarm when he dismissed Sencer's proposed reforms as politically unfeasible, seemed open to an effort.[55] The city's new health commissioner, Stephen Joseph, who had adopted a much more aggressive stance on AIDS than that of his predecessor, promised to develop a model program for approval by the state health authorities.[56] Once again the *New York Times* gave its editorial approval to the planned innovation.[57] But in mid-1987, several months after the city had submitted its expected protocol, the state health department rejected it as "scientifically unsound."[58] Whatever the merits of the technical objections, it was apparent that state officials had once again retreated from a plan that, no matter how delimited, was bound to stir political controversy. One state health official thus declared that it would be "exceedingly difficult" for the city to submit a plan that would satisfy the states' "scientific requirements."

It was not until the winter of 1988, in the wake of reports that one in sixty-one women who had given birth in New York City during a survey period was infected with the AIDS virus, that the state relented, granting the city permission to conduct a trial needle exchange program.[59] Heterosexual and perinatal transmission of HIV infection had become a reality in New York City as male addicts infected their female partners, who then went on to have children. In light of that epidemiological development, state health officials were apparently more willing to acknowledge the possibility of an experiment that would meet "scientific requirements."

The pattern of interaction witnessed in New York between reform-minded health officials and politicians sensitive to the fears and concerns of constituents with more conventional perspectives on drug abuse was repeated in New Jersey and San Francisco. Inspired by what he had learned about the needle exchange program in Amsterdam, John Rutledge, New Jersey's assistant health commissioner, fashioned a proposal that would have sought to determine on an experimental basis whether such an effort would work in his state.[60] "These are people who are going to shoot up anyway and we want to get rid of . . . contaminated needles . . . and have a chance to counsel the addict about the disease and drug problems."[61] Backed by the *New York Times,* which declared it a "bold experiment [that] offers a rare chance to halt the wildfire spread of AIDS among addicts and their contacts,"[62] and supported indirectly by James Curran,[63] head of the CDC's AIDS program, the proposal was thwarted by New Jersey's governor.[64] Commenting on the defeat of the "Amsterdam model," New Jersey health commissioner Molly Coye acknowledged that it had been a "poor strategy" to publicly entertain such an idea "without having first involved political leaders in the state."[65]

In San Francisco, the idea of providing addicts with sterile needles and syringes was aborted before much more than preliminary discussions had occurred. Aware of the discussions taking place in New Jersey, the press called on local health officials to explain whether they too were ready to launch a needle exchange program to meet the challenge posed by increasing levels of HIV infection among addicts.[66] The very suggestion that such an idea was under consideration provoked a sharp denunciation from Mayor Dianne Feinstein. In a letter to the city's director of health, she wrote, "In my opinion, it is a terrible and truly offensive idea, which would put the health department in the position of aiding and abetting drug addiction. . . . How can we consider spending the public's money for drug paraphernalia?"[67] The city's health director, David Werdegar, backed by the president of the Health Commission, joined the mayor, asserting that education, counseling, and treatment would remain his department's strategy for combatting AIDS among drug users. Though the department distributed vials of bleach so that addicts could clean their needles, it would not provide sterile equipment. "There is no evidence that the distribution of clean needles could reduce the spread of AIDS; but there is evidence that the distribution of needles can increase drug use."[68] In this way, the voice of reform was silenced.

The Limits and Promise of Education

The limits imposed on education by social conservatism and timidity have been the target of repeated reformist assault. Gay leaders, advocates of civil liberties, the liberal media, the Institute of Medicine and the National Academy of Sciences, as well as the surgeon general, have all in one way or another indicated the folly of such self-imposed constraints on the struggle against AIDS. Passionately they have tried to demonstrate that however discomfiting direct education of drug users or gay men might be, however difficult it might be for some to witness the expenditure of public resources on efforts to portray safer homosexual practices and drug use, the alternative was far grimmer. But there are other limits on education that do not stem from political resistance and that will not yield, however grudgingly, to the force of political wisdom informed by the exigencies of the AIDS epidemic. These are limits imposed by the inherent difficulties that always confront efforts to motivate individuals to alter behaviors that, no matter how ultimately dangerous, are deeply rooted in biological and psychological pleasures and are often reinforced by cultural and social dynamics.

The commitment to education as the first line of defense against AIDS occurred against a background of controversy about the efficacy of efforts to modify personal behavior by health-promotion campaigns. Attempts to encourage changes in vehicular behavior, alcohol consumption, and smoking by education alone have had only the most limited impact. Campaigns to encourage the use of seatbelts in automobiles in the United States, Canada, Great Britain, and France all faltered, ultimately necessitating the enactment of statutes mandating their use.[69] Antismoking campaigns have demonstrated some impact, though only after more than two decades, yet tens of millions continue to smoke.[70] Sex education programs have been a great disappointment to those who viewed them as a way of reducing the levels of teenage pregnancy in many urban centers. Finally, efforts to control venereal disease through moral education in the period before penicillin left a legacy of failure.[71] From a broad review of the literature on public health campaigns, Richard Bonnie has concluded that though "some experts are optimistic about the potential efficacy of such efforts *if they are based* on sound principles of mass communication theory, others are more dubious, doubting that such efforts can have much impact on attitudes and motivation, even if they improve the level of knowledge."[72]

Given this record it was stunning to find that in the face of the AIDS epidemic volunteer efforts undertaken by community organizations and funded in the most limited way by public agencies had apparently produced dramatic, even unprecedented changes in the sexual behavior of gay men. The shock wave sent through the gay communities of San Francisco, Los Angeles, and New York by the rising toll of the epidemic, the brute recognition that a pattern of sexual behavior involving multiple anonymous partners and anal intercourse without the use of condoms could well result in a fatal illness, and the extraordinary and inventive efforts undertaken by gay groups to reach large numbers with information about safer sex had created the conditions for a profound change in the culture of gay sexual behavior. One early indication that sexual behavior was changing was the rapid decline in certain sexually transmitted diseases associated with homosexuality. In New York City, for example, there was a 59 percent decline in the incidence of rectal and pharyngeal gonorrhea among males from 1980 to 1984.[73] Those declines paralleled reports from other cities in the United States, England, and northern Europe.[74] Detailed epidemiological studies provided more direct evidence of marked behavioral changes. In San Francisco, for example, several analyses found a decline in both the reported number of sexual partners and the extent to which men engaged in high-risk sexual acts like anal intercourse.[75]

Enthusiastically embraced by those who demanded ever greater efforts on behalf of risk-reduction education programs and those who had argued that coercive measures such as bathhouse closure and mandatory screening were neither justifiable nor necessary, these findings often masked the extent to which some gay men continued to engage in high-risk sexual activity. In New York and San Francisco, as well as other cities, substantial fractions of the gay men enrolled in longitudinal studies were found to be engaging in high-risk sexual acts, despite their awareness of the dangers involved. And in many ways those enrolled in such studies, because of education, income, and ethnicity, were unrepresentative of the broader gay community.

In New York City a study conducted by the New York Blood Center, which asked respondents to compare their sexual behaviors at three points—1976–1980, 1981–1982 (just prior to awareness of AIDS), and 1984—found dramatic declines in the number of sexual partners, as well as in the practice of oral-rectal and anal receptive sex.[76] The percentage that engaged in anal receptive intercourse had dropped from 80 to 46 percent. Though dramatic, these data showed that just under half the men in one sample continued to engage in a form of sexual behavior universally deemed unsafe. Furthermore, the use of condoms in this cohort "was too infrequent" to assess their effectiveness as a barrier to HIV infection. Later studies of gay men in New York were only marginally more encouraging. In one cohort just less than half of those interviewed indicated that they engaged in anal receptive intercourse, but the use of condoms was far more frequent than in the Blood Center's study.[77] Nevertheless, at least half the sample never used condoms.

A similar pattern was found in San Francisco. As of May 1985, approximately 25 percent of the men in one large sample continued to engage in at least one "high risk sexual act" *per month,* even though approximately 90 percent of the men in the study could correctly identify "safe sex behavior."[78] Underscoring the chasm between the almost universally successful effort to provide an understanding of the hazards of HIV transmission in San Francisco and the more limited achievement in attaining behavioral changes, the investigators commented, "Between May 1984 and May 1985, health education programs were conducted by a variety of community and government-based organizations. Saturation coverage of the epidemic by the local straight and gay media made it difficult for a member of the gay community to miss the message of the health education campaigns. Nonetheless, a significant proportion of gay men in our cohort did not adopt safe sex practices as of May 1985."[79]

What was true of the two cities most profoundly affected by AIDS was even more pronounced in the cities with relatively few cases. In Pittsburgh, for example, 65 percent of the men in one sample continued to engage in anal intercourse.[80] And though 90 percent agreed that the use of condoms could reduce the risk of

AIDS, 62 percent stated that they "hardly ever" or "never" used them. Thus, almost 40 percent of this study population continued to engage in the most risky of sexual behaviors.

The largest prospective study of the natural history of HIV infection, involving close to five thousand gay males from Los Angeles, San Francisco, Chicago, Pittsburgh, and Washington/Baltimore, provided striking corroboration of the very mixed picture of dramatic changes in sexual behavior and of a persistence in the willingness of many men to engage in life-threatening acts.[81] Interviewed at four six-month intervals beginning in April 1984, those surveyed indicated a rise in celibacy from 2 to 12 percent, and in monogomy from 12 to 27 percent. The proportion that did not engage in anal receptive intercourse had risen from 26 to 49 percent. Though the use of condoms had doubled over the four visits, fewer than one third of the respondents used them regularly. Hence, in this study of highly motivated participants, 51 percent still engaged in anal receptive intercourse, two-thirds of them without the protection afforded by condoms—in all, one-third of the entire sample.

Commenting on the significance of the mixed patterns of behavior change among gay men, Dean Echenberg of the San Francisco Health Department warned, "The lesson is clear. Even though we've seen a dramatic decrease in the level of sexual activity . . . it's simply not enough to cut back on the number of one's sexual partners. The only way for gay and bisexual men in San Francisco [where the level of HIV infection is 50 percent] to avoid infection is to practice 'safe sex' all of the time or to be celibate."[82] This perspective was reinforced by the city's director of AIDS activity: "Reducing unsafe sex is not enough any more, people must stop having unsafe sex altogether."[83]

Despite the reports of continued high-risk sexual behavior among gay men and the warnings about the implications of resistance to change, there was nevertheless unmistakable evidence that the occurrence of new infections with the AIDS virus was declining dramatically in gay communities across America. San Francisco provided the sharpest evidence. There the rate of infections with HIV among cohorts being studied by epidemiologists had fallen to a negligible level by 1987.[84] Whether these findings reflected the success of education or of saturation (had virtually all those at risk for infection become infected?) some were ready to proclaim that the epidemic of new infections had ended among gay men in that city. But such success had come at a very high price. The anticipated deaths of those already infected—more than 50 percent of its gay men—will decimate San Francisco's homosexual population in the next years.

Much less is known about the willingness of intravenous drug users—most of whom are men—to modify their sexual behavior, since they have been less frequently studied. But one survey in New York City found that while 69 percent of intravenous drug users had reported a reduction in the use of needles, only 32 percent acknowledged that they had modified their sexual practices to include the use of condoms or that they had reduced the number of their sexual partners.[85] With more than half of New York's addicts presumed to be infected, and with most addicted men having as their partners nonaddicted women, the implications were ominous for HIV transmission to the broader black and Hispanic ghetto communities.

Without minimizing the enormous contribution made by those who have sought to educate and counsel about the risk of AIDS, there can be no question but that the palpable presence of AIDS in communities across America has been an important teacher, perhaps *the* teacher. Amplifying the warnings of the safer sex literature have been the personal knowledge of those who are sick and dying, the visits to hospitals, the provision of care and comfort, the funerals and burial ceremonies, the obituaries. To the extent that educational efforts in the face of AIDS have been strikingly more effective than other health promotion campaigns it is very possible that the immediacy of disease and death has made the difference. If this is so, it may be that education will be most effective in those communities where the silent epidemic of HIV infection has already taken hold, producing an ever-rising toll of illness and death. But in those communities where relatively few are infected and still fewer clinically ill, education may have a more modest impact. In short, education may be most effective when it is almost too late to protect the communal good.

Education and the Culture of Responsibility

That more innovative and intensive anti-AIDS campaigns will be necessary in the next years is not a matter of dispute, though conservative resistance to the public funding of efforts directed at gay men and drug users will doubtlessly hinder such undertakings. What is clear, however, is that such efforts will be far more complex and difficult than the mere conveyance of information about risk reduction. Though pockets of ignorance about the risks of HIV transmission remain, the challenge is not primarily cognitive. Rather, it is psychological, social, and cultural. Involved in the effort to limit the spread of HIV infection will be nothing less than a profound transformation in the way men, women, and adolescents choose to behave in the face of risks to themselves and those with whom they have sexual relations.

Although as a practical matter individuals will be compelled to bear a great burden in learning how to protect themselves from AIDS, it would be a grave mistake to confine the foundations of social policy and communal expectations to the narrow premises of private self-defense. Repeatedly during the epidemic, fear of moralism and the dread of coercive state authority have resulted in assertions that because HIV infection is transmitted in private, individuals must be their own guardians. But the importance of vigilance does not eliminate the moral claims that can be made on those who pose a threat because of their infectious state. In the case of AIDS, precisely because the transmission of a lethal agent occurs in private, in the most intimate settings, those moral claims are all the more powerful.

The goals of education are clear. Those who are uninfected will have to insist that condoms be used in sexual intercourse with infected or possibly infected partners. Some will choose not to have intercourse, under any circumstances, with the infected. Uninfected addicts will have to give up the ritual of needle sharing. The most difficult changes to foster and sustain over time will be those that impose restrictions and imperatives on individuals who are already infected. Their motivation will be weaker than that of persons who can still protect themselves. They will have to warn their sexual partners about their HIV status even at the risk of rejection. And they will have to give up pleasures, some more difficult to yield than others—sexual intercourse without the use of condoms and the option of procreation, for example—solely on the basis of a sense of moral responsibility.

The fundamental challenge to public health officials is a collective one. It is to foster the emergence of a culture of restraint and responsibility that would inform sexual behavior, childbearing, and drug use.

Only such a transformation can affect the private choices that will determine the future of AIDS in America. Impeding that transformation will be the psychological capacity for denial in the face of dreadful situations, moral indifference, and the social factors that give rise to and sustain patterns of behavior linked to the transmission of the AIDS virus—most critically the poverty that is at the root of intravenous drug use and teenage pregnancy in America's ghettos. Without an assault on the socioeconomic roots of those behaviors linked to the spread of HIV infection, emphasis on the importance of a culture of restraint and responsibility will inevitably take on the tones of a moralistic crusade. Contempt for those who fail to conform their behavior to stipulated standards will be one consequence. More critically, without the understanding that far more is required to stop the AIDS epidemic than lessons in rectitude, any campaign of education for behavior modification is bound to end in failure. But if in the long run an assault on the social factors that make it so difficult for men, women, and adolescents to modify their behaviors will be necessary, the effort to foster change cannot await such broad-scale structural transformations.

Public health officials cannot create a culture of restraint and responsibility; they can only facilitate its development. Funding educational programs, both broadly directed and, especially, targeted at those most at risk for HIV infection, will be essential. So too will public policies that make clear the social interest in interrupting the transmission of HIV infection while protecting the rights of the infected. Ultimately, however, the culture of restraint and responsibility must take hold and be reinforced among those at risk for acquiring AIDS if it is to shape their private acts. It cannot be imposed upon them from above. Power has its limits.

Normally the pace of cultural change is measured in years. The transmission of HIV infection, however, occurs according to a biological tempo. In the struggle to alter the trajectory of the AIDS epidemic, time is not an ally.

Chapter 8

AIDS and the Politics of Public Health

At the conclusion of *Plagues and People,* his magisterial account of epidemics and their impact on history, William McNeill asserted, "Ingenuity, knowledge and organization alter but cannot cancel humanity's vulnerability to invasion by parasitic forms of life. Infectious disease, which antedates the emergence of humankind, will last as long as humanity itself, and will surely remain as it has been hitherto one of the fundamental parameters and determinants of human history."[1] Written in the mid-1970s, these observations seemed, at the time, somewhat overdrawn, especially in relation to the advanced technological societies. Now, in the midst of the AIDS epidemic, as American political and social institutions seek to fashion a response to the AIDS retrovirus, McNeill's observations seem prescient.

In the face of a new infectious and deadly disease, one whose etiological agent has already infected one to two million Americans, there has been an understandable popular tendency to believe that the public health response ought to reflect the gravity of the situation. A deadly disease demands a forceful, and, some have believed, a Draconian response. In fact, however, public health departments across the country—and especially those in New York City and San Francisco—have responded during the first years of the AIDS epidemic with remarkable restraint. What better indication of the efforts to avoid even the appearance of excess and to balance a commitment to public health with an appreciation of the political complexities of trying to control an epidemic spread in the context of intimate settings among groups deeply suspicious of governmental authority than the lengthy, even tortured, discussion of whether or not to shut the bathhouses? At the federal level, recommendations of the Centers for Disease Control that dealt with schools, the workplace, and hospitals in 1985 were designed to limit the impulse toward rash and unfounded acts of discrimination against those with HIV infection.

Indeed, in response to social anxiety about the threat of AIDS, public health officials have sought repeatedly to provide an antidote to panic. In a 1983 speech to the United States Conference of Mayors on the second anniversary of the first reports of AIDS, Margaret Heckler, secretary of the Department of Health and Human Services, declared, "My subject is a disease—a disease with two names. One is AIDS . . . the other is 'fear.' Not 'concern.' Not 'caution.' But unreasoned and unsubstantiated fear. . . . I am concerned that all of us . . . might be confronted with an unnecessary and unjustified level of fear, if misunderstanding of AIDS is allowed to grow. Such a level of fear could actually impede us in our real tasks—to understand and conquer the disease and to care for its victims. . . . The facts alone are an antidote to fear . . . and the facts are telling us more and more clearly . . . that the risk of AIDS is confined to identifiable factors. For the overwhelming majority of Americans, there appears to be little or no risk of falling victim to this disease—in particular through normal daily social contacts."[2] Writing in the fall of the same year, James Curran of the Centers for Disease Control lamented the "unwarranted hysteria" over AIDS.[3] He found especially distressing reports that some medical institutions had failed to provide appropriate levels of care to those with AIDS and were using "the syndrome as an excuse to justify discrimination." Such hysteria was grounded, argued Curran, in the public's perception that little was known about AIDS and its transmission. To such concerns, the director of the CDC's AIDS effort responded reassuringly about the very limited ways in which AIDS was transmitted.

In 1986 the surgeon general,[4] and the National Academy of Sciences and the Institute of Medicine added their voices to the chorus of appeals for calm and reason.[5] Amplifying the antialarmist message of these public health officials and institutions were the media—the TV networks, the weekly news magazines, and most strikingly, the *New York Times* and the Los Angeles *Times*.

Integral to the attempt to contain social anxiety and prevent social disruption was the effort to inform the public that the merely theoretical risks of HIV transmission posed no calculable hazard. How different was this effort at reassurance from what historian David Rothman has termed the apocalyptic thinking that has often characterized the response of public health officials to situations marked by some degree of uncertainty. "Public health practitioners generally tend . . . to treat unknowns as unfavorable outcomes. When in doubt, they assume that the risks are maximal, and they recommend doing everything possible to avert them."[6] Had such thinking dominated the response to AIDS, it would have provided the rationale for the wide-scale adoption of compulsory measures and subverted the very prospect for an ordered and socially effective response to the new disease. James Curran himself acknowledged in 1984 that a desire to avert disorder might well have played a role in the early characterization of AIDS. "I think to some extent we have underestimated the problem. . . . The reason is probably a strong subconscious urge for it not to be as bad as it could be. . . . [We haven't wanted] to disrupt society from the point of view of blood donations, blood banking, and a variety of other things."[7]

Certainly in New York City a desire to control irrational fears and to prevent social disruption produced an official climate within which an extraordinary effort was made to judge both public statements and policies in terms of how they might contribute, however inadvertently, to alarm. This effort was all the more striking since it was David Sencer, the city's health commissioner, who as director at the CDC had begun mobilizing for universal vaccination for a swine flu epidemic, on the basis of an outbreak involving a handful of cases. In that instance, in what has since been termed "the epidemic that never was," Sencer behaved precisely the way David Rothman's "apocalyptic" public health official might have been expected to respond.[8] How different he was with AIDS! Sencer had done just what Richard Neustadt and Harvey Fineberg had warned about in their study of the swine flu vaccine fiasco. He had "learned the lesson too well—too literally—producing stalemate in the face of the next out-of-routine threat."[9] Only it was not the flu but a virulent retroviral infection that had tested Sencer's judgment. Indeed, Roy Goodman, the state senator who was to mobilize legislative support for New York's innovative plan to create an AIDS Institute that would fund both research into AIDS and community efforts directed at prevention, said, "I am deeply disturbed at the fact that you [David Axelrod] as health commissioner of [New York] state and Dr. Sencer as health commissioner of the City, have been exceedingly low-key, to the point, in my judgment, of insufficiency of response to what medical experts have told us is a rapidly spreading syndrome."[10]

Opponents of the antialarmist and restrained posture of public health officials saw in their response to AIDS a failure of professional responsibility and public duty. The unwillingness to characterize every theoretical risk as a public danger, to put forth "tough" policies on AIDS, was not a sign of wisdom but of timidity, an unconscionable capitulation to gay political pressure and a subversion of the ethos of public health by that of civil liberties. Others, ironically, saw it as an act of collaboration with politicians who would not devote the resources necessary to combat an epidemic that afflicted primarily gay men and intravenous drug users.

Accusations against public health officials for their failure to move aggressively against disease and their capitulation to special interests are not new. Charles Rosenberg has noted that, in the nineteenth century, physicians who were too quick to discover the presence in their communities of epidemic diseases were often the targets of censure.[11] Since such diagnoses could well produce financial disaster for local commercial interests, public health officers, who were typically beholden to political leaders, sometimes sought to silence those who warned of the imminence of epidemics and to restrain the overzealous. A contemporary critic said of the New York Board of Health that "it was more afraid of merchants than of lying."[12]

In the case of AIDS—despite the professionalization in the twentieth century of those responsible for public health—anxiety surfaced over whether political motivations had colored not only the willingness to press for forceful measures, but also official antialarmist pronouncements about the threats posed by the AIDS virus. These anxieties were fueled by the very efforts to limit the impact of what had been termed early in the history of AIDS the "secondary epidemic"—the epidemic of fear. Reassuring statements about the risks of HIV transmission, no matter how sound, provoked questions about the scientific basis for judgments in the face of inevitable uncertainty. To the extent that some public health officials had relentlessly challenged data with socially discomfiting implications—the possibility of transmission from HIV-infected females to their male sexual partners, for example—they had inadvertently contributed to the disquiet. How much more had they refused to acknowledge? Similarly, refusals to adopt standard venereal disease control measures like sexual contact notification provoked concerns about whether arguments against other aggressive measures represented a capitulation to the demands of those who failed to give the public health the priority it warranted.

Ironically, public health officials were also charged with exaggerating the extent to which AIDS posed a threat to the American social mainstream. Here too they had contributed to a climate of distrust. To underscore the biologically incontestable point that HIV transmission could occur within both homosexual and heterosexual relations, that AIDS had no sexual preference, some public health leaders had asserted that there were no high-risk *groups*, only high-risk *acts*. But in terms of the epidemiological risk of contracting AIDS, such an appealingly universal formulation, which shifted the onus of attention from gay men and intravenous drug-users to all sexually active individuals, was misleading. It mattered who one was *as well as* what one did. Sexual acts like intercourse without the use of condoms posed a calculable danger among individuals who were at increased risk of infection. Where HIV infection was very rare or almost nonexistent, the same acts represented only a theoretical hazard. To those who were always ready to suspect the motives of public health officials, emphasis on the common threat of HIV infection—so prominent in both the surgeon general's report and the Institute of Medicine–National Academy of Science's *Confronting AIDS*—was nothing but a scientifically dishonest act of collaboration with gay leaders who had an understandable political interest in dehomosexualizing AIDS. How better to encourage massive expenditures on research and treatment than to destigmatize the epidemic by making it a challenge to the communal fate, rather than to the fate of the socially marginal? Motivated by antialarmist concerns, rather than by an animus toward gay men and intravenous drug users, the *New York Times*, too, cast doubt upon the motives of those who sought to stress the epidemic's universal threat.

Such AIDS-specific doubts merged with an undercurrent of populist distrust for scientific authority that had been amplified in recent years by politically charged debates among scientists over environmental and occupational health policy.[13] If committed experts could do battle over the threats posed by environmental or workplace toxins and if governmental standards for exposure to such substances could shift with Washington's administrations, what could guarantee that the American people were not being manipulated by scientists whose statements were inspired by partisan considerations? Certainly it was such suspicions that permitted Lyndon LaRouche's Prevent AIDS Now Committee to capture 29 percent of the vote on a California referendum opposed by the state's public health and scientific leadership.

The lessons of Proposition 64 were clear. The social basis for the support of groundless, drastic measures is created when popular perceptions take hold of a failure by public health officials to pursue a course deemed adequate to protect communal well-being. Writing about the Black Death, William McNeill noted, "In northern Europe, the absence of well-defined public quarantine regulations and administrative routines—religious as well as medical—with which to deal with plagues and rumors of plagues gave scope for violent expression of popular hates and fears provoked by the disease. In particular, long-standing grievances of poor against rich often boiled to the surface."[14] We have, thus far, not experienced the kind of anomic outbursts described by McNeill, though reported increases of assaults on gay men and strikes by parents seeking to keep schoolchildren with AIDS from the classroom may be viewed as functional, but pale, equivalents.[15] More to the point, however, have been the calls in the press, in state legislatures, and from insurgent candidates for elective office—still restricted to the extreme right-wing of American politics—for the quarantine of all antibody-positive individuals, despite the opposition of the public health establishment.

Rarely do those who propose mass quarantine suggest how all antibody-positive individuals would be identified, how they would be removed to quarantine centers, how they would be fed and housed, how they would be forcibly contained. Indeed, it is one of the remarkable features of proposals for mass quarantine as a public health response to AIDS, and an indication of the profound irrationality of such suggestions, that they treat with abandon matters of practicality and history. Because proponents of quarantine speak of mass removal as if it were an antiseptic surgical excision, it is possible for them to suggest that their ends could be achieved without grave social disruptions. A vision of benign quarantine measures is informed by memories of health officers imposing isolation on those who suffered from diseases such as scarlet fever. But when quarantine has been imposed upon those who viewed themselves as unfairly targeted by the state's actions, the story has at times been quite different. Judith Leavitt's description of how German immigrants in Milwaukee responded to efforts at the forced removal and isolation of those with smallpox provides ample evidence of what might be expected if even local and confined efforts to isolate large numbers of HIV-infected individuals were undertaken: "Daily crowds of people took to the streets, seeking out health officials to harass."[16]

Even if the vast and thoroughgoing rejection of our fundamental constitutional and moral values that would be entailed in such mass quarantine were tolerable, and even if it were possible to gather broad-based political support for such measures, the inevitable chaos and social burdens that would attend such an approach to containing the epidemic make such a move unlikely. Nevertheless, despite the irrationality and potentially destructive dimensions of mass quarantine, impulsive efforts to move in such a direction might be made if social anxiety over AIDS were to intensify dramatically in the next years.

Of a very different order are proposals for the quarantine of individuals—male or female prostitutes, for example—who, though infected with the AIDS virus, continue to behave publicly in ways that expose others to the possibility of HIV infection. Though moral, legal, and constitutional impediments to the imposition of state control over all antibody-positive individuals do not arise in such cases, it is abundantly clear that the strategy of isolating such persons could have very little direct impact on the spread of HIV infection. An examination of the more finely tuned attempts to impose isolation or quarantine upon "recalcitrant" tuberculosis patients ("careless consumptives"), for example, reveals the administrative burden created when even a modicum of procedural fairness is employed. More important, such efforts, directed as they are at the most obvious sources of infection, would fail to identify and restrict the many hundreds of thousands of infected individuals who in the privacy of their bedrooms might be engaged in acts that could involve the spread of HIV infection. If the quarantine of all antibody-positive individuals would be overinclusive—imposing deprivations upon those who had modified their behaviors in order to reduce the risk of HIV transmission—the quarantine of public "recalcitrants" would be underinclusive. That is the price that must be paid for living in a constitutional society with even a rudimentary commitment to the principles of law, privacy, and civil liberties. It is also a restriction placed upon us by reality.

To some who recoil from the notion of mass quarantine, the possibility of broad-scale mandatory screening to identify the infected seems a more practical and tolerable intervention, one that could with only "limited" intrusions upon privacy compel individuals to confront their own infectious status, thus permitting them to make responsible adjustments in their sexual and drug-using behavior as well as in their procreative choices. Generally, proposals for mass screening target those deemed to be at increased risk for AIDS. But since it is impossible to know who is, in fact, a member of a "high-risk group," such proposals would inevitably require universal screening. Such a program would, in turn, require the registration of the entire population to assure that none escaped the testing net. Since one-time screening would be insufficient to detect new cases of infection, it would be necessary to track the movements of all individuals so that they might be tested repeatedly. Finally, to make such an effort worthwhile, pressure would mount for a system of behavioral surveillance of those found to be infected. Thus, a "limited" intrusion would lead ineluctably to an extraordinary invasion of privacy and would entail the creation of a bureaucratic health apparatus at enormous social expense. And there is little reason to believe that such a venture into coercion would benefit the public health in a significant way.

Closer to the trend that began to emerge in 1987 are proposals to use virtually every encounter with the health care system as an occasion for mandatory or routine testing without informed consent. Such proposals have won popular support and the enthusiastic endorsement of some politicians. Virtually all such suggestions, however, lack any appreciation of how such testing would set the stage for behavioral modifications that are, in the absence of an effective therapeutic agent, crucial to the struggle against AIDS. Indeed, there is rarely even the beginning of a thoughtful consideration of whether programs of coercive testing are compatible with the difficult task of motivating individuals to give up behaviors that are the source of psychological and biological pleasures, and of creating a political climate within which a culture of restraint and responsibility could take hold among those at risk for transmitting HIV infection. Thus the defense of the public health is invoked to justify invasions of privacy with little evidence that the public health would be protected by such intrusions. In fact, there is reason to believe that such intrusions would, because of their social consequences, impair efforts to advance the cause of public health.

It is in the light of the very limited rational role that coercive measures might play in the control of AIDS that public health officials have so universally argued in favor of education as the preeminent line of social defense against the epidemic. It is, however, the disjunction between an epidemic that has been portrayed as representing the major public health challenge of the last part of the twentieth century and interventions that must ultimately rely on persuasion that is so disconcerting, that provokes questions about whether public health officials have the will to do everything that needs to be done to control so grave a threat.

In the next years public health officials will be confronted with repeated challenges to their characterization of the threat posed by AIDS and HIV transmission and to their proposed policies for controlling the epidemic's spread. It will take considerable effort and political skill to win popular support for the proposition that broad-scale recourse to coercive state power not only would be socially disruptive and inimical to the preservation of the values and institutions of a liberal democracy, but would subvert the very possibility of developing programs to foster change in those private behaviors linked to the spread of HIV infection. Popular support for such a strategy will depend on the capacity of public health officials to convey a sense of both urgency and the importance of restraint in the exercise of public health powers, and on their capacity to demonstrate why restraint is critical to the protection of the public health rather than a capitulation to the demands of those who place privacy above the communal good.

It will be all the more difficult to argue effectively for restraint in the next years as the number of AIDS cases rises dramatically, with the rapid spread of HIV infection in the black and Hispanic ghettos among intravenous drug users and their sexual partners. As antihomosexual social instincts were tapped in the early years of the AIDS epidemic, racism and disgust for the underclass will inevitably affect the responses in the years ahead. The ghettoization of HIV transmission may simultaneously weaken the commitment to the expenditure of the vast resources needed to combat AIDS and serve as an invitation to reliance on repressive public health interventions. The awful predicability of an increasing number of babies with AIDS will contribute to the temptation to employ coercive measures. Whether the political culture of the AIDS epidemic, forged in the first years of the disease when gay leaders so forcefully articulated the importance of a voluntarist strategy that respected privacy, will prevail cannot be predicted. But the ease with which it might be subverted should not mask the fact that essential features of that strategy will be crucial to the struggle against AIDS, however the epidemiological pattern changes. The fundamental task for public health in the next years will remain that of fostering a culture of restraint and responsibility among those who can transmit the AIDS virus through sexual behavior, drug use, and childbearing. That challenge will not be met if those at risk are given reason to view public health officials as agents of repression.

In the face of this challenge, what is to be done? Through education freed from the strictures of moralism and conveyed in forceful and imaginative ways, public health officials can disseminate not only knowledge but an appreciation of the moral claims imposed by the threat of HIV infection. By demanding that no drug user in search of treatment be denied access to care they can demonstrate that social neglect is incompatible with a vigorous campaign against AIDS. By undertaking bold experiments, including needle exchange programs designed to reach drug users uninterested in or refractory to treatment, they can underscore the willingness to place the prevention of HIV transmission above the dictates of convention. By promoting confidential as well as anonymous screening programs that reach out aggressively to those in need of testing to encourage the adoption of responsible behavior, they can advance the public health while simultaneously protecting the privacy of those who come forward. By defending the social rights of the infected, they can create a climate of trust among those who are so vulnerable to irrational acts of discrimination. By creating contact notification programs they can underscore the public commitment to warning those who might not otherwise know they had been exposed to the AIDS virus. And by supporting carefully delimited legislation to control those who are infected but who recklessly and maliciously place others at risk they can establish the moral priority of protecting the public health as a social norm.

Each of these measures, some with greater impact than others, will contribute to the interruption of the spread of HIV infection. But it is as an ensemble that these measures will make a contribution to the emergence of a culture of responsibility, the most enduring contribution that public health officials can make to the struggle against the AIDS epidemic.

In moving to enact such measures public health officials will be compelled to face the legacy of their own past efforts to control infectious diseases, the pressure of elected officials responding to social anxieties produced by the AIDS epidemic, and the fears of those most at risk for HIV infection. The history of public health is an authoritarian history rooted in the experience of confronting epidemics in a fundamentally different sociopolitical milieu. Public health officials will have to recognize that interventions deemed appropriate early in the twentieth century will now arouse profound opposition. More, they will need to tailor their interventions to the features of the AIDS epidemic that make virtually all recourse to coercion counterproductive. Inevitably, such efforts will provoke the ire of those politicians who will demand that the state's power be used in more aggressive ways. On some occasions the mistaken judgment of elected officials will prevail. Under such circumstances it will be especially critical for public health officials to preserve, publicly if possible, their distinctive perspectives, not only to bring about the reversal of unwise decisions, but to retain the prospects of collaborative relationships with those most at risk for AIDS. But the importance of fostering and preserving such relationships should not be confused with the assumption that agreement about how to combat AIDS invariably will exist between health officials and those who represent the populations at risk. Indeed, given the characteristically individualistic political ideologies of those who speak on behalf of gay men and women at risk, conflicts will be inevitable. The great challenge under such circumstances will be to argue openly for the requirements of public health while moving prudently. Failure to pursue such a course would rightfully provoke accusations of the betrayal of the public health by those charged with the responsibility for its defense.

However successful public health officials are in traversing the terrain of the politics associated with AIDS, however wise their policies in seeking to transform the social context within which HIV transmission occurs, and however attentive they are to the importance of developing interventions that are both just and effective, their efforts will have little impact on the course of AIDS in the near future. The contours of the epidemic in the next few years have been all but determined. The situation may get worse. There is little chance that it will get better. In the absence of a remarkable therapeutic breakthrough, a high proportion of those who are already infected will, with a grim inevitability, fall victim to AIDS. Almost all will die.

But even for the more distant future great difficulties lie ahead. Instead of the grand public health vision of stopping AIDS, it will be necessary to settle for the more modest goal of shaping the public context within which the struggle to limit the spread of HIV infection will occur. That struggle will be waged at a popular level by ordinary men, women, and adolescents as they seek to carve out private lives in the face of a biological challenge that has joined the intimate and the lethal. It is only to the extent that a culture of responsibility emerges from that struggle, and a recognition of the profound moral responsibilities imposed by AIDS takes hold, that the trajectory of morbidity and mortality will be altered. The epidemic will force a sharp confrontation with the individualistic self-interest that is so important a component of American social ideology.

As we pursue the circumscribed but critical goal of informing the public culture of the AIDS epidemic, we will have to understand at each juncture the limits on our capacity to fight an infectious disease like AIDS, even as we press against those limits. What will be required is a posture of social stoicism. Not to be confused with defeatism, such a stance would make possible the economic, scientific, clinical, and human exertions over the long haul that AIDS will demand. It will also provide the grounds for restraint against the impulse to embrace coercive solutions to the AIDS epidemic. Stoicism is the social antidote to unreasonable, illusory optimism as well as to despair.

We are, in the end, hostage to the advances of virology and immunology, and will be so for many years. In the interim, during this protracted encounter with the microparasitic threat posed by the AIDS virus it will be crucial to fashion policies that are both effective and protective of human dignity, policies that reflect a recognition of the fact that how we seek to interdict the spread of HIV infection, how we care for those who fall ill, and how we protect the infected from the social burdens of stigma will have fundamental consequences for the fabric of American social life. Wise policies may be subverted by those who rashly press for coercive measures as well as by those who denounce every public health intervention as a harbinger of repression. Health officials at municipal, state, and federal levels will play a central role in charting the course of America's response to AIDS. Ultimately, however, their efforts and the policies they pursue will be determined by how America as a political community faces the challenge of AIDS. Failure before this challenge not only will hinder the effort to limit the exactions taken by the epidemic, but will have dire social consequences. The history of earlier epidemics should serve as a warning.

Afterword

Entering the Second Decade

The Politics of Prevention, the Politics of Neglect

With 1991, the AIDS epidemic in the United States enters its second decade. More than 200,000 people have been diagnosed with AIDS; 140,000 are dead. It is a time of great promise but also of great risk. The remarkable advances in the biomedical realm and the formulation of public policies designed to limit the spread of HIV infection and protect the rights of those who are infected or at risk of infection stand as singular accomplishments, all the more so since they have come as a consequence of intense political conflict, spurred by the demands of those who have borne the burden of disease and their allies.

But these achievements also set the stage for new controversies in public health, some centering on matters that received only passing attention in *Private Acts, Social Consequences*, prepared for publication in mid-1988. The central political and ethical question of privacy that provided the core theme of political debate in the epidemic's first phase has now been joined, although not displaced, by that of equity. How America responds to the new set of issues surrounding access to potentially life-prolonging therapies will have a profound impact on the shape and course of the epidemic in the next years. The situation will be, however, far different in the Third World, where because of the international maldistribution of resources, both professional and economic, access to new therapeutic regimes will be all but beyond reach. A single virus may thus create two very different epidemic patterns—one that permits increasingly effective clinical responses; another where men, women, and children continue to succumb, with an enormous toll in human suffering and social dislocation.

Inevitably, public policy will be affected by changing perceptions of the dimensions of the epidemic. Estimates of the number of infected individuals made in 1986 were, it is now clear, too high. Indeed, figures presented in late 1989 suggest that no more and perhaps fewer Americans were infected at that time than were assumed to be infected three years earlier.[1] As important, epidemiological trends first noticed in the last years of the 1980s have made it clear that while heterosexual transmission of HIV does occur, the spread of infection has remained largely confined to those groups first identified as being at increased risk. The prospect of a rapid spread of HIV among the general population, which served as a specter haunting public policy and which fueled public anxieties, is not currently considered likely. Gay and bisexual men, intravenous drug users, their typically female sexual partners and their offspring will continue to bear the great preponderance of the epidemic's burden of disease, suffering, and death. Sexual orientation and the lines of social cleavage that tend to limit sexual contact between the poor, urban underclass and the broader society have served thus far to contain the epidemic.

Many have feared that because it appeared more marginalized, the epidemic of HIV infection might elicit fewer resources at a time when major infusions of funds for care would be needed. It is in that light that Michael Fumento's *Myth of Heterosexual AIDS* must be read, its polemical thrust directed at those who appealed for resources to meet the challenge of AIDS.[2] The angry reaction from gay groups such as Gay Men's Health Crisis, and especially ACT-UP, in the summer of 1988 when the New York City Health Department revised downward by 50 percent the estimated number of infected New Yorkers, must be understood in that light.[3] At the same time the increasing association of AIDS with the underclass may fundamentally weaken the political alliance that underlay the voluntarist consensus that dominated public discourse about prevention policies in the epidemic's first decade.

Even more critical to an understanding of the evolving political debates about AIDS and the public health are recent clinical developments. The therapeutic impotence of the early years of the epidemic has begun to yield. A sober yet more optimistic perspective has begun to emerge. There has been progress not only in meeting the challenge posed by opportunistic infections, but in slowing the progression of disease in those who are infected but still asymptomatic. While it is still too soon to speak of AIDS itself as a chronic disease, HIV infection will increasingly require the kind of long-term clinical management associated with such conditions. As a consequence, the importance of identifying those who are infected has undergone a fundamental transformation. No longer is the question before public health officials solely a matter of preventing the further spread of infection. Rather it is the task of creating the necessary medical infrastructure to assure that the million or more infected Americans are provided with appropriate clinical supervision. It is within this changed context that screening, reporting, and partner notification—issues that figured so prominently in the early days of AIDS prevention—have taken on new significance and have provoked fresh debates about the appropriate role of the state. The traditional approaches of public health officials to epidemic disease, so vigorously challenged in the early and mid-1980s, have found new support from those who had earlier found them inadequate or ethically unacceptable.

No issue has consumed more attention in the debates over public policy and AIDS than the use of the antibody test to identify those infected with HIV. In the period following the test's development, controversy centered on the role of testing in supporting the radical modifications of behavior that were universally deemed to be critical to altering the epidemic's course. Out of these debates emerged a broad consensus, often codified in state statutes, that testing should be conducted only with the informed voluntary and specific consent of individuals. Despite that standard, and the carefully defined, though always contested, exceptions to its scope, many clinicians and hospitals undertook surreptitious testing of patients, justifying their practices by the belief that the protection of health care workers and sound diagnostic work required such screening.[4] In Illinois, organized medicine went further, successfully pressing the governor and legislature, despite the opposition of the state's chief health official, to permit testing at the discretion of the clinician.[5] In New York State, four medical societies including the New York Medical Society unsuccessfully took the commissioner of health to court because of his failure to designate AIDS a sexually transmitted disease, a determination that would have permitted testing without consent.[6]

With the announcement in mid-1989 that clinical trials had revealed the efficacy of early therapeutic intervention in slowing the course of illness in asymptomatic but infected persons and in preventing the occurrence of *pneumocystis carinii* pneumonia, the political debate about testing underwent a fundamental change. Gay groups such as Project Inform in San Francisco and the Gay Men's Health Crisis in New York began to encourage those they had formerly warned against testing to determine whether or not they were infected.[7] Physicians pressed more vigorously for the "return of AIDS to the medical mainstream" so that testing might be routinely done under conditions of presumed consent.[8] Public health officials, most notably in New York and New Jersey, which had borne so much of the burden of AIDS, launched aggressive testing campaigns.

Although physicians and public health officials have typically avoided the language of compulsion, stressing instead routine testing, the threat of coercion loomed before gay activists, their liberal political allies, and proponents of civil liberties. So too did the risk of increased stigmatization and discrimination.

With the promise of early therapeutic intervention came the unraveling of the alliances that had been forged in the first phase of the epidemic. Nowhere was this clearer than in the emergence of a powerful movement supported by obstetricians and pediatricians for the routine screening of pregnant women who could transmit HIV to their offspring and the mandatory screening of infants at high risk for infection. In the case of the former, the public health practice of testing for syphilis and hepatitis B served as a model. In the latter instance, it was the wide-scale and broadly accepted tradition of screening for congenital conditions such as PKU that served as the standard. The promise—with little evidentiary base—that early intervention might protect the fetus or at least enhance the life prospects of babies at risk for HIV infection had begun to override ethical concerns about the coercive identification of infected women, most of whom were black or Hispanic, as well as about the potential burdens of exclusion from housing, social services, and health care itself that might be imposed on those so identified.

The erosion of the alliance that had resisted the application of traditional public health practices could be seen also in the shifting trends on the issue of reporting the names of those infected with HIV to confidential public health department registries. Such reporting requirements had been fiercely resisted by gay groups and their allies because of concerns about privacy and confidentiality and opposed by public health officials in areas with large numbers of AIDS cases because of the potential impact on the willingness of individuals voluntarily to seek HIV testing and counseling. As a consequence, they had become policy in only a handful of states. It was thus a great setback for those who opposed reporting that the Presidential Commission on the HIV Epidemic —appointed by President Reagan and skillfully chaired by Admiral James D. Watkins—urged in its mid-1988 final report the universal adoption of a policy first chosen by Colorado three years earlier.[9] That decision was all the more distressing since so much of the Commission's final report contained proposals broadly applauded by liberal critics of the Reagan administration's failure to commit either sufficient resources or political leadership to the struggle against AIDS.

Ultimately more significant were the fissures that had begun to appear in the alliance opposing named reporting in those states where the prevalence of HIV infection was high and where gay communities were well organized. In New York, for example, the same suit brought by the medical societies that sought to compel the commissioner of health to declare AIDS a sexually transmitted disease demanded that HIV infection be made a reportable condition.[10] What made the (ultimately unsuccessful) suit so remarkable was the posture of the opposing sides. Historically, clinicians had resisted efforts by public health officials to require the reporting by name of individuals with infectious diseases, arguing that such policies represented an intrusion upon the doctor-patient relationship. In this instance the representatives of clinical medicine were asserting that reporting was critical to the public health while the state's chief health official resisted such a perspective. That apparent paradox can be explained only by the unique political alliances that had been created early in the epidemic between gay organizations, civil liberties groups, and public health officials.

But by June 1989, even that feature of the political landscape of public health had begun to change. In an address that was met with cries of protest, Stephen Joseph, commissioner of health in New York City, told the Fifth International Conference on AIDS that the prospect of early clinical intervention necessitated "a shift toward a disease control approach to HIV infection along the lines of classic tuberculosis practices."[11] A central feature of such an approach would be the "reporting of seropositives" to assure effective clinical follow-up and the initiation of "more aggressive contact tracing." Joseph's proposals opened a debate that was only temporarily settled by the defeat of New York's Mayor Edward Koch in his bid for reelection. When newly elected Mayor David Dinkins selected Woodrow Myers, formerly commissioner of health in Indiana, to replace Joseph, his appointment was almost aborted, in part because he had supported named reporting.[12] The festering debate was ended only by a political decision on the part of the mayor, who had drawn heavily on support within the gay community, to stand by his appointment while promising that there would be no named reporting in New York.

In New Jersey, which shares with New York a relatively high level of HIV infection, the commissioner of health also supported named reporting, but in that case the politics which surrounded the issue were very different. There both houses of the state legislature endorsed without dissent a confidentiality statute that included named reporting of cases of HIV infection.[13] New Jersey simply exemplified a national trend. For, although only nine states at the end of 1989 required named reporting without any provision for anonymity, states increasingly were adopting policies that required reporting in at least some circumstances.[14] And always the arguments were the same. New therapeutic possibilities provided the warrant for reestablishing a standard of traditional public health practice.

Ironically, pressure to provide Medicaid coverage for early treatment and to expand government-funded clinics to treat those with HIV infection will inevitably result in the creation of records on growing numbers of infected individuals regardless of whether states adopt mandatory reporting requirements. The move toward early clinical intervention is, then, incompatible with the preservation of anonymity. As a result, the importance of creating and enforcing regimes to protect the rights of infected persons from acts of discrimination will assume greater importance than in the epidemic's first years. In this context, not only state-level protections for individuals with HIV infection will be crucial. More important will be the enforcement of the Americans with Disabilities Act by the Congress, legislation that extends to those with HIV infection rights guaranteed to those with other impairments.

The move toward reporting was linked only in part to the argument that state health departments needed the names of individuals to assure adequate clinical follow-up. As important was the assertion from public health officials that effective contact tracing, now more critical than ever because of the need for early clinical intervention, could be undertaken only if those with HIV infection, but who were not yet diagnosed as having AIDS, could be interviewed. Despite its central and well-established role in venereal disease control, the notification of the sexual and needle-sharing partners in the context of AIDS had been a source of ongoing conflict between gay groups and civil liberties organizations on the one hand, and public health officials who had proposed such a strategy in the early years of the epidemic on the other. Always predicated on the willingness of those with sexually transmitted diseases to provide public health workers with the names of their partners in exchange for a promise of anonymity, this standard disease control measure had been viewed by AIDS activists as a threat to confidentiality, and as a potentially coercive intervention. Indeed, opponents of contact tracing typically denounced it as "mandatory."

With time and a better understanding of how contact tracing functioned in the context of sexually transmitted diseases, some of the most vocal opponents of tracing yielded their principled opposition at least in private meetings and discussions, and instead centered their concerns about the cost of so labor-intensive an intervention. Support for voluntary contact tracing was ultimately to come from the Institute of Medicine and the National Academy of Sciences, the Presidential Commission on the HIV Epidemic, the American Bar Association, and the American Medical Association.[15] Indeed, it was the AMA's support for tracing, justified by its executive director, James Sammons, as having "the potential in the heterosexual society to substantially reduce the proliferation and spread of AIDS," that provided the grounds for the group's support for mandatory HIV reporting.[16]

Most influential in pressing for the adoption of contact tracing programs at the state level, where all such programs are organized and funded, has been the Centers for Disease Control.[17] Critically involved in the training of STD workers and in the funding of local venereal disease programs, the CDC had from the outset urged the adoption of this standard public health approach to AIDS and HIV infection. In February of 1988, the federal agency took on a more aggressive posture, making the adoption of partner notification by the states a condition for the receipt of funds from its HIV Prevention Program.[18] Despite such pressure, the response on the part of the states was variable. Those that were most heavily burdened by AIDS continued to favor programs that encouraged infected individuals to notify their own partners. Of the states that stressed the role of professional public health workers—the "provider referral" model—most tended to have relatively modest AIDS case counts.[19] Thus, local epidemiological factors as well as political forces continued to influence the course of public health policy.

In part, both the early and the lingering resistance to partner notification can be explained by the conflation of the standard public health approach to sexually transmitted disease control with policies and practices which are rooted in a very different tradition, entailing a "duty to warn" or protect those who might be threatened by individuals with communicable conditions. In the early part of this century courts and legislatures adopted legal norms that imposed upon those with infectious diseases a duty to inform those they might place at risk through contact. Physicians who knew that their patients could place family members or neighbors in danger could be held civilly liable for failure to warn those at risk.[20] With the decline of infectious disease as a social threat, this legal tradition fell into disuse. It was given new life, however, with the 1976 case of *Tarasoff* v. *Regents of California*, which held that psychotherapists had a duty to protect the identifiable potential victims of their patients' violent acts. While some state courts have rejected *Tarasoff*, others have handed down rulings that placed limits on the principle of the inviolability of physician-patient communications, holding that clinicians had a duty to either protect or warn identifiable individuals who might be harmed by those under their treatment.[21] It was that line of cases that set the stage for the debate over whether physicians could be held liable for failing to warn the partners of those who, though infected with HIV, planned to act in a way that posed a risk of viral transmission.

The early and strict confidentiality rules surrounding HIV screening and medical records all but precluded physicians from assuming their *Tarasoff*-like duties, especially in New York and California. In recent years, the recognition that such limitations placed physicians in a position that sometimes violated professional ethical norms, the realization that some patients could pose a grave threat to unsuspecting partners, and the increasing importance of early therapeutic intervention have led to modifications of early confidentiality restrictions. Although often opposed on principled grounds by those who believed that physician-patient communications should never be violated and by those who argued that such breaches of confidentiality would have the counterproductive consequence of reducing patient candor, thus limiting the capacity of clinicians to effectively counsel and persuade individuals who might harm their partners, such modifications in the standard of strict confidentiality have been given strong support in a number of state legislatures, and by the American Medical Association and the Association of State and Territorial Health Officials.[22]

As of 1990, no state had imposed upon physicians a duty to warn unsuspecting partners. But about a dozen had adopted legislation granting physicians a "privilege to warn or inform," thus freeing physicians from liability for either warning or not warning those at risk.[23] Reflecting profound concerns about the centrality of confidentiality to the struggle against AIDS, New York's 1989 confidentiality statute went further and, borrowing from the tradition of contact tracing, stipulated that the identity of the threatening party not be revealed to those being warned.[24] To those—the American Bar Association, for example[25]—who believed that adequate warnings required the identification of the infected party to the individuals placed at risk, such compromises represented an undue limitation imposed by a mistaken interpretation of the ethics of confidentiality.

The question of how to respond to individuals whose behavior represented a threat to unknowing partners inevitably provoked continued discussion of the public health tradition of imposing restrictions on liberty in the name of communal welfare. The specter of quarantine has haunted all such discussions, not because there was any serious consideration in the United States of the Cuban approach to AIDS—which mandates the isolation of all persons infected with HIV[26]—but because of fears that even a more limited recognition of the authority to quarantine would lead to egregious intrusions upon privacy and invidiously imposed deprivations of freedom.

Although fierce opposition has surfaced to all efforts to bring AIDS within the scope of state quarantine statutes, more than a dozen states did so between 1987 and 1990, typically using the occasion to modernize their disease control laws to reflect contemporary constitutional standards which detail procedural guarantees, and to require that restrictions on freedom represent the "least restrictive alternative" available to achieve a "compelling state interest."[27]

Soon after he resigned as commissioner of health in New York City at the end of 1989, Stephen Joseph bluntly made the case for the careful exercise of the power of quarantine. He did so on the occasion of the continuing uproar surrounding the appointment of Woodrow Myers as his successor. Gay and civil liberties groups opposed Myers, in part, because he had supported quarantine legislation in Indiana and had reportedly exercised the authority then granted him under state law. They demanded that such policies never be pursued in New York. No such pledge could or should be made, stated Joseph in an editorial written for the *New York Times*.[28] Among his last formal acts had been the signing of a detention order for a woman with infectious tuberculosis because of her continued unwillingness to take the medication that would render her noninfectious. "It is virtually certain that at some point, a New York City Health Commissioner will be faced with an analogous situation concerning the transmission of the AIDS virus. When all lesser remedies have failed, can anyone doubt what would be the proper course of action for the Commissioner to take, faced with . . . an infected individual who knowingly and repeatedly sold his blood for transfusion?" When and if a treatment became available that would render HIV-infected persons less infectious, "would there not then be a clear obligation to take all reasonable measures to ensure that the infected take their medication, thus protecting others?" In characteristically vigorous form Joseph reasserted the traditional claims of public health, the former commissioner's language emboldened by the freedom to speak without the constraints of office. It was a boldness reinforced by the belief that with advances in therapy AIDS and its control would follow the model established by earlier infectious diseases.

With the exception of the few notable cases that have received press attention, there is no well-documented review of the extent to which newly revised quarantine statutes have been applied to the AIDS epidemic. There are, however, data to suggest that the power vested in public health officials by such laws has been used more often to warn those whose behavior has posed a risk of HIV transmission than to incarcerate. But in any case the numbers have been small. It is clear therefore that the enactment of revised quarantine laws has been responsive to political pressures and the belief in the efficacy of symbolic bulwarks.

The enactment of statutes criminalizing behaviors linked to the spread of AIDS has paralleled the political receptivity to laws extending the authority of public health officials to control individuals whose behavior posed a risk of HIV transmission. Such use of the criminal law, broadly endorsed by the Presidential Commission on the HIV Epidemic, called upon a tradition of state enactments that made the knowing transmission of venereal disease a crime.[29] Though they almost never were enforced, the existence of these older laws served as a rationale for new legislative initiatives. Between 1987 and 1989, twenty states enacted such statutes, the vast majority of which defined the proscribed acts as felonies despite the fact that older statutes typically treated knowing transmission as a misdemeanor.[30] As important, aggressive prosecutors have relied on laws defining assaultive behavior and attempted murder to bring indictments even in the absence of AIDS-specific legislation.

Any effort to determine the extent to which prosecutions for HIV-related acts have occurred must confront the difficulty of monitoring the activity of local courts when there is neither a guilty verdict nor an appeal to a higher state tribunal. One survey, relying on newspaper accounts as well as official court reports, estimated that between fifty and one hundred prosecutions had been initiated involving acts as diverse as spitting, biting, blood splattering, blood donation, and sexual intercourse with an unsuspecting partner.[31] Though small in number these cases have drawn great attention. In the vast majority there was either an acquittal or the prosecution was dropped. In the small number of cases that produced guilty verdicts, there have been some unusually harsh sentences. In Nevada, where prostitution is both legal and regulated, a woman was sentenced to twenty years' imprisonment in 1989 under a statute that made solicitation by those who tested positive for HIV a felony. In the same year, an Indiana appeals court upheld a conviction for attempted murder against an individual who had splattered blood on emergency workers seeking to prevent him from committing suicide.[32]

Whatever the allure of such measures and of the rediscovery of traditional public health approaches in the effort to combat the spread of HIV infection, it has remained clear that the future course of the AIDS epidemic will be determined by the creation of a social and institutional milieu within which radical voluntary changes in behavior can occur and be sustained. Educational campaigns and counseling programs, most effectively undertaken by groups linked to the populations at risk, have remained the centerpiece of that preventive effort. Such efforts are, however, still limited by moralistic trends in American society, and especially by those reflecting the abhorrence of homosexuality. The most striking failure in the preventive realm, however, is rooted in the unwillingness to commit the resources necessary for the provision of drug abuse treatment.

The dimensions of that failure were underscored in the 1988 preliminary report of the Presidential Commission on the HIV Epidemic.[33] A vast expansion in government efforts was needed. One and a half billion dollars a year would be necessary for drug abuse treatment and education. Only such an investment could make possible the provision of immediate treatment to all drug users who might seek such help. For the Reagan administration, which had placed its emphasis on a moral appeal to abstinence and which had entertained the idea of a return to harsh street-level enforcement of drug use and possession statutes, the call for the massive funding of drug abuse treatment programs must have seemed the siren call of a discredited liberalism. For those who were all too familiar with the inadequacy of available services, and the difficulties that would follow even were there a commitment of resources, the commission's declaration provided some reason for hope.

The call for greater attention to the problem of drug abuse in the light of the AIDS epidemic was repeated by the Institute of Medicine and the National Academy of Sciences. In the 1988 update to its earlier report, *Confronting AIDS*, the IOM-NAS painted a bleak picture linking intravenous drug use, heterosexual transmission, and the birth of infants with HIV infection. "The Committee believes that the gross inadequacy of federal efforts to reduce HIV transmission among IV drug users, when considered in relation to the scope and implications of such transmission, is now the most serious deficiency in current efforts to control HIV infection in the United States."[34] Relying on the report of the Presidential Commission, the IOM-NAS too called for an annual expenditure of $1.5 billion. But despite these appeals, little has been done. In its first report to President George Bush, issued in December 1989, the National Commission on Acquired Immune Deficiency Syndrome lamented the failure of the White House National Drug Control Strategy to give appropriate attention to AIDS. Like its predecessor, the National Commission, chaired by June Osborn, a well-known critic of federal AIDS policy, and vice-chaired by David Rogers, a persistent voice for increased federal support to the cities most severely affected by the epidemic, called for the availability of treatment "on request" for all drug users.[35]

Concern about budgetary deficits, ten years of ideological opposition to welfare state–like programs by conservative national administrations, and the absence of a strong political constituency capable of effectively clamoring for the needs of the underclass have resulted in the politics of neglect. It is in this context that opposition, or suspicion, on the part of black and Hispanic community leaders to the halfway measures of needle exchange and education about the use of bleach to cleanse drug injection equipment must be understood.[36] In the absence of a strong commitment to treatment, such measures appear to write off the needs of the poor. Thus, there has emerged the tragic alliance of the moralistic right and those who speak in the name of the dispossessed. It was the first black commissioner of health in New York City acting at the behest of the city's first black mayor who terminated a small and politically hobbled needle exchange program soon after assuming office.[37] More stunning, the commissioner sought to cancel a municipal contract that funded a community-based group to provide drug users with bleach and education about how to sterilize injection equipment.[38]

The failure to fund drug abuse services was but a portion of a much deeper problem: the failure of the federal government to plan for and assist those localities that were compelled to bear the burden of providing care for large numbers of patients with AIDS. And such patients were but a fraction of those who would increasingly be defined as in need of care. In mid-1989, the Public Health Service announced that chemoprophylaxis could dramatically affect the likelihood of developing *pneumocystis carinii* pneumonia.[39] Soon thereafter, clinical investigators announced that the use of AZT could retard the onset of disease in asymptomatic individuals whose immune systems had already begun to show the impact of HIV infection.[40] Writing in the *Journal of the American Medical Association*, researchers predicted that "rather than a fulminant disease treated primarily inside the hospital, the disease will become a largely chronic condition requiring years of outpatient monitoring and pharmacologic intervention."[41] To meet the challenge of chronic HIV infection it would be necessary to create and fund an infrastructure capable of providing ongoing clinical services to more than half of those with HIV infection. Some predicted that soon such care would be necessary for a million individuals.

Here then was a paradox not new to the American health care system. Extraordinary advances in medicine must inevitably confront the social reality of the most inequitable system of medical care among advanced democratic societies. Thirty to forty million Americans have no health insurance at all. Of those who are insured, many are inadequately protected. Virtually the whole cost of prescription drugs must be borne by those for whom they are prescribed. Could such a health care system meet the challenge of providing between 500,000 and 1,000,000 persons, many of whom are impoverished, with the outpatient clinical services they would need and with the expensive drugs they would require? Would it be possible for a health care system so fundamentally unjust to fashion a just response to those infected with HIV? Before these questions, the earlier important debates about discrimination by private medical insurers paled.

Emergency federal programs to assist the states in paying the cost of AZT for those without insurance, Medicaid reimbursement policies and a host of patchwork programs in the states provided some relief but were clearly inadequate.[42] In its December 1989 report to the President, the National Commission on Acquired Immune Deficiency Syndrome warned that medical breakthroughs would "mean little unless the health care system can incorporate them and make them accessible to people in need."[43] The existence of a medically disenfranchised class meant that for many, access to care was almost solely through the "emergency room door of one of the few hospitals in the community that treats people with HIV infection and AIDS." Hardly the foundation for the kind of care HIV infection would require in the 1990s.

These were the conditions under which ACT-UP, which had rejected conventional political styles of protest for the methods of direct action reminiscent of the 1960s, turned its attention to the shape of the American health care system, going beyond its earlier bold challenge to the bureaucratic structure of new drug development. It was the context in which President George Bush's first address on AIDS, in the spring of 1990, was greeted as so hollow by many AIDS activists. No longer was it enough to declare that those who were ill had a right to be treated with "dignity, compassion, care and confidentiality and without discrimination."[44] Certainly federal exclusionary policies in the military, the Foreign Service, and the Job Corps, as well as restrictions on the rights of foreign travelers with HIV infection, made such a declaration seem less than honest. But as important was the failure to guarantee that those with HIV infection would have access to the full range of needed clinical and social services.

The situation that prevailed in New York, the epicenter of the American AIDS epidemic, was extreme because of the existence of a number of concurrent socio-medical and economic crises including drug abuse, homelessness, and dire fiscal conditions. Nevertheless, it revealed how a failure to commit sufficient resources, itself a consequence of federal default, could have catastrophic results, not only for those with HIV-related disorders and the poor—so dependent on publicly provided medical services—but for the system of health care more generally.

As early as the spring of 1988, investigators writing in the *Bulletin of the New York Academy of Medicine* could write that "to ignore the possibilities inherent in the empirical evidence available is to create a social calamity even greater than the one already perceived. . . . One can imagine bitter competition for hospital beds. . . . The AIDS epidemic threatens not only individual lives but the city's health care, education and research environment as well. The time is short, the need is great, and is likely to grow rapidly."[45] Within a year three separate reports by public or voluntary sector groups detailed how far New York was from being able to meet the demands of the epidemic.[46] Community-based organizations, typically within the gay community, had provided an extraordinary range of services to those with HIV infection and AIDS. They could not, however, meet the needs that public bodies and large private-sector agencies were responsible for meeting. Volunteerism was no substitute for the institutional response that was demanded. Three to five hundred new acute care hospital beds would be needed each year for five years in order to meet requirements of those who would become ill. In addition, hundreds of nursing home beds and special housing units would be needed for those requiring less intensive medical care. The capital costs alone for meeting these demands would be over $700 million. And if only one-half of those who could benefit from ambulatory care for HIV infection were to seek it, the city's already overburdened clinic system would have to absorb an additional 800,000 visits a year. Commenting on the care and attention to detail revealed in each of the report projections, Kenneth Raske, president of the Greater New York Hospital Association, said, "This is the biggest amount of planning for an epidemic with the least amount of action to go along with it."[47]

It was not too soon to start thinking of worst-case scenarios.[48] Middle-class patients together with their physicians might increasingly flee the city in search of medical care in the suburbs. If they remained, and were able to protect their own interests by insulating themselves from the critical shortage of hospital beds, those institutions forced to bear the burden of caring for the poor would be compelled to restrict even further access to in-patient care for "elective" procedures. While middle-class patients would continue to receive increasingly effective outpatient care from their overworked physicians, the poor would face growing delays and waiting lists as they sought out the benefits of early therapeutic intervention. Many, discouraged, would simply not seek care at all.

Shortages would impose the need for rationing, and in the political economy of a city like New York competition among the desperate would ensue. In what Bruce Vladek termed the "calculus of misery," it would become increasingly necessary to choose between AIDS cases and the frail elderly for admission to nursing homes; between single adults with AIDS and homeless families with young children for access to newly renovated apartments; between homeless persons dying of AIDS or children for access to transitional shelter; between HIV-infected pregnant women and women not yet infected for admission to drug abuse treatment programs.

The looming crisis in health care for those with HIV disease set the stage for congressional action that could scarcely have been imagined a short time earlier, the fruit of dogged efforts on the part of AIDS activists, their allies, and some political leaders from the cities and states that had borne the disproportionate share of AIDS cases. In the winter of 1990, Senator Edward Kennedy, the exemplar of Democratic party liberalism, and Senator Orrin Hatch, a Republican whose stance on abortion often cast him in the role of a conservative, jointly sponsored legislation—the Comprehensive AIDS Resource Emergency Act of 1990—that would provide a major infusion of federal assistance to those localities most severely burdened by AIDS. As the government has responded to natural disasters, the Kennedy-Hatch Bill asked it to respond to the medical disaster of AIDS. "The Human Immunodeficiency Virus constitutes a crisis as devastating as an earthquake, flood or drought. Indeed, the death toll of the unfolding AIDS tragedy is already a hundredfold greater than any natural disaster to strike our nation in this century."[49]

As remarkable as the joint sponsorship of this legislation, which promised to provide $2.9 billion over five years in a complex political formula to the cities and states most severely struck by AIDS, was the overwhelming support the legislation received in the Senate, where the vote in favor was 95–4.[50] When similar legislation, with even greater resource commitments, was voted on by the House of Representatives, the vote was 408–14.[51]

However late in coming, this legislation represented on both symbolic and practical levels an important act of national solidarity. But the hopes of early summer were dashed by the fall as the Congress, confronted with a severe budgetary crisis, slashed funds for the now renamed Ryan White Act. What allocations will be made in successive years cannot be foretold. It is certain, however, that such an emergency act cannot be a substitute for the fundamental change in the organization and financing of health care in the United States that will be required by the chronic management of the medical and social needs of all HIV-infected persons at a moment when so many other medical needs of the nation's poor remain unmet.

Written at a time when the therapeutic picture was exceedingly bleak, *Private Acts, Social Consequences* made only passing reference to the reciprocal relationship between the culture of responsibility so crucial to the modification of behaviors linked to the spread of HIV and the obligations of government to provide care for those who would become ill.

With the rapid development of therapies, the link between the provision of care and the strategy of prevention has assumed critical importance.[52] Public health officials have used the occasion of new therapeutic prospects as a justification for rethinking policies adopted in the epidemic's first years. But the prospect of new therapies is not enough. They must be available to those who need them if lives are to be prolonged and if the public health goal of preventing the further spread of HIV infection is to be achieved. The possibility of engaging those with HIV infection in ongoing clinical care provides a crucial opportunity to sustain behavioral change where it has occurred, to encourage and support such change where it has not yet taken place. A failure to provide care and counseling, especially to the poor among whom intravenous drug use plays so critical a role in HIV transmission, will entail not only a sentence of needlessly foreshortened life, but a lost opportunity to intervene in the epidemic's epidemiological course.

In 1988 I wrote about the culture of responsibility, primarily in terms of the behavior of those infected with HIV or at risk of infection. New therapeutic possibilities now require that the standard of social responsibility be vigorously applied as a measure against which to judge the actions of those officials with the authority to assure access to care for those who need it and of the public to whom they are ultimately accountable. Unlike the Third World, where absolute scarcity imposes limits upon what can be done to meet the challenge of HIV infection, in the United States restrictions on governmental efforts will be the consequence of social decisions. History will judge us by the choices we make at this moment, when the possibilities are greater than at any point since HIV first made its appearance.

Notes

Chapter 1 Private Acts, Social Consequences

1. "Pneumocystis Pneumonia-Los Angeles," *Morbidity and Mortality Weekly Report* (June 5, 1981), 250–52. This journal hereafter is referred to as *MMWR*.
2. *Ibid.*
3. "Kaposi's Sarcoma and Pneumocystis Pneumonia Among Homosexual Men—New York City and California," *MMWR* (July 3, 1981), 305–8.
4. "Update on Kaposi's Sarcoma and Opportunistic Infections in Previously Healthy Persons—United States," *MMWR* (June 11, 1982), 294–301.
5. "A Cluster of Kaposi's Sarcoma and Pneumocystis Carinii Pneumonia Among Homosexual Male Residents of Los Angeles and Orange Counties, California," *MMWR* (June 18, 1982), 305–7.
6. United States Public Health Service, "Public Health Service Plan for the Prevention and Control of AIDS and the AIDS Virus," *Public Health Reports* (July-August, 1986), 341–48.
7. *Ibid.*
8. National Academy of Sciences-Institute of Medicine, *Confronting AIDS* (Washington, DC: Academy Press, 1986), 91.
9. Thomas Quinn, "Perspectives on the Future of AIDS," *Journal of the American Medical Association* (January 11, 1985), 247–49.
10. June Osborn, "The AIDS Epidemic: Multidisciplinary Trouble," *New England Journal of Medicine* (March 20, 1986), 780.
11. *Confronting AIDS*, 8.
12. *New York Times* (January 30, 1987), A24.

13. Stephen J. Gould, "The Terrifying Normalcy of AIDS," *New York Times Sunday Magazine,* (April 19, 1987), 33.
14. 381 U.S. 479 (1965).
15. *Eisenstadt v. Baird,* 405 U.S. 438 (1972).
16. *Stanley v. Georgia,* 394 U.S. 557 (1969).
17. Laurence Tribe, *American Constitutional Law* (Mineola, N.Y.: Foundation Press, 1978), 948.
18. *Ibid.,* 985.
19. Kenneth L. Karst, "The Freedom of Intimate Association," *Yale Law Journal* (1980), 624–92.
20. *Ibid.,* 894.
21. *Bowers v. Hardwick,* 85–140 (June 30, 1986).
22. *Ibid.*
23. *Ibid.*
24. *Ibid.*
25. *Ibid.*
26. Sanford Kadish, "The Crisis of Overcriminalization," *American Criminal Law Quarterly* (1968), 17–34.
27. Edwin Schur, *Labeling Deviant Behavior* (New York: Harper and Row, 1971).
28. Edwin Schur, *Crimes Without Victims* (Englewood Cliffs, NJ: Prentice Hall, 1971).
29. William Curran, Larry Gostin, and Mary Clark, "AIDS: Legal and Regulatory Policy," (U.S. Public Health Service, July 1986), 244.
30. *Kirk v. Wyman,* cited in Larry Gostin, "Traditional Public Health Strategies," *AIDS and the Law,* eds., Harlon Dalton, Scott Burris, and the Yale Law Project (New Haven: Yale University Press, 1986), 50–51.
31. *Kirk v. Board of Health* in Deborah Jones Merritt, "The Constitutional Balance Between Health and Liberty," *Hastings Center Report* (December 1986), 5.
32. Allan Brandt, *No Magic Bullet: A Social History of Venereal Diseases in the United States from 1880* (New York: Oxford University Press, 1985).
33. Wendy Parmet, "AIDS and Quarantine: The Revival of an Archaic Doctrine," *Hofstra Law Review* (Fall, 1985), 70–71.
34. Deborah Jones Merritt, "Communicable Disease and Constitutional Law: Controlling AIDS," *New York University Law Review* (November, 1986), 739–99.
35. Curran, Gostin, and Clark, "AIDS," 242.

36. *Ibid.*, 251.
37. *In re Holko* cited in Merrit, "Communicable Disease," *NYU Law Review*, 754.
38. Gostin, "Traditional Public Health," *AIDS and the Law.*
39. *New York State Association for Retarded Children v. Carey*, cited in Merritt, "Communicable Disease," 763–64.
40. Tribe, *Law*, 891.
41. Cited in Merritt, "The Constitution Basis," *Hastings Center Report*, 3.
42. Richard Mohr, "AIDS, Gay Life, State Coercion," *Raritan* (Summer 1986), 41.
43. For a discussion of these studies, see *Confronting AIDS*, 69.
44. Lewis Kuller and Lawrence Kingsley, "The Epidemic of AIDS: A Failure of Public Health Policy," *Milbank Quarterly*, Supplement 1 1986(1), 61.
45. *Confronting AIDS*, 69.
46. *New York Times*, (January 13, 1988), 13.
47. This discussion is taken from Ronald Bayer and Jonathan Moreno, "Health Promotion: Ethical and Social Dilemmas of Government Policy," *Health Affairs* (Summer, 1986), 72–85.
48. Marc Lalonde, A *New Perspective on the Health of Canadians*, (Ottawa: Government of Canada, 1975), 15.
49. *Ibid.*, 36.
50. John Knowles, "The Responsibility of the Individual, "*Daedalus* (Winter 1979), 80.
51. U.S. Department of Health, Education and Welfare, *Healthy People: the Surgeon General's Report on Health Promotion and Disease Prevention* (Washington, DC: U.S. Government Printing Office, 1979).
52. *Ibid.*
53. Robert Crawford, "You Are Dangerous to Your Health," *Social Policy* (January/February, 1978), 10–20.
54. Washington Post (September 8, 1985) Section II, 5.

Chapter 2 Sex and the Bathhouses

1. Gerald Oppenheimer, "In the Eye of the Storm: The Epidemiological Construction of AIDS," *AIDS and the Burden of History* (Berkeley, CA: University of California Press, 1988).

2. James Foege, "The National Pattern of AIDS," in *The AIDS Epidemic*, ed. Kevin M. Kahill (New York: St. Martin's Press, 1983), 9.
3. *New York Native* (July 27–August 9, 1981), 1.
4. *New York Native* (August 24–September 6, 1981), 13.
5. *Advocate* (March 18, 1982), 6.
6. *Advocate* (April 15, 1982), 12.
7. *New York Native* (March 29–April 11, 1982), 15.
8. *New York Native* (June 21–July 4, 1982), 11.
9. *New York Native* (September 13–26, 1982), 49.
10. *New York Native* (November 8–21, 1982), 29.
11. *Ibid.*, 22.
12. *New York Native* (January 3–16, 1983), 23.
13. Cited in Jonathan Lieberson, "Anatomy of an Epidemic," *New York Review of Books* (August 18, 1983), 19.
14. *New York Native* (December 6–19, 1982), 27.
15. *New York Native* (January 12–30, 1983), 5.
16. *New York Native* (March 14–27, 1983), 1.
17. *Advocate* (January 6, 1983), 20.
18. American Association of Physicians for Human Rights, February 19, 1983, Mimeo.
19. San Francisco Department of Public Health, "AIDS in Gay Men," May 1983.
20. *Advocate* (March 18, 1982), 6.
21. *New York Native* (July 16–29, 1984), 23.
22. *New York Native* (August 16–29, 1982), 32.
23. *New York Native* (January 17–30, 1983), 25.
24. Francis FitzGerald, "A Reporter at Large: The Castro," *The New Yorker* (July 28, 1986), 52.
26. Mervyn Silverman, Interview, San Francisco, August 21, 1986.
27. *Ibid.*
28. Mervyn Silverman, Letter to Larry Littlejohn, May 10, 1983.
29. Mervyn Silverman, Letter to Larry Littlejohn, September 12, 1983.
30. *Advocate* (August 18, 1983), 53.
31. *Advocate* (October 27, 1983), 8.
32. *Advocate* (March 20, 1984), 17.
33. San Francisco *Chronicle* (February 3, 1984), 4.

34. FitzGerald, "Reporter at Large," *The New Yorker,* 53.
35. *California Voice* (April 5–11, 1984), 3.
36. *Ibid.*
37. *California Voice* (April 5–11, 1984), 2.
38. *Coming Up* (April 1984), 8, 10.
39. California Voice (April 5–11, 1984), 2.
40. National Gay Task Force, *NGTF Update,* March 28, 1984.
41. Wardell Pomeroy *et al.*, Letter to Mervyn Silverman, March 29, 1984.
42. Mervyn Silverman, Interview, San Francisco, August 21, 1986.
43. California Voice (April 5–11, 1984), 2.
44. *Coming Up* (April 1984), 10.
45. *Bay Area Reporter* (April 5, 1984), 7.
46. Neil Schram, Letter to Mervyn Silverman, April 2, 1984.
47. *Coming Up* (April 1984), 9.
48. *Ibid.*
49. *Ibid.*
50. Mervyn Silverman, Interview, San Francisco, August 21, 1986, but see Burk E. Deleventhal, Deputy City Attorney, Memorandum to Mervyn Silverman, June 2, 1983.
51. Mervyn Silverman, Interview, San Francisco, August 21, 1986.
52. Mervyn Silverman, Memorandum to Mayor Dianne Feinstein, May 30, 1984.
53. Mervyn Silverman, Press Statement, April 9, 1984, Mimeo.
54. *Bay Area Reporter* (November 29, 1984), 3.
55. Mervyn Silverman, Press Statement, April 9, 1984, Mimeo.
56. *New York Native* (May 21–June 3, 1984), 10.
57. *New York Native* (April 23–May 6, 1984), 6.
58. *Advocate* (May 1, 1984), 15.
59. *Advocate* (May 15, 1984), 7.
60. *New York Native* (April 23–May 6, 1984), 3.
61. *New York Native* (July 16–29, 1984), 21.
62. Thomas Stoddard, Letter to Dorothy Ehrlich, April 10, 1984.
63. Northern California Gay Rights Chapter, ACLU *Bulletin,* No. 1 (1984). 2.
64. Northern California Branch, American Civil Liberties Union, Board of Directors, Minutes, May 10, 1984.

65. Northern California Gay Rights Chapter, *Bulletin,* No. 1, (1984), 2.
66. Mervyn Silverman, Interview, San Francisco, August 21, 1986.
67. William Darrow, Letter to Dean Echenberg, July 10, 1984.
68. Dean Echenberg, Interview, New York City, Oct. 15, 1986.
69. Harold Jaffe and William Darrow, Letter to Mervyn Silverman, October 15, 1984.
70. *Bay Area Reporter* (November 29, 1984), 1.
71. Phillip S. Ward, Memorandum to Mervyn Silverman, September 27, 1984.
72. Files of Mervyn Silverman, San Francisco.
73. Mervyn Silverman, Press Statement, October 9, 1984.
74. Files of Mervyn Silverman, San Francisco.
75. Brett Cassons, Letter to Mervyn Silverman, October 10, 1984.
76. *Bay Area Reporter* (November 1, 1984), 3.
77. *People of the State of California v. Ima Jean Owen et al.*, Memorandum of Points and Authorities in Support of Application for Preliminary Injunction and for Temporary Restraining Order.
78. Dean Echenberg, Interview, New York City, October 15, 1986.
79. *People of the State of California v. Ima Jean Owen et al.* [Defendant Response] (November 7, 1984).
80. Roy Wonder, Preliminary Injunction, *People of the State of California v. Ima Jean Owen et al.* (November 28, 1984).
81. San Francisco *Examiner* (November 30, 1984).
82. San Francisco *Chronicle* (November 30, 1984), 70.
83. *Coming Up* (December 14, 1984), 7.
84. *Ibid.*
85. Mervyn Silverman, Interview, San Francisco, August 21, 1986.
86. Judge Roy Wonder, Modified Preliminary Injunction, *People of the State of California v. Ima Jean Owen et al.* (December 21, 1985).
87. *New York Native* (December 17–30, 1984), 9.
88. *Advocate* (September 1, 1983), 20.
89. Lieberson, "Anatomy," *New York Review of Books,* 21.
90. *New York Native* (September 12–25, 1983), 8.
91. Peter J. Millock, Memorandum to David Axelrod, July 25, 1983.
92. *New York Native* (January 16–29, 1984), 8.
93. *Advocate* (February 7, 1984), 17.

94. John Boring, Memorandum to Ginny Apuzzo, February 15, 1984.
95. Thomas Stoddard, Letter to Peter Vogel, November 20, 1984.
96. Michael Callen, Interview, New York, September 9, 1986.
97. Michael Callen, "The Case for Temporary Closure of Commercial Sex Establishments During the AIDS Crisis," December 3, 1984, Mimeo.
98. *Village Voice* (December 8, 1984), 24.
99. John Boring, Memorandum to Virginia Apuzzo, December 11, 1984.
100. Michael Callen, Interview, New York, September 9, 1986.
101. Stephen Caiazza, Letter to David Nimmons, January 24, 1985.
102. Virginia Apuzzo and Timothy Sweeney, Letter to Bathhouse Owners, February 1, 1985.
103. *Advocate* (April 16, 1985), 10.
104. New York State AIDS Institute, Advisory Council, Transcript.
105. *Ibid.*
106. *Ibid.*
107. *New York Times* (October 30, 1985), B4.
108. *New York Times* (October 2, 1985), B1.
109. *New York Times* (October 5, 1985), 25.
110. Coalition for Sexual Responsibility, "Interim Report," October 1985.
111. Mervyn Silverman, Interview, San Francisco, August 21, 1986.
112. Alan Kristal, Memorandum to David Sencer, October 9, 1985.
113. Lambda Legal Defense and Education Fund, Letter to David Axelrod, October 18, 1985.
114. *New York Times* (October 19, 1985), 26.
115. David Sencer, Memorandum to Mayor Edward Koch, October 22, 1985.
116. *New York Times* (October 25, 1985), B3.
117. State of New York, Public Health Council, Minutes, October 25, 1985.
118. *Ibid.*
119. *New York Times* (October 30, 1985), B4.
120. *Advocate* (December 24, 1985), 24.
121. *New York Times* (November 9, 1985), 29.
122. *Newsday* (November 18, 1985), 3.
123. *Coalition of Lesbian and Gay Rights v. Mario Cuomo, David Axelrod, Public Health Council* and *Robert Abrams*, (December 2, 1985).

124. State of New York, Public Health Council, Minutes, December 20, 1985.
125. Affirmation in Support of Plaintiff's Motions for a Temporary Closing Order, Restraining Order and a Preliminary Injunction, in *City of New York v. the St. Marks Baths,* Index #46340/85 (December 6, 1985).
126. Plaintiff's Memorandum of Law, in *ibid.* (December 26, 1985).
127. Defendant's Memorandum in Opposition to Motion for Preliminary Injunction and in Support of a Cross Motion to Dismiss the Complaint, in *ibid.*
128. Richard W. Wallach in *ibid.* (January 6, 1986).
129. Public Health Service, Executive Task Force on AIDS, Minutes, October 7, 1985.
130. Donald Hopkins, Memorandum to State and Territorial Health Officials, November 7, 1985.
131. San Francisco *Examiner* (October 3, 1985).
132. William Dannemyer, Letter, Los Angeles *Times* (December 10, 1985), Section II, 4.
133. *Medical World News* (July 28, 1986), 31.
134. William Curran, Larry Gostin, and Mary Clark, "AIDS," 363–64.
135. *Commissioner of Health of the County of Erie v. Morgan Inc., et al.,* (May 29, 1986).
136. *New York Times* (August 30, 1986), 26.
137. *Advocate* (March 4, 1986), 22.
138. Oregon, HIV AIDS Policy Committee, February 1987.
139. Michael Osterholm, Telephone Interview, October 24, 1986.

Chapter 3 Blood, Privacy, and Stigma

1. "Pneumocystis Carinii Pneumonia Among Persons with Hemophilia A," *MMWR* (July 16, 1982), 365–67.
2. *Ibid.,* 366.
3. National Hemophilia Foundation, *Hemophilia Newsnotes,* "Hemophilia Patient Alert #1" (July 14, 1982).
4. *New York Native* (August 16–29, 1982), 32.
5. *New York Native* (August 2–15, 1982), 11.
6. *New York Native* (September 13–26, 1982), 22.

7. Charles Carman and Louis Aledort, Letter to William Dolan, November 2, 1982.
8. *Ibid.*
9. Working Group on the Evaluation of Stored Blood, Blood Products Advisory Committee, Food and Drug Administration, Meeting Minutes, December 4, 1982.
10. "Update on Acquired Immune Deficiency Syndrome (AIDS) Among Patients with Hemophilia A," *MMWR* (December 10, 1982), 644–52, and "Possible Transfusion-Associated Acquired Immune Deficiency Syndrome (AIDS)—California," *Ibid.*, 652–54.
11. *Ibid.*, 654.
12. Alfred Katz, Executive Director Red Cross Services, Memorandum to All Blood Centers, December 10, 1982.
13. *CCBC Newsletter* (December 10, 1982).
14. William Dolan, Letter to Louis Aledort, December 20, 1982.
15. *New York Native* (December 20, 1982–January 2, 1983), 13.
16. *Advocate* (February 16, 1983), 15.
17. William Check, "Preventing AIDS Transmission: Should Blood Donors Be Screened," *Journal of the American Medical Association* (February 4, 1983), 569.
18. *The Advocate* (February 17, 1983), 9.
19. Check, "Preventing AIDS Transmission," *JAMA*, 568.
20. *Ibid.*
21. James Allen, Interview, Briarcliff Manor, NY, March 31, 1988.
22. Check "Preventing AIDS Transmission," *JAMA*, 570.
23. Philadelphia *Inquirer (January 9, 1983), 1.*
24. *Check "Preventing AIDS Transmission," JAMA*, 568.
25. *Ibid.*, 569.
26. Philadelphia *Inquirer* (January 9, 1983), 1.
27. *New York Native* (January 31–February 13, 1983), 23.
28. *Ibid.*
29. Committee on Transfusion Transmitted Diseases, American Association of Blood Banks, "Acquired Immune Deficiency Syndrome" January 6, 1983, Mimeo.
30. National Gay Task Force, Press Release, January 10, 1983.
31. American Association of Blood Banks, American Red Cross, and Council Community Blood Centers, "Joint Statement on Acquired

Immune Deficiency Syndrome (AIDS) Related to Transfusion," January 13, 1985, Mimeo.

32. National Hemophilia Foundation, Medical and Scientific Advisory Committee, Statement, January 14, 1983, Mimeo.
33. National Gay Task Force, Press Release, January 27, 1983.
34. Coordinating Committee of Gay and Lesbian Health Services, cited in National Gay Task Force Press Release, January 10, 1983.
35. Bay Area Physicians for Human Rights, *BAPHRON* (January 1983), [emphasis supplied].
36. Files of American Association of Physicians for Human Rights, Mimeo.
37. Johanna Pindyk, Interview, November 17, 1986.
38. American Association of Physicians for Human Rights. "The AAPHR Statement on AIDS and Blood Donation," February 19, 1983, Mimeo.
39. "Prevention of Acquired Immune Deficiency Syndrome (AIDS) Report of Interagency Recommendations," *MMWR* (March 4, 1983), 101–3.
40. *Ibid.*, 102.
41. *Ibid.*
42. *Ibid.*
43. *Ibid.*
44. Virginia Apuzzo, Letter to Edward Brandt, March 22, 1983.
45. *New York Native* (March 14–27, 1983), 11.
46. *Advocate* (April 14, 1983), 9.
47. Director, Office of Biologics, National Center for Drugs and Biologics, Memorandum to All Establishments Collecting Blood for Transfusions, March 24, 1983.
48. Alfred J. Katz, Memorandum to All Blood Service Regions, April 7, 1983.
49. Virginia Apuzzo, Letter to James Curran, October 11, 1983.
50. American Association of Physicians for Human Rights, "The AAPHR Statement on AIDS and Healthful Gay Male Activity," "AIDS and Blood Donations," December 17, 1983, Mimeo.
51. James Curran *et al.*, "Acquired Immunodeficiency Syndrome (AIDS) Associated with Transfusions," *New England Journal of Medicine* (January 12, 1984), 69–75.
52. *Ibid.*, 73.

53. *Ibid.*
54. *Ibid.*, 74.
55. Joseph Bove, "Transfusion Associated AIDS: A Cause of Concern," *New England Journal of Medicine* (January 12, 1984), 115–16.
56. American Association of Blood Banks, American Red Cross, Council of Community Blood Centers, "Joint Statement on AIDS and Blood Transfusions," January 3, 1984, Mimeo.
57. *Advocate* (April 17, 1984), 16.
58. *New York Times* (April 24, 1984), C1.
59. *AMA News* (May 25, 1984), 1.
60. Neil Schram, Letter to Edward Brandt, April 23, 1984.
61. Jeff Levi, Memorandum to Interested Parties, July 3, 1984.
62. James Curran, Memorandum to State and Territorial Epidemiologists, July 20, 1984.
63. Neil Schram, Letter to James Mason, August 13, 1984.
64. Neil Schram, Dear AAPHR Member, September 1984.
65. Acting Director, Office of Biologics, Research and Review, Memorandum to All Establishments Collecting Blood, Blood Components and Source Plasma and All Licensed Manufacturers of Plasma Derivatives, December 14, 1984.
66. Jeff Levi, Memorandum to Ginny Apuzzo, December 19, 1984.
67. Conference on AIDS, Ethics and the Blood Supply, *Proceedings*, eds., Ronald Bayer, Nancy Holland, and Ernest Simon (American Blood Commission, 1985).
68. Marsha Goldsmith, "HTLV-III Testing on Donor Blood Immanent; Complex Issues Remain," *Journal of the American Medical Association* (January 11, 1985), 179.
69. *Ibid.*, 173.
70. "Provisional Public Health Service Inter-Agency Recommendations for Screening Donated Blood and Plasma for Antibody to the Virus Causing Acquired Immunodeficiency Syndrome," *MMWR* (January 11, 1985), 1–5.
71. *Ibid.*, 3.
72. Public Health Service, Executive Task Force on AIDS, Summaries of Meetings Held on January 14, 1985, Mimeo.
73. *MMWR* (January 11, 1985), 3.
74. Virginia Apuzzo, Letter to Lowell Harmenson, January 18, 1985.

75. Association of State and Territorial Health Officials, "Screening Position Paper," n.d., Mimeo.
76. Director, Office of Biologics, Research and Review, to All Registered Blood Establishments, February 19, 1985.
77. Frank Young, Dear Doctor, n.d.
78. Working Group on Medical, Social, and Health Policy Aspects of Screening Tests for AIDS, New York Blood Center, Minutes, July 17, 1985, Mimeo.
79. David Axelrod, Dear Colleague, March 22, 1985.
80. New York Blood Center, Information for Donors with HTLVIII Antibody, July 17, 1985.
81. Charles Marwick, "Blood Banks Give HTLVIII Test Positive Approval at Five Months," *Journal of the American Medical Association* (October 4, 1985), 1681.
82. *Ibid.*, 1683.
83. *Ibid.*
84. Public Health Service Executive Task Force on AIDS, Minutes, October 8, 1985.
85. *New York Times* (June 20, 1986).
86. Thomas Zuck, "Future Tasks for the Protection of the Nation's Blood Supply," prepared for presentation at the Public Health Service Conference on Prevention and Control of AIDS: Planning for 1991, June 4–6, 1986.
87. Joint Statement of the American Association of Blood Banks, the American Red Cross, and the Council of Community Blood Centers, June 7, 1985.
88. *AMA News* (April 18, 1986), 1.
89. State of New York, Department of Health, Memorandum, Notification of Transfusion Recipients, July 18, 1986.
90. Gene Dodds, Personal Communication, October 1, 1986.

Chapter 4 Testing, Reporting, and Notifying

1. *New York Native* (October 8–21, 1984), 5.
2. Stephen Caiazza, *New York Native* (October 8–21, 1984), 7.
3. American Association of Physicians for Human Rights, "Position Paper on HTLVIII Testing and Alternative Test Sites" (January 20, 1985), Mimeo.

4. Philadelphia Health Department, Letter to Margaret Heckler, March 6, 1985.
5. *New York Native* (May 6–19, 1985), 8.
6. Cited in Association of State and Territorial Health Officials, *Guide to Public Health Practice* (Kensington, MD: ASTHO Foundation, 1985), 3.
7. *Ibid.*, 5.
8. "Human T-Lymphotropic Virus Type III/Lymphadenopathy-Associated Virus and Acquired Immunodeficiency Syndrome Testing at Alternative Test Sites," *MMWR* (May 2, 1986), 284–87.
9. *New York Native* (March 25–April 7, 1985), 13.
10. AIDS Action Council, *AIDS Action Update* (March 1985).
11. Franklin Judson, Dear Collegue, March 25, 1985.
12. *Advocate* (May 14, 1985), 9.
13. *Ibid.*
14. *Advocate* (April 30, 1985), 5.
15. *New York Native* (May 6–19, 1985), 20.
16. Stephen Caiazza, Letter, *New England Journal of Medicine* (October 31, 1985), 1158.
17. American Association of Physicians for Human Rights, *Newsletter* (November 1985).
18. American Association of Physicians for Human Rights, (November 12, 1985).
19. Neil Schram, "Open Letter to the Gay and Lesbian Community" January 14, 1986, Mimeo.
20. *New York Native* (February 3–9, 1986), 4.
21. Association of State and Territorial Health Officials, *ASTHO Guide to Public Health Practice: HTLVIII Antibody Testing and Community Approaches* (Washington, DC: Public Health Foundation, 1985), 16.
22. *Ibid.*
23. CDC, "Recommendations for Assisting in the Prevention of Perinatal Transmission of Human T-Lymphotropic Virus Type III/Lymphadenopathy-Associated Virus and Acquired Immunodeficiency Syndrome," *MMWR* (December 6, 1985), 721–26, 731–32.
24. *Ibid.*, 721.
25. *Ibid.*, 725.
26. Committee on Perinatal Transmission of HTLVIII/LAV, New York

City Department of Health, Bureau of Maternity Services and Family Planning, *Report*, n.d.

27. Sheldon Landesman, Interview, New York, February 20, 1987.
28. James Chin, Memorandum to California Health Officers, AIDS Surveillance and Epidemiology Personnel, August 14, 1985.
29. CDC, "Additional Recommendations to Reduce Sexual and Drug Abuse-Related Transmission of Human T-Lymphotoropic Virus Type III/Lymphadenopathy-Associated Virus," *MMWR* (March 14, 1986), 152–55.
30. *Ibid.*, 152.
31. *Ibid.*
32. Jeff Levi, Letter to James Mason, January 10, 1986.
33. Neil Schram, Letter to James Mason, reprinted in AAPHR *Newsletter* (April 1985).
34. American Association of Physicians for Human Rights, Press Release, March 18, 1986.
35. National Hemophilia Foundation, *AIDS Update, Medical Bulletin* (March 19, 1986).
36. National Hemophilia Foundation, *AIDS Update* (April 16, 1987).
37. Coalition Statement on HTLVIII Testing and Related Issues, May 30, 1986, Mimeo.
38. Daniel Fox, "From TB to AIDS: Value Conflicts in Reporting Disease," *Hastings Center Report* (December 1986), 11–16.
39. Odin Anderson, *Syphilis and Society: Problems of Control in the United States*, 1912–64, (Chicago: Center for Health Administration Studies, 1965), 12.
40. AAPHR *Newsletter* (July 1983).
41. James Allen, Interview, Briarcliff Manor, NY, March 31, 1988.
42. AMA *News* (October 7, 1983), 1.
43. *Ibid.*
44. *New York Native* (June 3–16, 1985), 17.
45. United States Conference of Local Health Officers, Letter to Ronald Altman, May 8, 1985.
46. *New York Native* (June 3–16, 1985), 17.
47. *Ibid.*
48. *Ibid.*, 18.
49. Fisher Broadcasting, Broadcast Transcript of May 15, 1985.

50. Jeff Levi, Letter to James Mason, May 18, 1985.
51. Thomas Vernon, Interview, Denver, Colorado, November 14, 1986.
52. Amendment to the Rules and Regulations Pertaining to Communicable Disease Control to Require the Reporting of HTLVIII Antibody Tests, submitted to Colorado Board of Health, Meeting, August 21, 1985.
53. Colorado Board of Health, Minutes, August 21, 1985.
54. Colorado Board of Health, Minutes, September 18, 1985.
55. *Rocky Mountain News* (October 13, 1985), 55.
56. Julian Rush, Interview, Denver, Colorado, November 14, 1986.
57. Thomas Vernon, Interview, Denver, Colorado, November 14, 1986.
58. Thomas Vernon, "Remarks," *AIDS: Impact on Public Policy*, eds., Robert Hummel, William Leavy, Richard Rampola, and Sherry Chorost (NY: Plenum Press, 1986).
59. Julian Rush, Interview, Denver, Colorado, November 14, 1986.
60. James Mason, Letter to State and Territorial Health Officers, December 6, 1985.
61. Gary MacDonald, Letter to Russel Havlok, January 13, 1986.
62. Jeff Levi, Letter to James Mason, January 10, 1986.
63. "Additional Recommendations," *MMWR* (March 14, 1986), 154.
64. U.S. Conference of Mayors, *AIDS Information Exchange* (February 1986).
65. Christopher Collins, Letter to Kathleen Hoerner, March 24, 1986.
66. Kristine Gebbie, Interview, Portland, Oregon, November 13, 1986.
67. Kristine Gebbie, Telephone Interview, July 23, 1988.
68. Oregon, HIV/AIDS Policy Committee, "The AIDS Epidemic: Policy Recommendations for Oregon's Response" (February 1, 1987), 32–33.
69. Dean Echenberg, "A New Strategy to Prevent the Spread of AIDS Among Heterosexuals," *Journal of the American Medical Association* (1985), 2129–30.
70. *Newsday* (November 16, 1985), 7.
71. Philadelphia *Gay News* (October 25–November 1, 1985), 24.
72. Brandt, *No Magic Bullet*, 150.
73. CDC, Recommended Additional Guidelines for HIV Antibody Counseling and Testing in the Prevention of HIV Infection and AIDS, April 30, 1987, Appendix IV, Mimeo.

74. Brandt, *No Magic Bullet,* 151.
75. CDC, "Recommendations," April 30, 1987, Appendix IV, Mimeo.
76. Brandt, *No Magic Bullet,* 151.
77. CDC, "Recommendations," April 30, 1987, Appendix IV, Mimeo.
78. Willard Cates, Interview, Atlanta, Georgia, November 4, 1986.
79. Jeff Levi, Letter to James Mason, January 10, 1986.
80. National Coalition of GAY STDS, *Newsletter,* n.d.
81. Jeff Levi, Letter to Elizabeth Rains, November 19, 1985.
82. Northern California Branch, American Civil Liberties Union, Board of Directors, Minutes, January 16, 1986.
83. Northern California Branch, American Civil Liberties Union, "AIDS and Civil Liberties" March 1986.
84. Privacy Committee, American Civil Liberties Union, Memorandum to Board of Directors, Proposed Policies on Communicable Diseases and AIDS, February 12, 1986.
85. Board of Directors, American Civil Liberties Union, Minutes, April 12–13, 1986.
86. Minnesota Department of Health, Task Force on AIDS, Minutes, January 7, 1986.
87. Minnesota Department of Health, Task Force on AIDS, Minutes, January 28, 1986.
88. *Equal Times* (January 22, 1986), 1.
89. Minneapolis *Star and Tribune* (February 16, 1986), 12A.
90. *Ibid.*
91. *GLC Voice* (February 17, 1986), 3.
92. Minnesota Department of Health, Task Force on AIDS, Minutes, May 13, 1986.
93. Minnesota Department of Health, Protocol for Notification of Referral of Sexual and Needlesharing Partners of HIV Antibody Positive Persons, November 17, 1986.
94. "Contact Notification Services," Mimeo.
95. Jeff Levi, Letter to James Dimos, March 14, 1986.
96. Wendy Wertheimer, Letter to Kristine Gebbie, n.d.
97. Association of State and Territorial Health Officials, *Guide to Public Health Practice: State Health Agency Programmatic Response to HTLVIII Infection* (Washington, DC: Public Health Foundation, June 1986), 24.

98. *New York Times* (October 15, 1987), B1.
99. *Surgeon General's Report on Acquired Immune Deficiency Syndrome* (October, 1986), 33.
100. *Ibid.*, 30.
101. Institute of Medicine and National Academy of Sciences, *Confronting AIDS* (Washington, DC: National Academy Press, 1986), 96.
102. *Ibid.*
103. *Ibid.*, 129.
104. *Ibid.*, 125.

Chapter 5 Compulsory Screening

1. Dorothy Nelkin and Stephen Hilgartner, "Disputed Dimensions of Risk: A Public School Controversy Over AIDS," *Milbank Quarterly,* Supplement 1 (1986), 118–142.
2. *Ibid.*, 121.
3. *District 27 Community School Board and Samuel Granier v. Board of Education of the City of New York et al.*, Index #14940/85, Judge Harold Hyman (February 11, 1986).
4. "Education and Foster Care of Children Infected with Human T-Lymphotropic Virus type III/Lymphadenopathy-Associated Virus," *MMWR* (August 30, 1985), 517–21.
5. *Ibid.*, 519.
6. *Ibid.*
7. *Ibid.*, 520.
8. Dennis Altman, *AIDS in the Mind of America* (Garden City, NY: Anchor Books, 1986), 60–62. See also Mark Rothstein, "Screening Workers for AIDS," *AIDS and the Law,* eds., Harlan Dalton, Scott Burris, and the Yale Law Project (New Haven, CT: Yale University Press, 1987), 126–141, and Arthur S. Leonard, "AIDS in the Workplace," *ibid.*, 109–25.
9. *Weekly News* (June 19, 1985), 1.
10. Washington *Post* (September 20, 1985), A6.
11. *Advocate* (December 10, 1985), 20.
12. *New York Times* (October 10, 1985), A25.
13. Detroit *Free Press* (October 18, 1985), 15A.
14. "Recommendations for Preventing Transmission of Infection with

Human T-Lymphotropic Virus Type III/Lymphadenopathy-Associated Virus," *MMWR* (November 15, 1985), 681–86, 691–95.

15. *Ibid.*, 682.
16. "Recommendations for Preventing Transmission of Infection with Human T-Lymphotropic Virus Type III/Lymphadenopathy-Associated Virus during Invasive Procedures," *MMWR* (April 11, 1986), 221–23.
17. *MMWR* (November 15, 1985), 683.
18. *Ibid.*, 686, 691.
19. *Ibid.*, 682.
20. Los Angeles *Times* (November 15, 1985), 6.
21. Mark Rothstein, "Screening Workers," *AIDS and the Law*, 135–36.
22. *Ibid.*, 136.
23. Office of the Legal Counsel, Department of Justice, Memorandum June 20, 1986.
24. Rothstein, "Screening Workers," *AIDS and the Law*, and *New York Times* (September 17, 1986), A20.
25. *LaRocca v. Dalshein*, 120 Misc ed. 697, 467 NYS 2d 302, Supreme Court (1983).
26. Philadelphia *Inquirer* (March 4, 1986), A4.
27. CDC, "Recommendations for Preventing Transmission of Infections with HTLVIII/LAV in Correctional Facilities," December 14, 1985, Draft.
28. Philadelphia *Inquirer* (March 4, 1986), A4.
29. Urvashi Vaid, "Prisons," *AIDS and the Law*, 239.
30. *AIDS, Policy and Law* (February 12, 1986), 4.
31. CDC, "Acquired Immunodeficiency Syndrome in Correctional Facilities: A Report of the National Institute of Justice and the American Correctional Association," *MMWR* (March 28, 1986), 195–99.
32. Vaid, "Prisons," *AIDS and the Law.*
33. ABT Associates, AIDS and Correctional Facilities.
34. Robert Cohen, Interview, Hastings-on-Hudson, NY, May 19, 1986.
35. Yehudi Felman, "Repeal of Mandated Premarital Tests for Syphilis: A Survey of State Health Officers," *American Journal of Public Health* (February 1981), 155–59.
36. Brandt, *No Magic Bullet*, 138–54.
37. *Washington Post* (October 17, 1985), 66.

38. Kristine Gebbie, Interview, Portland, Oregon, November 13, 1986. Thomas Vernon, Interview, Denver, Colorado, November 14, 1986.
39. Paul Cleary *et al.*, "Compulsory Premarital Screening for the Human Immunodeficiency Virus," *Journal of the American Medical Association* (October 2, 1987), 1757–62.
40. *New York Times* (July 7, 1987), A18.
41. Hilary Lewis, "Acquired Immune Deficiency Syndrome," State Legislative Activity, *Journal of the American Medical Association* (November 6, 1987), 2413.
42. *Surgeon General's Report on Acquired Immune Deficiency Syndrome,* 21.
43. Khrusho Ghandhi and Brian Lantz, Letter to Attorney General State of California, October 23, 1985.
44. San Francisco *Chronicle* (June 25, 1986), 7.
45. Washington *Post* (October 9, 1985), C5.
46. Oakland *Tribune* (June 22, 1986), D5.
47. "Initiative Measure to be Submitted Directly to the Voters," Mimeo.
48. *Wall Street Journal* (August 11, 1986), 38.
49. Southern California Branch, American Civil Liberties Union, Memorandum, "AIDS Carriers Initiative," December 13, 1985.
50. Orange County Chapter, American Civil Liberties Union, "LaRouche Initiative and Existing Laws," April 10, 1986.
51. "Rebuttal Argument Against Proposition 64," Mimeo.
52. *New Scientist* (September 25, 1986), 19.
53. California, AIDS Task Force, Minutes, August 13, 1986.
54. *Ibid.*
55. No on 64—Stop LaRouche, "Partial List of Opponents of Proposition 64," n.d., Mimeo.
56. Los Angeles *Times* (August 24, 1986), part 5, 4.
57. San Francisco *Chronicle* (June 27, 1986), 76.
58. San Francisco *Examiner* (June 29, 1986), A12.
59. San Diego *Union* (July 28, 1986), B6.
60. San Francisco *Chronicle* (July 20, 1986), 8.
61. San Francisco *Chronicle* (July 19, 1986).
62. Oakland *Tribune* (June 22, 1986), D5.
63. Los Angeles *Times* (August 24, 1986), 30.
64. William Dannemyer, Press Release, n.d.

65. William Dannemyer, Letter, "Dear Elected Official," July 10, 1986.
66. California, Legislative Analyst, Acquired Immune Deficiency Syndrome (AIDS), Initiative (Proposition 64), July 21, 1986, Mimeo.
67. No on 64, "Campaign Report," November 30, 1986, 26.
68. *New York Times* (February 4, 1987), 1.
69. Conference on the Role of AIDS Virus Antibody Testing in the Prevention and Control of AIDS (February 24–25, 1987), Closing Plenary Sessions: Reports from the Workshops; Transcript of the Proceedings, n.d., Mimeo.
70. CDC, Recommended Additional Guidelines for HIV Antibody Counseling and Testing in the Prevention of HIV Infection and AIDS, April 30, 1987, Mimeo.
71. *Ibid.*, 1.
72. CDC "Recommendations" (April 30, 1987), Appendix III.
73. "Recommendations" (April 30, 1987), 7.
74. *Ibid.*, 4.
75. *Ibid.*, 6.
76. *Ibid.*, 8.
77. *Ibid.*, 6.
78. *Ibid.*, 9.
79. *Ibid.*, 12.
80. *Ibid.*, 15.
81. J. Jarret Clinton, Memorandum for the Executive Secretary, Armed Forces Epidemiological Board, "HTLVIII Antibody Positivity," June 10, 1985.
82. William Taft, IV, Memorandum, "HTLVIII Testing," August 30, 1985.
83. Washington *Post* (August 31, 1985), 1.
84. Theodore Woodward and Robert Wells, Memorandum to Assistant Secretary of Defense (Health Affairs), September 19, 1985.
85. Caspar Weinberger, Memorandum, "Policy on Identification, Surveillance, and Disposition of Military Personnel Infected with Human T-Lymphotropic Virus Type III (HTLVIII)," October 24, 1985.
86. *New York Times* (September 14, 1986), 37.
87. Rhonda Rivera, "The Military," *AIDS and the Law,* 230.
88. *New York Times* (November 29, 1986), A10.
89. Office of Medical Services, "Policy Paper: AIDS and the Foreign Service," n.d.

90. Personal Communication, Paul A. Goff, March 15, 1987.
91. *New York Times* (November 29, 1986), A10.
92. *New York Times* (December 17, 1986), B19.
93. "Medical Examination of Aliens: AIDS," *Federal Register* (April 23, 1986), 15354–55.
94. *New York Times* (March 27, 1987), A14.
95. *New York Times* (May 1, 1987), A18.
96. *Ibid.*
97. *New York Times* (April 9, 1987), B8.
98. *New York Times* (May 22, 1987), A20.
99. *Ibid.*
100. *New York Times* (May 28, 1987), B5.
101. *New York Times* (June 1, 1987), A1.
102. Washington *Post* (June 1, 1987), 1.
103. *New York Times* (June 3, 1987), B8.
104. *New York Times* (June 7, 1987), Sec. IV, 28.
105. *New York Times* (July 2, 1987), A28.
106. *New York Times* (July 13, 1987), B3.
107. *New York Times* (March 13, 1987), A21.
108. *New York Times* (July 11, 1987), A1.

Chapter 6 Isolating the Infected

1. *New York Times* (June 15, 1987), 3.
2. *New York Times* (June 12, 1987), B4.
3. Erwin Ackerknecht, "Anticontagionism Between 1821 and 1867," *Bulletin of the History of Medicine* (1948), 562–93.
4. Charles Rosenberg, *The Cholera Years* (Chicago: University of Chicago Press, 1962), 79.
5. Charles Mullet, "A Century of English Quarantine (1709–1825)," *Bulletin of the History of Medicine,* (November–December 1949), 536.
6. Gunther Rotenberg, "The Austrian Sanitary Cordon and the Control of the Bubonic Plague 1710–1871," *Journal of the History of Medicine* (January 1973), 15–23.
7. David Musto, "Quarantine and the Problem of AIDS," *Milbank Quarterly,* Supplement 1 (1986), 98.

8. *Ibid.*, 108.
9. *New York Native* (January 31–February 13, 1983), 23.
10. Larry Gostin, "The Future of Communicable Disease Control: Toward a New Concept in Public Health Law," *Milbank Quarterly* Supplement 1, (1986), 80.
11. Wendy Parmet, "AIDS and Quarantine: The Revival of an Archaic Doctrine," *Hofstra Law Review* (Fall 1985), 53–90.
12. Musto, "Quarantine," *Milbank Quarterly*, 112.
13. Parmet, "AIDS and Quarantine," *Hofstra Law Review*, 61.
14. Gostin, "Traditional Public Health," *AIDS and the Law*, 93.
15. Michael Mills, "Legal Aspects of Infectious Disease Control," *Medical Times* (August 1983), 83–86.
16. *Balderas v. County of Los Angeles.*
17. *Balderas v. County of Los Angeles.* Stipulated Judgment and Permanent Injunction.
18. David Musto, *The American Disease: Origins of Narcotics Control* (New Haven, CT: Yale University Press, 1973).
19. Brandt, *No Magic Bullet.*
20. Ohio, House Bill 704 (1986).
21. Washington, House Bill 1977 (1986).
22. J. F. Grutsch and A. D. J. Robertson, "The Coming of AIDS: It Didn't Start with Homosexuals and It Won't End with Them," *American Spectator* (March 1986), 12.
23. James Mason, "Speech Before the Republican Study Committee of the House of Representatives" (November 7, 1985), Mimeo.
24. *Medical Information Network* (July 31, 1985).
25. Larry Gostin, "Traditional Public Health," *AIDS and the Law*, 60.
26. *Ibid.*
27. These studies are reported in Eleanore Singer and Theresa Rogers, "Public Opinion about AIDS," *AIDS and Public Policy Journal* (1986), Vol. 1, 8–13.
28. Conference of Local Health Officers Report to U.S. Conference of Mayors, Task Force on AIDS, January 1986, Mimeo.
29. Alvin Novick, "Quarantine and AIDS," *Connecticut Medicine* (February 1985), 81–83.
30. David Black, "The Plague Years," *Rolling Stone* (April 25, 1985), 60.
31. *Ibid.*

32. James Chin, Interview, Berkeley, California, August 18, 1986.
33. James Chin, Memorandum to Ramon Perez, Office of Legal Services [State of California], December 1, 1983.
34. Sharon Mosley [Office of Legal Services, State of California], Memorandum to James Chin, February 16, 1984.
35. James Chin, Interview, Berkeley, California, August 18, 1986.
36. Gostin, "Traditional Public Health," *AIDS and the Law,* 61.
37. Parmet, "AIDS and Quarantine," *Hofstra Law Review,* 87.
38. Oregon, HIV/AIDS Policy Committee, "The AIDS Epidemic: Policy Recommendations," 42.
39. *Ibid.*
40. Parmet, "AIDS and Quarantine," *Hofstra Law Review,* 85–86.
41. Washington *Post* (December 6, 1985), A27.
42. Ronald Bayer, "Crime, Punishment, and the Decline of Liberal Optimism," *Crime and Delinquency* (April 1981), 189–90.
43. *Moral Majority Report* (June 1985), 1.
44. Idaho, House Bill 662 (1986).
45. *New York Native* (November 25–December 1, 1985), 8.
46. William Curran, Larry Gostin, and Mary Clark, "AIDS: Legal and Regulatory Policy" (U.S. Public Health Service, July 1986), 347.
47. *New York Times* (April 12, 1987), 29.
48. *New York Times* (May 8, 1987), B9.
49. *Fulton County [Georgia] Daily Report* (June 16, 1987), 1.
50. Brandt, *No Magic Bullet,* 85.
51. *Ibid.*
52. Allan Brandt, "A Historical Perspective," *AIDS and the Law,* 40.
53. *Ibid.*
54. *AIDS, Policy and Law* (March 12, 1986), 6.
55. New York *Daily News* (September 28, 1985), 5.
56. "Antibody to Human Immunodeficiency Virus in Female Prostitutes," *MMWR* (March 27, 1987), 160.
57. *New York Times* (January 2, 1987), A12.
58. Robert Bernstein, Telephone Interview, January 5, 1987.
59. *Gazette Telegraph* [El Paso County, Colorado] (November 4, 1986), 1.
60. *New York Times* (November 5, 1985), C8.

61. *New York Native* (April 8–21, 1985), 25.
62. *Ibid.*
63. William Curran, "Venereal Disease Detection and Treatment: Prostitutes and Civil Rights," *American Journal of Public Health* (February 1975), 180–81.
64. Mary Guinan and Ann Hardy, "Epidemiology of AIDS in Women in the United States," *Journal of the American Medical Association* (February 17, 1987), 2039.
65. Robert Redfield *et al.*, "Heterosexually Acquired HTLVIII/LAV Disease (AIDS-Related Complex and AIDS)," *Journal of the American Medical Association* (October 18, 1985), 2094–96.
66. See Letters, *Journal of the American Medical Association* (April 4, 1986), 1702–6.
67. See, for example, Nancy Padian and John Pickering; and Richard Pearce, Letters, *Journal of the American Medical Association* (August 1, 1986), 590–91.
68. *MMWR*, (March 27, 1987).
69. Rand Stoneburner *et al.*, Letter, *New England Journal of Medicine* (November 20, 1986), 1355.
70. *New York Times* (November 5, 1985), 68.
71. U.S. Public Health Service Executive Task Force on AIDS, Minutes, March 25, 1985.
72. *Rocky Mountain News* [Colorado] (November 16, 1986), 11.
73. *New York Times* (January 2, 1987), A12.
74. *MMWR* (March 27, 1987), 159.
75. "Public Health Service Guidelines for Counseling and Antibody Testing to Prevent HIV Infection and AIDS," *MMWR* (August 14, 1987), 513.
76. Northern California Branch, American Civil Liberties Union, "AIDS and Civil Liberties," March 1986.
77. Northern California Branch, American Civil Liberties Union, Board of Directors Meeting, Minutes, January 16, 1986.
78. New York Civil Liberties Union, Legislative Department, "Proposed ACLU Policy on AIDS," n.d.
79. Privacy Committee, American Civil Liberties Union, Memorandum to the Board of Directors, "Proposed Policies on Communicable Diseases and AIDS," April 2, 1986.
80. American Civil Liberties Union, Board of Directors, Minutes, April 12–13, 1986.

81. American Civil Liberties Union, Board of Directors, Minutes, June 21–22, 1986.
82. Privacy Committee, American Civil Liberties Union, Memorandum to the Board of Directors, January 9, 1987.
83. *Ibid.*
84. American Civil Liberties Union, Board of Directors, Minutes, January 24–25, 1987.
85. Robert Bernstein, Telephone Interview, January 5, 1987.
86. Dallas *Morning News* (October 22, 1985), 1A.
86. *Ibid.*
87. *Ibid.*
88. Dallas *Times Herald* (October 23, 1985), 21.
89. C. N. Rothe, Letter to John Doe, October 14, 1985.
90. Gara La Marche, Letter to Sam Millsap, October 9, 1985.
91. Dallas *Morning News* (October 19, 1985), 32A.
92. Dallas *Morning News* (October 22, 1985), 1A.
93. Washington *Post* (October 23, 1985). A2.
94. *Advocate* (January 21, 1986), 16.
95. Houston *Chronicle* (October 22, 1985), 6.
96. *Ibid.*
97. *Ibid.*
98. Dallas *Times Herald* (November 27, 1985), 1.
99. Dallas *Morning News* (November 27, 1985), 1A.
100. Lesbian/Gay Rights Advocates, "To All AIDS-Related Organizations, Re: November 24 Meeting with Commissioner Bernstein, and December 14, Meeting with State Board of Health," n.d., Mimeo.
101. *Ibid.*
102. Jeff Levi, Austin *American Statesman* (November 30, 1985), A15.
103. Jeff Levi, Letter to Ronald Anderson, December 10, 1985.
104. Gary MacDonald, Letter to Ronald Anderson, December 10, 1985.
105. Mary B. Duffy, Letter to Kris Lloyd, December 3, 1985.
106. Dallas *Herald News* (December 15, 1985), A17.
107. *Ibid.*
108. Dallas *Morning News* (December 15, 1985), A34.
109. Dallas *Times Herald* (January 14, 1986), 4A.
110. Jerome Greenberg, associate commissioner for preventable diseases

[Texas], Hearing on Proposed AIDS Rule, Memo for the Record, January 13, 1986.

111. Mathilde Krim, Interview, New York, September 29, 1986.
112. Houston *Post* (January 14, 1986), 1A.
113. Texas Department of Health, News Release, January 15, 1986.
114. Houston *Chronicle* (January 17, 1986), 1.
115. Ronald Anderson, Interview, Dallas, Texas, January 20, 1988.
116. Houston *Chronicle* (January 17, 1986), 1.
117. Texas Department of Health, News Release, January 15, 1986.
118. Dallas *Morning News* (January 17, 1986), 25A.
119. *Advocate* (February 18, 1986), 15.
120. *Ibid.*
121. Robert Bernstein, Telephone Interview, January 5, 1987.
122. Revision of the Communicable Disease Law, Draft, January 28, 1987.
123. Glen Maxey, Personal Communication, February 15, 1987.
124. Thomas Vernon, Interview, Denver, Colorado, November 14, 1986.
125. Dale Erickson, Letter to Governor Richard Lamm and Colleagues of the House and Senate, February 18, 1986.
126. Thomas Vernon, Interview, Denver, Colorado, November 14, 1986.
127. Thomas Vernon, "Remarks," *AIDS: Impact on Public Policy,* eds., Robert Hummel, William Leary, Michael Rampola and Sherry Chorost (New York: Plenum Press, 1986), 28.
128. *Ibid.*
129. Colorado, House Bill 1290 (1986).
130. *Rocky Mountain News* (March 13, 1986), 10.
131. Thomas Vernon, "Remarks," 128.
132. Colorado, House Bill 1177 (1987).
133. Tom Witte, Telephone Imterview, August 22, 1986.
134. *New York Native* (June 3–16, 1985), 14.
135. *Ibid.*
136. Washington *Post* (December 16, 1985), A26.
137. Epidemiology and Disease Control Committee, California Council of Local Health Officers, "California Local Health Jursidictions and the Management of Willful Agents of Infection with Human Immunodeficiency Virus" January 22, 1987, Mimeo.
138. *Bay Area Reporter* (February 12, 1987), 1.

139. Los Angeles *Times* (February 26, 1987), 1.
140. *Bay Area Reporter* (February 12, 1987), 1.
141. *Ibid.*
142. Los Angeles *Times* (February 26, 1987), 1.
143. Carl Smith and George Wolfe, "California Local Health Jurisdiction and the Management of Recalcitrant Patients with AIDS or AIDS Related Conditions," May 21, 1987, Mimeo.
144. "Frontline," WGBH, March 25, 1986.

Chapter 7 Prevention Through Education

1. G. Russel Havlak and Stephen Margolis, "Potential Strategies for the Control and Prevention of AIDS," prepared for the Public Health Service Conference, Prevention and Control of AIDS: Planning for 1991, June 4–6, 1986, Mimeo.
2. U.S. Congress, Office of Technology Assessment, Review of the Public Health Service's Response to AIDS (Washington, DC: Government Printing Office, 1985), 53.
3. *Ibid.*, 51.
4. *New York Native* (February 11–24, 1985), 8.
5. Los Angeles *Times* (June 23, 1986), part 2, 4.
6. Stephen Schultz, Interview, New York City, November 25, 1986.
7. *New York Native* (January 14–27, 1985), 11.
8. National Academy of Sciences and Institute of Medicine, *Confronting* AIDS, 92.
9. *Ibid.*, 97.
10. *Ibid.*, 133.
11. *Ibid.*, 96.
12. *Ibid.*, 231.
13. *Ibid.*, 96.
14. *New York Times* ((July 14, 1986), A16.
15. *Advocate* (October 1, 1985), 22.
16. Douglas Conway, "For the Sake of Words: Language Restrictions and AIDS Education," unpublished manuscript, 1986, Mimeo.
17. Washington *Post* (November 21, 1985), 11.
18. Alvin Novick, Telephone Interview, October 10, 1986.
19. CDC, CDC Guidance on Written, Pictorial and Audiovisual Materials

and Questionnaires or Survey Instruments Related to AIDS Risk Reduction and for Conducting Group Educational Sessions in CDC Funded Programs, n.d., Mimeo.

20. Los Angeles *Times* (January 20, 1986), 8.
21. Los Angeles *Times* (January 20, 1986), 8.
22. Interviews, Stephen Schultz, New York, November 25, 1986, and Alvin Novick, Hastings-on-Hudson, May 19, 1986.
23. *New York Native* (February 10–16, 1986).
24. *Surgeon General's Report on Acquired Immune Deficiency Syndrome,* 4.
25. *Ibid.*, 27
26. *Ibid.*, 5.
27. *Ibid.*, 16.
28. *Ibid.*, 17.
29. *Ibid.*, 19.
30. *Ibid.*, 19.
31. *Ibid.*, 31.
32. William E. Dannemyer, Letter to Everett C. Koop, November 18, 1986.
33. *New York Times* (January 24, 1987), 1.
34. *Ibid.*
35. *New York Times* (January 31, 1987), A6.
36. Edwin Meese III, Memorandum for the Domestic Policy Council, February 11, 1987.
37. *Congressional Record* (October 14, 1987).
38. *New York Times* (April 29, 1988), B4.
39. Los Angeles *Times* (August 22, 1985), Part 2, 1.
40. John Rutledge, Interview, New York, October 11, 1986.
41. U.S. Public Health Service, Executive Task Force on AIDS, Minutes, April 8, 1985.
42. Don Des Jarlais, Samuel Friedman, and William Hopkins, "Epidemiology and Risk Reduction for AIDS Among Intravenous Drug Users," *Annals of Internal Medicine* (November 1985), 758.
43. *Ibid.*
44. John Black, *et al.*, "Sharing of Needles Among Users of Intravenous Drugs," *New England Journal of Medicine* (February 13, 1986), 447.

45. John French and Joyce Jackson, "Needle Sharing and AIDS" (July 1985), Mimeo.
46. David Sencer, Interview, New York City, October 21, 1986.
47. David Sencer, Memorandum to Edward Koch, August 13, 1985.
48. *New York Times* (September 15, 1985), 20.
49. *Ibid.*
50. *New York Times* (May 30, 1986), B3.
51. U.S. Public Health Service Executive Task Force on AIDS, Minutes, September 23, 1985.
52. *New York Times* (May 30, 1986), B3.
53. *New York Times* (November 8, 1986), A8.
54. *Confronting AIDS*, 110.
55. *New York Times* (October 8, 1986), 8.
56. *New York Times* (November 10, 1986), B5.
57. *New York Times* (November 11, 1986), 24.
58. *New York Times* (May 17, 1987), 38.
59. *New York Times* (January 13, 1988), 1.
60. John Rutledge, Interview, New York City, October 11, 1986.
61. *New York Times* (July 24, 1986), A12.
62. *New York Times* (August 24, 1986), A16.
63. *New York Times* (May 30, 1986), B3.
64. John Rutledge, Interview, New York, October 11, 1986.
65. Molly Coy, Interview, New York City, October 21, 1986.
66. San Francisco *Chronicle* (July 25, 1986), 1.
67. San Francisco *Chronicle* (July 26, 1986), 2.
68. San Francisco Department of Public Health, Press Release, July 25, 1986.
69. Kenneth Warner, "Bags, Buckles, Belts: The Debate over Mandatory Personal Restraints in Automobiles," *Journal of Health Policy, Politics and Law* (1983), 44–75.
70. U.S. Public Health Service, *The 1990 Health Objectives for the Nation: A Midcourse Review* (November, 1986), 177–192. See also Harvey Fineberg, "Education to Prevent AIDS: Prospects and Obstacles," *Science* (February 5, 1988), 596.
71. Brandt, *No Magic Bullet*, 23–31.
72. Richard Bonnie, "The Efficacy of Law as a Paternalistic Instrument," *Nebraska Symposium on Motivation* (1985), 156.

73. "Declining Rates of Rectal and Pharyngeal Gonorrhea Among Males-New York City," *MMWR* (June 1, 1984), 295–97.
74. M. C. A. Gellan and C. A. Ison, Letter, *The Lancet* (October 18, 1986), 920.
75. "Self-Reported Behavioral Changes Among Gay and Bisexual Men-San Francisco," *MMWR* (October 11, 1985), 613–15.
76. Cladd Stevens *et al.*, "Human T-Cell Lymphotropic Virus Type III Infection in a Cohort of Homosexual Men in New York City," *Journal of the American Medical Association* (April 25, 1986), 2167–72.
77. John Martin, "The Impact of AIDS on Gay Male Sexual Behavior Patterns in New York City," *American Journal of Public Health* (May, 1987), 578–81.
78. Thomas Coates *et al.*, "Prevention of HIV Infection Among Gay and Bisexual Men: Two Longitudinal Studies," *Abstracts: III International Conference on AIDS* (1987), 213.
79. Ron Stall *et al.*, "Alcohol and Drug Use During Sexual Activity and Compliance with Safe Sex Guidelines for AIDS: the AIDS Behaviorial Research Project," *Health Education Quarterly* (Winter 1986), 365.
80. Ronald Valdiserri *et al.*, "Condom Use in a Cohort of Gay and Bisexual Men," *Abstracts: Third International Conference on AIDS* (1987), 213.
81. Robin Fox *et al.*, "Changes in Sexual Activities Among Participants in the Multicenter AIDS Cohort Study," *Abstracts: Third International Conference on AIDS* (1987), 213.
82. *New York Native* (October 7–13, 1985), 12.
83. *Ibid.*
84. "Human Immunodeficiency Virus Infection in the United States: A Review of Current Knowledge," *MMWR* (December 18, 1987), 38.
85. *New York Times* (June 4, 1987), A1.

Chapter 8 *AIDS and the Politics of Public Health*

1. William McNeill, *Plagues and People* (Garden City, NY, Anchor Press, 1976), 291.
2. Margaret Heckler, Speech to United States Conference of Mayors, July 14, 1983, Mimeo.
3. James Curran, "Two Years Later," *New England Journal of Medicine* (September 8, 1983), 610.
4. *Surgeon General's Report on Acquired Immune Deficiency Syndrome* (October 1986).

5. National Academy of Sciences and Institute of Medicine, *Confronting AIDS.*
6. David Rothman, "Public Policy and Risk Assessment in the AIDS Epidemic," *AIDS: Public Policy Dimensions* (New York: United Hospital Fund, 1987), 59.
7. *New York Native* (November 19–December 2, 1984), 14.
8. Richard Neustadt and Harvey Fineberg, *The Epidemic That Never Was* (New York: Vintage Books, 1983).
9. *Ibid.*, xxvi.
10. *New York Native* (July 4–17, 1983), 62.
11. Charles Rosenberg, *The Cholera Years* (Chicago: University of Chicago Press, 1962), 27.
12. *Ibid.*, 19.
13. Leon Eisenberg, "The Genesis of Fear: AIDS and the Public Response to Science," *Law, Medicine and Health Care* (December 1986), 243–49.
14. McNeill, *Plagues and People,* 172.
15. *New York Times* (November 16, 1985), 31.
16. Judith Leavitt, "Politics and Public Health: Smallpox in Milwaukee, 1894–5," *Bulletin of the History of Medicine,* (1976), 559.
17. David Musto, "Quarantine and the Problem of AIDS," *Milbank Quarterly,* Supplement 1, (1986), 97–117.

Afterword Entering the Second Decade

1. "CDC Estimates of HIV Prevalence and Projected AIDS Cases: Summary of a Workshop, October 31–November 1, 1989," *MMWR* (February 23, 1990), 110–119.
2. Michael Fumento, *The Myth of Heterosexual AIDS* (New York: Basic Books, 1990).
3. Expert Panel on HIV Seroprevalence Estimates and AIDS Cases Projection Methodologies, *Report* (February 15, 1989); Richard Dunne, Letter to Stephen Joseph, August 18, 1988.
4. *New York Times* (February 17, 1990), 1.
5. *Windy City Times* (September 8, 1988), 1.
6. *New York State Society of Surgeons, New York State Society of Orthopoedic Surgeons, New York State Society of Obstetricians and Gynecologists, and the Medical Society of New York* v. *David Axelrod.*
7. *PI Perspective* (April 1988), 7; *New York Times* (August 16, 1989), 1.

8. Frank S. Rhame and Dennis A. Maki, "The Case for Wide Use of Testing for HIV Infection," *New England Journal of Medicine* (1989), 1248–1254.
9. Presidential Commission on the Human Immunodeficiency Virus Epidemic, *Report* (June 1988), 76.
10. *New York State Society of Surgeons, New York State Society of Orthopoedic Surgeons, New York State Society of Obstetricians and Gynecologists, and the Medical Society of New York* v. *David Axelrod.*
11. Stephen C. Joseph, "Remarks at the Vth International Conference on AIDS" (June 5, 1989), Mimeo.
12. *New York Times* (January 19, 1990), B-1.
13. *Newark Star Ledger* (January 5, 1990).
14. Intergovernmental Health Policy Project, "HIV Reporting in the States," *Intergovernmental AIDS Reports* (November–December 1989).
15. Institute of Medicine and National Academy of Sciences, *Confronting AIDS: Update 1988* (Washington, DC: National Academy Press, 1988), 82; Presidential Commission, *Report*, 76; American Bar Association, AIDS Coordinating Committee, *ABA Policy on AIDS* (August 1989); *American Medical News* (July 8–15, 1988), 4.
16. *American Medical News* (July 8–15, 1988), 4.
17. Kathleen Toomey and Willard Cates, "Partner Notification for the Prevention of HIV Infection," *AIDS* (1989): Supplement 1, 557–562.
18. *Federal Register* 53, No. 24 (February 1988), 3554.
19. Kathleen Toomey, "Partner Notification for HIV Prevention: Current State Programs and Policies in the United States," Paper Presented at the Vth International AIDS Conference, Montreal, Canada, June 7, 1989.
20. Donald H. J. Hernann, "AIDS: Malpractice and Transmission Liability," *University of Colorado Law Review* (1986–1987), 63–107.
21. Vanessa Merton, "Confidentiality and the 'Dangerous' Patient: Implications of *Tarasoff* for Psychiatrists and Lawyers," *Emory Law Journal* (Spring 1982), 263–343.
22. Board of Trustees, American Medical Association, December 1989; Association of State and Territorial Health Officials, National Association of County Health Officials, U.S. Conference of Local Health Officers, *Guide to Public Health Practice: HIV Partner Notification Strategies* (Washington, DC: Public Health Foundation, 1988).
23. Intergovernmental Health Policy Project, "1989 Legislative Overview," *Intergovernmental AIDS Reports* (January 1990), 3.
24. New York State, Public Health Law, Article 27-F.
25. American Bar Association, House of Delegates, *Report* No. 124 (February 12–13, 1990).

26. Ronald Bayer and Cheryl Healton, "Controlling AIDS in Cuba," *New England Journal of Medicine* (April 1989), 1022–1024.
27. Based on a review of all AIDS-related legislation in the files of the Intergovernmental Health Policy Project, Washington, DC.
28. *New York Times* (February 10, 1990), 25.
29. Presidential Commission, *Report*, 130–131.
30. Based on a review of all AIDS-related legislation in the files of the Intergovernmental Health Policy Project, Washington, DC. See, generally, Martha A. Field and Kathleen M. Sullivan, "AIDS and the Criminal Law," *Law, Medicine and Health Care* (Summer 1987), 46–60.
31. Lawrence O. Gostin, "The AIDS Litigation Project: A National Review of Court and Human Rights Commission Decisions, Part 1: The Social Impact of AIDS," *Journal of the American Medical Association* (April 11, 1990), 1963.
32. Larry Gostin, "The Politics of AIDS: Compulsory State Powers, Public Health, Civil Liberties," *Ohio State Law Journal* (1989), 1041.
33. *New York Times* (February 25, 1988), 1.
34. Institute of Medicine and the National Academy of Sciences, *Confronting AIDS: Update 1988* (Washington DC: National Academy Press, 1988), 84.
35. National Commission on Acquired Immune Deficiency Syndrome, *Report Number One* (December 5, 1989), Mimeo.
36. Harlan Dalton, "AIDS in Black Face," *Daedalus* (Summer 1989), 205–227.
37. *New York Times* (February 14, 1990), B-1.
38. *AMA News* (May 25, 1990), 5.
39. Public Health Service, "Guidelines for Prophylaxis Against *Pneumocystis Carinii* Pneumonia for Persons Infected with Human Immunodeficiency Virus," *MMWR* (June 16, 1989), Supplement 5.
40. Paul Volberding *et al.*, "Zidovudine in Asymptomatic Human Immunodeficiency Virus Infection: A Controlled Trial in Persons with Fewer than 500 CDR-Positive Cells per Cubic Milliliter," *New England Journal of Medicine* (April 5, 1990), 941–949.
41. Peter S. Arno *et al.*, "Economic and Policy Implications of Early Intervention in HIV Disease," *Journal of the American Medical Association* (September 15, 1990), 1494.
42. Intergovernmental Health Policy Project, "AZT: Who will Pay?" *Intergovernmental AIDS Reports* (May-June 1989), 4; Intergovernmental Health Policy Project, "State Financing for AIDS: Options and Trends," *Intergovernmental AIDS Reports* (March-April 1990).

43. National Commission, *Report Number One*.
44. *New York Newsday* (March 30, 1990), 1.
45. Michael Alderman *et al.*, "Predicting the Future of the AIDS Epidemic and Its Consequences for the Health Care System of New York City," *Bulletin of the New York Academy of Medicine* (March 1988), 181.
46. New York City AIDS Task Force, *Report* (July 1989); Citizens Commission on AIDS, *The Crisis in AIDS Care* (March 1989); Mayor's Task Force on AIDS, *Assuring Care for New York City's AIDS Population* (March 1989).
47. *New York Times* (April 23, 1989).
48. United Hospital Fund, "President's Letter" (February 1990).
49. Senator Edward Kennedy, Letter, February 1990, Mimeo.
50. *New York Times* (May 17, 1990), B-10.
51. *New York Times* (June 14, 1990), B-9.
52. Donald Francis *et al.*, "Targetting AIDS Prevention and Treatment Toward HIV-1–Infected Persons: The Concept of Early Intervention," *Journal of the American Medical Association* (November 10, 1989), 2572–2576.

Index